DIAGNOSTIC INTERVIEWING

DIAGNOSTIC INTERVIEWING

Edited by
Michel Hersen
and
Samuel M. Turner

Western Psychiatric Institute and Clinic
University of Pittsburgh School of Medicine
Pittsburgh, Pennsylvania

PLENUM PRESS • NEW YORK AND LONDON

Library of Congress Cataloging in Publication Data

Main entry under title:

Diagnostic interviewing.

Includes bibliographies and index.
1. Interviewing in psychiatry. 2. Mental illness—Diagnostic. I. Hersen Michel. II. Turner, Samuel M., 1944–   . |DNLM: 1. Interview, Psychological. 2. Mental Disorders—diagnosis. WM 141 D536|
RC480.7.D5 1985   616.89′075   85-19298
ISBN 0-306-42050-3

© 1985 Plenum Press, New York
A Division of Plenum Publishing Corporation
233 Spring Street, New York, N.Y. 10013

Printed in the United States of America

Contributors

Hagop S. Akiskal, Department of Psychiatry, University of Tennessee, Memphis, Tennessee

H. E. Barbaree, Department of Psychology, Queen's University, Kingston, Ontario, Canada

Judith V. Becker, New York State Psychiatric Institute, New York, New York

Glenn R. Caddy, Department of Psychology, Nova University, Fort Lauderdale, Florida

Margaret A. Chesney, SRI International (formerly Stanford Research Institute), Department of Behavioral Medicine, Menlo Park, California

Larry W. Dupree, Florida Mental Health Institute, University of South Florida, Tampa, Florida

John P. Foreyt, Diet Modification Clinic, Baylor College of Medicine and The Methodist Hospital, Houston, Texas

Alan M. Gross, Department of Psychology, Emory University, Atlanta, Georgia

Michel Hersen, Department of Psychiatry, Western Psychiatric Institute and Clinic, University of Pittsburgh School of Medicine, Pittsburgh, Pennsylvania

Stuart L. Keill, State University of New York, VA Medical Center, Buffalo, New York

Albert T. Kondo, Diet Modification Clinic, Baylor College of Medicine and The Methodist Hospital, Houston, Texas

W. L. Marshall, Department of Psychology, Queen's University, Kingston, Ontario, Canada

Jesse B. Milby, Veterans Administration Medical Center and Department of Psychiatry, University of Alabama, Birmingham, Alabama

Roger L. Patterson, Veterans Administration Medical Center, Tuskeegee, Alabama

Joseph A. Rice, Veterans Administration Medical Center and Department of Psychiatry, University of Alabama, Birmingham, Alabama

Renate H. Rosenthal, Department of Psychiatry, University of Tennessee, Memphis, Tennessee

Linda J. Skinner, Department of Psychology, University of Hartford, West Hartford, Connecticut

Paul H. Soloff, Department of Psychiatry, Western Psychiatric Institute and Clinic, University of Pittsburgh School of Medicine, Pittsburgh, Pennsylvania

Susan Stewart, Department of Psychiatry, Western Psychiatric Institute and Clinic, University of Pittsburgh School of Medicine, Pittsburgh, Pennsylvania

Herman V. Szymanski, VA Medical Center, Pittsburgh, Pennsylvania

Samuel M. Turner, Department of Psychiatry, Western Psychiatric Institute and Clinic, University of Pittsburgh School of Medicine, Pittsburgh, Pennsylvania

Charles VanValkenburg, Department of Psychiatry, University of Minnesota School of Medicine, Minneapolis, Minnesota

Marcia M. Ward, SRI International (formerly Stanford Research Institute), Department of Behavioral Medicine, Menlo Park, California

Preface

Over the years, in our teaching of diagnostic interviewing to graduate students in clinical psychology, psychology interns, medical students, and psychiatric residents, we have searched for appropriate reading materials that encompass theoretical rationale, clinical description, and the pragmatics of "how to." However, surprising as it may seem, there is no one work that includes the theoretical, the clinical, and the practical under one cover. This being the case, we thought it would be useful to us in our pedagogic efforts if we could put together such a text. And it is to this end that we developed the outline for our multiauthored text and presented it to Plenum Press for their review. We felt then, as we do now, that the material in this book simply does not represent "the cat being skinned in yet another way." We sincerely believe that our students really do need this one, and it is to them that we dedicate *Diagnostic Interviewing*.

Our book is divided into three parts. In the first part (*General Issues*), basic interviewing strategies and the mental status examination are covered. The bulk of the book (Parts II and III) is devoted to examination of diagnostic interviewing for the major psychiatric disorders and for special populations. Each of the chapters in Parts II and III have similar formats: (a) general description of the condition or population; (b) procedures for gathering information; (c) case illustrations with dialogue; and (d) critical information required to make the diagnosis, with illustration of the *do*'s and *dont*'s.

Many people have contributed to the development and production of this book. First, we are most grateful to the contributors for sharing with us their particular expertise and "special strategies" they have used in clinical practice. Second, we thank our secretaries and research assistants—Mary Newell, Kim Sterner, Felicia Zack, and Deborah

Berdel—for their technical assistance. And finally, but hardly least of all, we thank Eliot Werner at Plenum Press for his interest, encouragement, and patience.

MICHEL HERSEN
SAMUEL M. TURNER

Contents

I. **General Issues**

   1. The Interviewing Process   3
      Samuel M. Turner and Michel Hersen

   2. Mental Status Examination   25
      Renate H. Rosenthal and Hagop S. Akiskal

II. **Psychiatric Disorders**

   3. Anxiety-Based Disorders   55
      H. E. Barbaree and W. L. Marshall

   4. Affective Disorders   79
      Charles VanValkenburg and Hagop S. Akiskal

   5. Schizophrenia   111
      Herman V. Szymanski and Stuart L. Keill

   6. Personality Disorders   131
      Paul H. Soloff

   7. Alcoholism   161
      Glenn R. Caddy

8. Drug Abuse   183
   Jesse B. Milby and Joseph A. Rice

9. Sexual Dysfunctions and Deviations   205
   Linda J. Skinner and Judith V. Becker

10. Eating Disorders   243
    John P. Foreyt and Albert T. Kondo

11. Diagnostic Interviewing for Psychophysiological
    Disorders   261
    Marcia M. Ward and Margaret A. Chesney

III. Special Populations

12. Families   289
    Susan Stewart

13. Children   309
    Alan M. Gross

14. Assessing Deficits and Supports in the Elderly   337
    Larry W. Dupree and Roger L. Patterson

Index   361

Part **I**

General Issues

Chapter 1

The Interviewing Process

Samuel M. Turner and Michel Hersen

Introduction

Perhaps the most difficult milestone in a young clinician's career is the completion of the first interview. This endeavor is fraught with apprehension and with some degree of dread in the typical trainee. If the interview goes well, there is considerable rejoicing; but if it goes badly, much consternation results. Regardless of the amount of preparation that has taken place prior to the interview, the novice interviewer will remain apprehensive about this experience. However, having general guidelines to follow should prove to be of value. Thus, in this chapter, we will endeavor to delineate some of the issues related to interviewing and specify some of the behaviors that we think are important in the interview setting.

An effective initial interview in the therapeutic setting can pave the way for more fruitful exchange and lasting rapport with a patient. Similarly, knowledge of what and how to pose questions in the emergency setting may determine whether or not the information needed to reach a diagnostic decision and to make an appropriate disposition is obtained. We will discuss a number of issues confronting the clinician in the interview, such as type of setting, confidentiality, ethical and legal considerations, ethnic and racial considerations, methods of gathering information, therapist behavior affecting the interview, and special populations

SAMUEL M. TURNER and MICHEL HERSEN • Department of Psychiatry, Western Psychiatric Institute and Clinic, University of Pittsburgh School of Medicine, Pittsburgh, Pennsylvania 15213.

to be interviewed. It is our intent to discuss these issues in a "clinical fashion" that is liberally spiced with information from our own experience.

Clinical Issues in the Interview Setting

The setting in which an interview is conducted will have considerable impact on the manner in which it is carried out. Thus, if one is interviewing a patient in an emergency setting, the approach would be quite different than the one taken in the context of a private therapist's office. What will be some of the situational factors impinging upon the interview process? In order to answer that question, we will now examine some of the characteristics of patient populations seen in various types of settings.

Emergency Diagnostic Centers

Emergency diagnosis takes place in general hospital emergency rooms, diagnostic centers in psychiatric facilities, and intake centers in comprehensive mental health clinics. Such settings frequently serve as the first mental health contact for patients who decide on their own to seek mental health services, those who are brought for evaluation by law enforcement agencies, those who are persuaded to seek help by relatives, and those who are remanded by the courts through involuntary commitment procedures. A wide variety of disorders, including psychotic disturbances (e.g., schizophrenia, bipolar affective disorders), organic disorders, drug and alcohol problems, other affective disorders as well as a variety of anxiety and personality disturbances are evaluated. As an example of the types of disorders seen, Table 1 lists the distribution of diagnostic categories recorded in the Diagnostic and Evaluation Center at Western Psychiatric Institute and Clinic during a 1-year period.

In emergency settings, clinicians must be aware that patients are often frightened by their surroundings and may not be lucid enough to provide detailed histories. The task in such situations is to gain enough information to make a reasonable diagnostic decision in order to arrange for a rational disposition. Thus, it would be sufficient to determine that a patient is psychotic and in need of hospitalization without being certain of the exact nature of the psychosis. Similarly, it would be sufficient to know that one is having anxiety symptoms as a result of situational stress and that such an individual could be best served on an outpatient

Table 1. Distribution of Diagnostic Categories for a 1-Year Period in an Emergency Diagnostic Center

Axis I: Diagnostic category	Frequency of diagnosis
Mental retardation	36
Attention deficit disorders	28
Conduct disorders	99
Anxiety disorders of childhood or adolescence	19
Eating disorders	26
Stereotyped movement disorders	2
Other disorders with physical manifestations	5
Pervasive developmental disorders	23
Other disorders of childhood and adolescence	41
Senile and presenile dementia	48
Substance-induced organic mental disorders	36
Organic brain syndrome	72
Alcohol use disorders	145
Other substance abuse	88
Schizophrenic disorders	206
Paranoid disorders	16
Other psychotic disorders	118
Bipolar, manic	55
Bipolar disorder, mixed	26
Bipolar, depressed	30
Major depression, single episode	294
Major depression, recurrent	344
Dysthymic disorders	122
Other affective disorders	55
Phobic disorders	99
Anxiety states	76
Other anxiety disorders	18
Somatoform disorders	9
Dissociative disorders	2
Psychosexual disorders	14
Factitious disorders	1
Impulse control disorders	13
Adjustment disorders	280
Factitious disorder with physical symptoms	11
Unspecified mental disorders	9
Condition not a mental disorder	74
Deferred	209
No diagnosis	87

basis. Of particular importance in such interviews is the close examination of mental status as opposed to detailed social history and more formal psychological evaluations. Because patients may be frightened by the symptoms they are experiencing as well as the setting in which they find themselves, they should be approached firmly but in a supportive fashion. The conveyance of a calm and controlled demeanor may serve to reassure the patient and gain at least a minimum level of cooperation. In the emergency setting, it may be necessary to supplement information obtained from the patient with reports from significant others or from police or court records. Finally, an important source of information is the patient's behavior prior to and during the actual interview. Frequently, this will be the single most important source of information in the emergency room.

Outpatient Settings and Private Offices

Most patients examined in outpatient and private office settings are somewhat less severe than those seen in the settings described previously. Thus, the goal of the interview frequently is somewhat different. Although the mental status remains an important issue and diagnosis is still an objective, disposition is not normally a major concern. Therefore, the patient can be approached in a more inquiring manner, with sufficient time available for detailed questioning. The objective is to learn as much about the patient's psychiatric status as possible. Of course, such questioning will still be limited to what is perceived as tolerable for an individual patient. Thus, one would choose not to pressure a patient with paranoid features regarding his or her sexual behavior in an initial interview. In general, there is time during the initial contact for the interviewer to give greater attention to establishing rapport with the patient and to lay the groundwork for a smoother therapeutic relationship. Many patients seen in such settings are also more inquiring about the causes of their disorders and treatments that are available for remediation. Thus, the clinician will have to engage in much more of a social exchange process than is typical in the emergency setting. For example, in interviewing many patients suffering from the various anxiety disorders, it is quite common for them to want to engage in protracted discussion concerning their distress, why they developed the symptoms as opposed to someone else, what types of treatment can be used and what is the "cure" for their condition, how many people have their condition, what the prognosis is for them, and how much treatment will cost. Frequently, the manner in which such questions are answered will determine whether or not a patient will remain in treatment. Moreover, the manner in which such questions are answered is important in helping the patient to develop a "proper" perspective on his or her condition in terms of what can and cannot be done in treatment and what long-term prognosis entails.

Medical Settings

The interviewing of patients in a general medical setting presents a unique type of challenge. In many instances, medical patients have not requested to see a mental health professional. Rather, this is frequently a decision of the treating physician to obtain a psychological or psychiatric consultation. Thus, such patients will at times be reluctant to communicate and may refuse to be interviewed. It must be remembered in interviewing general medical patients that these individuals have defined their disorders as medical, and indeed they may have a ligitimate medical condition. Hence, they may not feel that they have need of a psychologist or psychiatrist. Similarly, such patients may be in considerable discomfort, which might well influence their ability to respond to questions as well as the type of response they might give. In approaching patients in medical settings, we have found it advisable to present oneself as an information gatherer, acknowledging the patient's physical condition without suggesting that there is a psychological disturbance, even if it is suspected. These patients may require a "cultivation period" before they are willing to discuss their emotional status. Thus, several brief visits may be required before the interview task can actually be completed.

A potential major problem in this setting can arise if interviewers allow themselves to be put into a position of siding with the patient against his or her physician or other care giver. A patient may complain about his or her doctor or nursing personnel to the mental health professional, or he or she may seek to prove his or her physician wrong by getting the therapist to agree with his or her conception of the presenting problem. It is crucial that the therapist assume no specific position in such interviews, maintaining the attitude of investigator with no paritcular point of view at that time. Consultants must remember that they are invited in by the treating physician to render their expert advice on a given problem. Statements regarding other aspects of the patient's care can have a negative impact on the doctor–patient relationship and can well reduce the credibility and effectiveness of the interviewer.

Confidentiality

The issue of confidentiality is one of the more critical in the interview setting. Guidelines for psychologists regarding confidentiality can be found in the *Ethical Principles of Psychologists* and the specialty guide-lines for *Delivery of Services of Clinical Psychologists* as well as in numerous other publications produced by the American Psychological Association. In addition, state laws regulating the practice of psychologists fre-quently have provisions regarding confidentiality and guidelines per-taining to the doctor–patient relationship.

The issue of confidentiality will arise in a number of ways. First, patients enter into the interview with the expectation that the informa-tion they divulge is done so in confidence. Thus, in many instances, whether patients feel they can divulge highly personal information will be determined by their perception that what they reveal will be held in confidence. The setting, to some extent, will dictate the level of confi-dentiality. For example, patients being interviewed in an emergency setting may be seen by more than one person, and the interviewer might involve other individuals—such as significant others—in the interview-ing process. There are a number of dimensions that impinge upon the confidentiality issue.

Age. The age at which one can assume responsibility for himself or herself varies among the different states. Thus, adolescents seeking mental health services at the age of 15 may be able to obtain treatment without informing their parents in one state but not in another. There-fore, in a state where it is legal to provide services to adolescents at the age of 15 without informing their parents, all confidentiality laws would apply. On the other hand, such persons would be considered minors for this purpose in other states, and the clinician might be required to in-form the parents that their child was seeking treatment. In such in-stances, the clinician should inform the patient of this requirement be-fore services are rendered. The interviewing of minors normally requires parental consent, and the parents have a legal right to the results of such an interview and/or assessment.

Confidentiality of Records. Written records of psychological inter-views are also confidential. Such records may be released to others (including other professionals) only after written consent is given by the patient. Confidentiality is governed by APA ethical guidelines as well as by state laws. It is the responsibility of each professional to provide adequate safeguards for such material. Even though records are nor-mally considered privileged information, they are subject to court sub-poena in certain criminal cases. This is true even though the commu-nication between doctor and patient may be privileged information under state law.

Despite the enormous amount of time required for record-keeping activities, this should not be taken lightly for a number of reasons. First, records may be important to a patient for future treatment or third-party reimbursement. Second, information in the medical chart may prove helpful to the therapist in reviewing information provided by the patient as well as reviewing treatment plans and options. Third, records reflect the diagnosis and treatment given the patient. This information could prove to be highly important for reimbursement and also in any disagreement of malpractice claims arising from treatment. Thus, it behooves the clinician to maintain up-to-date, detailed, and accurate records of patient contact.

The security of patient records is the responsibility of everyone concerned, and in particular the clinician. Records often contain highly personal and intimate data and should never be treated lightly. Written information should not be left lying in open view for anyone to see and should be filed promptly. Records should be kept in locked files with limited access.

Ethnic and Racial Considerations

The relationships of ethnic and racial variables to psychopathological states, diagnosis, and the therapeutic accord remain poorly researched areas, and little attention is given these variables in training programs. Thus, mental health professionals are left to learn to cope with these issues with little knowledge and training. Perhaps they will be lucky enough to receive some tutelage on the job during their supervisory experiences. How important are ethnic and racial variables in the interview process? Because there have been so few studies, there is no real way to adequately address this question. However, if research pertaining to these variables is accurate, they are likely to be extremely important in certain instances. Indeed, race has been demonstrated to influence type of diagnosis (e.g., Adebimpe, 1982) and to be related to treatment decisions. Similarly, the perception of social behavior has been shown to be influenced by race (e.g., Turner, Beidel, Hersen, & Bellack, 1984). The most likely immediate problem presented to an interviewer with respect to race and ethnic considerations is that he or she will not understand (or misunderstand) culturally and racially specific behavior patterns. One extreme example of this is provided by Adebimpe (1982) when he noted the cultural relevance of various religious patterns and how they might be misinterpreted as psychotic behavior in a diagnostic interview.

When racial and ethnic issues arise during an interview, we have found it best to acknowledge them without dwelling on the topic and making this the focus of the interview. If racial or ethnic issues become that important, it is unlikely that the interview would prove to be useful. Interviewers must be prepared to acknowledge any racial or ethnic biases of their own as well as those that might be harbored by the interviewee. In some instances, it might be advisable to bring in an interviewer of the same race or ethnic background as the interviewee. That decision must be made by each individual clinician.

In recent years, a number of works have appeared addressing ethnic and minority issues with respect to interviewing as well as the therapeutic process itself. Those works have focused on such issues as race of interviewer and interviewee, black therapists and white patients, white patients and black therapists, and the particular psychology of the various minority groups. Issues regarding ethnicity and race are highly complex and poorly understood. Here we will focus on some of the issues related to interviewing and the gathering of data as well as the diagnostic process. Our intent is to simply alert the reader to potential problem areas. For more in-depth coverage, the interested reader is referred to a number of sources that cover this area more comprehensively. (See Block, 1984; Boyd-Franklin, 1984; Jones, 1984; Jones & Block, 1984; Jones & Korchin, 1982; Stewart, 1981; Turner & Jones, 1982; Willie, Kramer, & Brown, 1973).

Interview Process. A number of studies have examined racial variables as they affect the interview process. Most of these have been analog studies involving the use of college student populations. With respect to self-disclosure, such studies indicate that subjects tend to prefer counselors of their own race, whereas in others race did not prove to be a significant variable (e.g., Burrell & Rayder, 1971; Casciani, 1978). How much these analog studies reflect problems faced in the consulting room is unclear, although an early study involving a clinic sample tended to support the notion that clients most similar to the race of the counselor tended to explore themselves most (Banks, 1971; Carkhuff & Pierce, 1967). If self-exploration can be considered a positive behavior for successful outcome in therapy, then the studies would seem to suggest that same-race pairs of patients and therapists would probably be best. On the other hand, a similar study by Banks, Berenson, and Carkhuff (1967) raised the question that level of experience of the therapist and not race was the more crucial variable with respect to self-exploration, although the findings were not clear. This latter study points once again to what in most instances would be perceived as the obvious. That is to say, race is probably not a major factor in the majority of cases, just as other demographic variables are not, with respect to revealing significant information in the interview setting. In order to elucidate the significant variables, studies will have to be directed to specific behavior and/or characteristics and not the global concept of race.

Perhaps more crucial to the initial interview are factors that may impede communication. A number of possible variables have been noted to affect this process. One such variable is the perception that many blacks have about therapy. Psychological services are viewed in many instances by blacks as being available only to the white privileged classes (Mitchell, 1978). Moreover, the dominant culture pattern among the black population is toward self-help rather than help from mental health professionals (cf. Maultsby, 1982). Given this skepticism toward therapy and a cultural norm calling for self-resolution of difficulties, it can be seen that the clinician will many times confront a highly skeptical patient in the interview setting. Mitchell (1978) noted a second variable that can have a negative influence in the interview setting. Such is the language barrier, although this is partly a socioeconomic issue. Black patients are often noted to use the phrase *that's alright* when asked questions about their motives for engaging in certain behaviors. This is a phrase that is often used to mean that "although I know exactly how to answer you, I have no intention of doing so." Under such circumstances, direct questioning in an interrogative fashion may not be the best tack to pursue. Clinicians also should be alert to a tactic used by black patients that involves what appears to be nonverbal ability, inability to conceptualize, mumbling, or display of other negative behaviors that have sometimes been used to describe black patients. Jones and Seagull (1977) pointed out that this may well be a 300-year-old defense mechanism used by field slaves against their masters. The behavior pattern is referred to as *shucking*. Similar behavior among prisoners has been referred to as *dummying up* (Spewack & Spewack, 1953). Such behavior was also seen in concentration camp survivors (Bettelheim, 1960; Frankel, 1963). Thus, this behavior is a method of exerting control by individuals who do not have or who feel they are unable to control their destinies. We believe this is a particularly important point to remember when interviewing patients from lower socioeconomic groups. The level at which such behavior is displayed might well be a function of the patient's level of distrust. Hence, it may be wise for the clinician to engender some feeling of trust beyond the normal requirements when confronting this type of behavior. It may also mean that the interviewing strategy will need to be significantly altered. Highly personal and probing questions may have to take a back seat to more general and superficial questioning and discussion until some level of trust is obtained.

The cultural norm of self-sufficiency and denial of emotional problems mentioned previously is a significant factor when interviewing many black patients. Another way in which it is expressed can be seen in patients who verbally deny the depth of their problems and the need for help. Block (1984) noted that this is part of a coping style aimed at avoiding the appearance of being helpless and dependent. The fact that such patients are at a mental health facility is considered by them as a necessary enough expression of the need for help. Therefore, the clinician should not assume that the patient is unwilling or uninterested in receiving help. Moreover, the interviewer should not be dissuaded by such behavior and should proceed to complete a diagnostic assessment.

Diagnosis. That the cluster of symptoms usually associated with a given disorder varies from one culture to another has been well documented in the literature. Similarly, various groups within a particular culture may show a diversity of symptom patterns. Thus, Canadians of British origin differ from Canadians of French ancestry with respect to patterns of symptomatology and a host of other dimensions relevant to treatment (Murphy, 1974). In the United States, similar findings have been reported for ethnic and racial groups. That this is a particularly critical variable in the diagnostic enterprise has been amply demonstrated in a number of empirical studies. We will delineate a number of the differences here. However, for a more complete discussion, the reader is referred to Adebimpe (1982) and Singer (1977).

In the case of depression, it has been reported that blacks and lower-class patients do not primarily present with a depressed mood when they are in fact suffering from depression. Rather, multiple somatic complaints predominate (e.g., Carter, 1974; Schwab, 1975). How much of this different style of presentation is a function of race and how much is a function of socioeconomic status is not clear. It is clear, however, that the clinician must be able to recognize the potential importance of somatic complaints in these patient groups. It has also been observed that black patients who are depressed are likely to be more active, self-destructive, and to overeat as opposed to showing appetite loss. They are also less likely to have crying episodes and more likely to appear agitated (Block, 1984). It has also been noted that among black patients who commit suicide, there is a strong association with concomitant alcohol use (Thomas & Lindenthal, 1975), and that black homicides frequently result from interpersonal conflict in close relations, such as jealousy in marital partners (Thomas & Lindenthal, 1975). This is in contrast to what is seen in white populations.

Stress-related disorders occur at an alarmingly high rate among black Americans. Therefore, clinicians are likely to see many black patients with such disorders. These include hypertension and other associated cardiovascular diseases. In fact, hypertension has been described as the number one medical problem affecting blacks. Although the causes of hypertension are complex, a number of variables have been found to be highly correlated with the incidence and rising mortality rates. These include poor education and low occupational status (Jenkins, 1977). A large percentage of people meeting such criteria are indeed black and in many instances Hispanics. This issue is being raised here because when stress-related disorders are seen in blacks, the primary source of stress is often environmental as opposed to interpersonal. Hence, the clinician needs to be sensitive to such issues if a correct assessment is to be made.

It is not our purpose in this chapter to provide the necessary background material for one to adequately assess patients from different cultural or racial groups. Rather, our purpose is to alert the clinician to the importance of such issues. Training programs in psychiatry, psychology, and other mental health professions have not devoted the necessary attention to these variables in their curricula. Hence, black clinicians are often as inadequate in this regard as are their white counterparts. Most clinical psychology training programs give some lip service to the need for such training, but few ever implement serious curricular and experiential training. However, with the establishment of the Board of Ethnic and Minority Affairs within the American Psychological Association, a mechanism may have been created to push for the needed changes in the current accreditation standards for such programs.

Methods of Obtaining Information

In recent years, a plethora of *structured* and *semistructured* schedules has been used to enhance interrater reliability in the interview. These have been developed for interviewing children (Chambers, Puig-Antich, & Tabrizi, 1978: Kiddie SADS; Hodges, McKnew, Cytryn, Stern, & Klein, 1982: Child Assessment Schedule; Kovacs, 1983: Interview Schedule for Children) and adults (Endicott & Spitzer, 1978: Schedule for Affective Disorders and Schizophrenia; Hamilton, 1960: Rating Scale for Depression; Wing Birley, Cooper, Graham, & Isaacs, 1967: Present State Examination). The fully structured interview schedules enable the interviewer to follow an established format and sequence. In the semistructured schedules, the interviewer experiences considerable more latitude.

In contrasting the unstructured clinical interview with the schedules that now have been developed, Spitzer and Endicott (1975) noted that

> although valuable information can be obtained from the usual, relatively unstructured clinical interview, attempts have been made during recent years to improve the research value of a psychiatric interview by standardizing the interview techniques so that the variability associated with differences in interviewing methods and coverage is reduced. Interview schedules have been developed which combine the flexibility and rapport that are inherent in a clinical interview with the completeness of coverage and comparability of interviewing method that result from using a structured interview procedure. (p. 224)

Specific Techniques

If the final objective of the interview is to establish a formal diagnosis, some very specific material will have to be covered. Information of relevance would include but not be limited to (a) mental status; (b) presenting complaints; (c) psychiatric history; (d) psychiatric history of close relatives, if relevant; (e) medical history; (f) social history; (g) educational and/or military history; (h) work history; (i) dating or marital history; (j) alcohol or drug history; (k) vegetative functioning including sexual history; (l) interpersonal relationships; (m) legal history, if applicable; (n) hospitalizations, if applicable; and (o) leisure-time activities.

One of us (M.H.), in teaching interviewing to sophomore medical students, recalls presenting these 15 points to his class, with emphasis that they tended to be covered in a good diagnostic interview. In rather concrete response to such emphasis, one of the medical students proceeded to do a practice interview, with the 15 points listed on a sheet in front of him. Moreover, he followed each of the 15 points in sequence, irrespective of the flow of the patient's sequence.

We all know better, of course, that all of the 15 points can be dealt with in an interview without adhering to a rigid format, as did our sophomore medical student. Indeed, the experienced interviewer, through skillful manipulation, generally is able to weave the 15 points within the 60 to 90 minutes available. Specifically how this is done certainly is of considerable interest. Again, we wish to underscore that the type of patient and his or her responsiveness will dictate whether the interview is directed or free floating and whether open-ended questions or closed-ended questions predominate.

We can remember starting one interview in a rather existential framework, saying to our young schizophrenic patient: "How did you get here?" He responded in a most concrete fashion, "By taxicab, doctor." Although somewhat humorous, it is clear that with this kind of patient a clearer and more precise question was warranted: "What are the events that led to your being hospitalized on this psychiatric ward?" Of course, there is no guarantee that the new question would bear fruit, but at least a closer approximation of requisite historical information might emerge.

Some patients (e.g., severe obsessives, schizophrenics and manics not controlled pharmacologically) "need to be kept on track" and periodically "retracked" during the course of the interview. Thus, if the interviewer is nondirective and uses mainly open-ended questions, the specific information sought after might never surface. Nondirective interviewing with these kinds of patients invariably will lead to circumlocution and a morass of endless, albeit irrelevant detail. This in itself is diagnostic but does not fulfill the objective of the interview. With such patients, clear and direct questions (frequently closed ended) are a must!

By contrast, with defensive and highly suspicious patients, use of closed-ended questions invariably will result in rather terse replies (e.g., yes, no, maybe, I don't know, etc.). With such patients it generally is better to use open-ended questions (e.g., Tell me how things are going for you in recent weeks). Such a strategy *may* be helpful, but may also fail at times. Suspicious patients may retort, "What do you mean by that?" or "I don't understand what you are saying." When this happens, it is advisable for the interviewer to reflect the patient's concerns and to discuss them openly. However, sometimes when all of the techniques at hand have been tried, failure to "break through" the patient's defensive stance still may result.

Further, with some patients the open-ended approach may yield information that will not be reliable or valid. This especially happens when interviewing alcoholics and drug addicts. Generally, we instruct our students, when interviewing suspected alcohol or drug addicts, to say the following: "Tell me, how much alcohol [or the specific drug] are you using a day?" Or, going one step further: "What is your favorite bar in your neighborhood?" This strategy, of course, obviates the silly game playing (professionally referred to as *denial*) that often transpires between the alcoholic or drug addict and the interviewer.

A very critical element in the effective interview is the issue of timing. By *timing* we mean exactly when in the interview sequence a particular question or topic is introduced. Beginning interviewers tend to be awkward in this regard, postponing till later questions that need to be asked earlier, and conversely, presenting topics too early in the interview sequence. Again, the nature of the interview and its relative emergency valence will determine how quickly the interviewer "moves." In the emergency room situation, questions about suicide, aggressiveness, and sexual conduct cannot wait. That is not to say that the issue of suicide potential in the more leisurely paced interview can be delayed significantly. But with more time available and less of a press for decision making, greater interviewing finesse is possible.

Therapist Behavior Affecting the Interview

For too long a period of time, difficulties in obtaining relevant information in the interview have been attributed to patient and client characteristics. As graduate students and beginning clinicians, we often would hear such statements as (a) "He's being defensive and won't let his guard down. Therefore, he's not really telling you how he feels." (b) "She's lower class and not particularly verbal, so you're going to have a lot of trouble getting her to think in terms of psychological notions." (c) "His sullenness and terse replies reflect a 'negative transference' toward authority figures. You're going to have a hard time making him talk." (d) "Your adolescent patient is into drugs, sociopathic, and a chronic liar. Don't believe very much of what he says to you." (e) "She's hysterical and telling you all about that sexual material to keep you entertained. This all is part of her defensive structure to avoid her real problem of basic depression." (f) "He's only got an IQ of about 90 and will not be a terribly good psychotherapy candidate. He won't grasp the subtleties of what you're trying to do."

The preceding list of six items may be a bit of an exaggeration of the commentaries of some of the supervisors we may have experienced (and others still do), but they do reflect the pervasive trend of focusing on only one aspect of the interview equation (i.e., the client's behavior). Unfortunately, this narrow-band approach does not take into consideration the complicated interpersonal interactions that constantly are occurring during the course of the interview. Irrespective of whether we are dealing with an initial interview or one later in therapy, the interviewer's behavior critically affects how the client will respond (cf. Waterhouse & Strupp, 1984). Indeed, there is an extensive research literature clearly documenting how particular strategies carried out by the interviewer will alter interviewee behavior. An excellent review of this work is provided by Matarazzo and Wiens (1972), and the interested reader is referred to that source.

In looking at how therapist behavior can affect the interview process, let us consider the role of each of the following: (a) jargon, (b) empathy, (c) self-disclosure, and (d) humor. In so doing, we will provide examples from both our clinical experience and supervisory interactions with graduate students, psychiatric residents, and medical students.

Jargon

Use of jargon, irrespective of theoretical persuasion, is the mark of the inexperienced and naive interviewer. From our perspective, there is no justification for using technical language with clients at any point in the interview process. To say to a client that his or her behavior "reflects an unresolved Oedipal complex" or that she or he is "responding to a discriminative stimulus and not sufficiently reinforcing to her or his child" does not enhance the interview. First, unless the client is psychologically sophisticated, the meaning of such terminology will be lost. Second, even if the client is psychologically sophisticated and highly intelligent, the abstract nature of such jargon will interfere with the emotional understanding of the interviewer's points. Third, if the interviewer really is intent on using jargon, considerable effort would be expended in teaching the client the nature of the terms. We firmly believe that this represents a waste of valuable time. But moreover, it tends to inhibit the natural flow of a good interview.

Instead of using jargon and technical language, experience dictates that it is best for the interviewer to use clear behavioral descriptions of what clients do and how they respond. Again, we argue that this is so irrespective of whether the interviewer proceeds from a psychoanalytic stance or a behavioral position. The interviewer may think and conceptualize psychoanalytically or behaviorally, but he or she should speak in clear English. Also, the interviewer should never speak to clients at a level beyond their comprehension, nor should he or she underestimate their intellectual capacity. Indeed, the same question may be posed in different ways to clients of varying mental capacities. Thus, sophisticated interviewers learn to modulate their approach given the unique inherent mental capacities of their clients. But, as a rule of thumb, it is better to slightly underestimate than to overestimate.

Empathy

Many an interview has gone awry because the therapist has been intent on extracting information from a client but seemingly oblivious to his or her feelings. Or the interviewer may be pursuing a line of inquiry that is inconsistent with the client's most pressing problems at the time. For example, if a therapist is treating a height phobic, and she reports having just "broken up" with her boyfriend, it would be most insensitive to pursue original treatment and ignore the new crisis. To the contrary, it behooves this therapist to explore the client's feelings about her recent loss and the possible resulting depressive symptomatology. Indeed, the empathic interviewer must always be "in touch" with how the client feels. And, as a result, interview or therapeutic "shift of gears" may be necessary. Not only should the interviewer pay careful attention to what the client says, but he or she especially needs to be attuned to paralinguistic features, facial expressions, gestures, and general body language. This is what Reik (1948) referred to as *listening with the third ear*.

Being empathic, of course, requires much more than being a good listener. That is, interviewers must communicate to clients that they *understand* how they feel, that they *appreciate* their frustrations, and are *fully aware* of the intricacies of their lives. Empathy in the interviewer is a feature that, researchers now have shown, cuts across all theoretical persuasions (cf. Greenwald, Kornblith, Hersen, Bellack, & Himmelhoch, 1981; Sloane, Staples, Cristol, Yorkston, & Whipple, 1975). There is no one technical strategy to communicate such empathy to the client. To the contrary, there are many, including what line of questioning is to be pursued, the interviewer's affect and facial expressions, timing of comments, and the reflection of feeling in the Rogerian sense. How this is accomplished still is something of an art, but the key to it is that the client must experience the interviewer as genuine.

In the absence of empathy, the therapist not only will find the interview difficult to carry out, but he or she very well may lose the client altogether. When well-conducted taped interviews are played back, the empathic quality of the therapist is ever present.

Self-Disclosure

Early during the course of Hersen's clinical training, one of his "old-line" supervisors made the categorical statement that you never disclose any of your personal business to the patient or client. Consistent with his mentor's instruction, he maintained such distance from his clients. However, at the end of the 1-year treatment of the wife of a faculty member at the university, he "slipped" and let her know he was about to be married. One year later, he received a thank-you note from this patient for his therapeutic efforts. She apprised him that her marriage was much better and that she had just given birth to a baby girl (named Hope). She ended her note by saying that she really appreciated it when he informed her he was engaged to be married: "It made you seem more human and less remote to me."

That is not to say that a therapist should indiscreetly reveal highly personalized information (e.g., one's sex life, income, illnesses, fears, frustrations) to clients. But the occasional sharing of information, timed just right, certainly can have a facilitative effect on the interview process. A recent example that comes to mind is a client who was complaining about her 8-year-old stepson who needed to be "entertained" and "kept busy" on weekends. The interviewer, then, proceeded to say, "I can remember when my son was 8 and what that was like."

Again, we would like to underscore that self-disclosure, used sporadically and well placed, is useful to enhance the flow of the interview and to communicate empathic understanding to the client. But like sweets, "too much may not be a good thing." Thus, the interviewer must walk the proverbial "fine line" here. The caution is that the interviewer should be "friendly" but not a "friend" in the traditional sense of the word.

Humor

Use of humor (or bantering with the patient) is yet another one of the bugaboos of the old-line supervision that some of us received in the 1960s and 1970s. Somehow the notion was perpetrated that psychotherapy was serious business and that you never "cracked a smile." This undoubtedly is a holdover from psychoanalysis of the therapist conceptualized as a "blank mirror" to be projected upon by the patient. However, during the course of our practices and supervision of students, we have found that humorless interviewing and therapy are not effective. Even in the most difficult and trying situations, the perceptive patient and therapist can identify some humorous elements. We recall a very well-educated patient who was in his third marriage, and it too seemed to be headed for failure. When asked about how he might deal with the ensuing loneliness of possible separation, he replied, "Well, you know, the first one was hard; the second was a bit easier; this one should hurt even less."

There can be no doubt that some of the "lighter" therapeutic exchanges in the interview can have a beneficial effect. That is, they serve to release tension (for both the therapist and the client) from some of the more difficult material previously tackled. Humor also can be used to direct attention to required behavioral change from one session to the next. When some of our patients ask "When is my next appointment?" we often reply "Next week, same day, same time, same station, but a different story!"

As in the case of self-disclosure, humor has its place. It too should be used sparingly and needs to be timed properly. Moreover, the key is that one does not laugh *at his or her client*, but *with his or her client*.

Special Populations

In the previous sections, we have outlined some general guidelines that apply to the interviewing of a large variety of diagnostic categories. However, there are a number of diagnostic groupings where additional guidelines should prove useful, particularly for the beginning interviewer with a less broad exposure to special populations. Many of our recommendations are of a "common sense" nature, but unfortunately may be overlooked at times. Therefore, we will briefly comment on interviewing patients who are (a) intellectually deficient, (b) aggressive, (c) psychotic, (d) physically disabled, and (e) in pain.

When interviewing retarded individuals, it is *critical* that the therapist ensure that questions posed have been clearly understood. That is, language used by the interviewer should be consistent with the retarded individual's level of comprehension. However, the interviewer also should be warned that he or she can go too far in the opposite direction. Thus, it is important to avoid a line of questioning that is condescending and patronizing. One strategy to ensure that the retarded client has understood the question is to have him or her rephrase it or explain what is required. Furthermore, the sensitive interviewer should be aware that retarded people *do have feelings* and are subject to the same types of psychopathological responses as nonretarded individuals.

With highly aggressive individuals (who may be psychotic, organically impaired, or deranged as a function of illicit drug use), the safety of the interviewer may be at issue. We definitely do not recommend that the patient be interviewed when in a *highly agitated* state. This never proves to be productive in any way. However, when such individuals are sufficiently sedated or have "run the course" of an explosive episode, then interviewing may be attempted. For the interviewer secure in his or her abilities, such an interview will proceed without incident. If, however, the interviewee should evince signs of aggressivity, he or she needs to be warned that this *will not be tolerated*. When this kind of patient becomes visibly agitated, it is advisable to terminate questioning. Also, the sensitive interviewer will word questions such that they will evoke minimal arousal.

With highly psychotic patients, the interview process frequently proves to be difficult and tedious. The problem is that the interviewer must extract bizarre material without attempting to reinforce it and prolong its discussion (e.g., delusions, hallucinations). Also, an additional difficulty here is to keep the patient "on track" and *relevant*. Under such circumstances, the interviewer must be fully in charge and not allow the patient to ramble and become discursive. Short, directed questioning helps as does frequent interruption when the patient strays.

Novice interviewers, when dealing with the physically disabled, often ignore their disabilities during the course of the interview. This is as technically inadequate as totally focusing on the disability and ignoring psychopathology. Obviously a proper balance needs to be achieved. In our opinion, it is important for the interviewer to acknowledge the interviewee's physical disability in the attempt to understand how psychopathology may be related to its existence. Thus, the possible interplay between the two has to be carefully evaluated. Moreover, the interviewee's attitude toward his or her disability should be determined.

Finally, we should note that it is most difficult to interview patients who are experiencing severe *physical* pain, whether such pain is acute or of a chronic nature. In general, beyond a given pain threshold some interviews may not be possible: the patient may be totally preoccupied with such pain and its resolution. Even where pain is not that intense, the patient may have a limited attention span for the usual methods of interviewing. Our experience dictates that such interviews, if really necessary, should be brief (no more than 15 minutes at a time) and focused. If specific information is required, it can be obtained through serial interviewing. Once again, it behooves the interviewer to be exquisitely sensitive to the tolerance of his or her patient to diagnostic questioning.

Summary

In this chapter, we have looked at a number of variables that contribute to conducting a successful clinical interview. In so doing, we have highlighted our discussion with examples from our own clinical experience ina variety of inpatient and outpatient settings. In considering clinical issues in the interview setting, we have looked at the impact of the setting on the type of interview that is conducted. Specifically, we have differentiated the interviews that are conducted in emergency diagnostic centers, outpatient settings, and medical settings.

Irrespective of the setting, however, the importance of confidentiality has been underscored. Also, it is clear that the astute interviewer takes into consideration the critical impact of racial and ethnic variables of the interviewee. These variables certainly can affect the interview process and the ultimate diagnosis that is reached.

We then considered the various methods of obtaining information, including use of structured and semistructured schedules. Examples of difficult patients to interview were presented for illustration.

Next we discussed how the therapist's behavior can affect the interview process. We talked about the use of jargon, development of empathy in the interview, self-disclosure, and humor. The final section was devoted to a discussion of interviews with specific populations, such as the intellectually deficient, aggressive and psychotic patients, the physically disabled, and those individuals suffering from physical pain.

References

Adebimpe, V. (1982). Psychiatric symptoms in black patients. In S. M. Turner & R. T. Jones (Eds.), *Behavior modification in black populations: Psychosocial issues and empirical findings* (pp.57–69). New York: Plenum Press.

Bauhr, G. (1971). The effects of race on one-to-one helping interview. *Social Service Review, 45,* 137–146.

Banks, B., Berenson, B. G., & Carkhuff, R. R. (1967). The effects of counselor race upon counseling process with Negro clients in initial interview. *Journal of Clinical Psychology*, 23, 70–72.

Banks, W. M. (1971). The differential effects of race and social class in helping. *Journal of Clinical Psychology*, 28, 90–92.

Bettelheim, B. (1960). *The informed heart: Autonomy in a mass age*. Glencoe, IL: Free Press.

Block, C. B. (1984). Diagnostic and treatment issues for black patients. *The Clinical Psychologist*, 37, 52–54.

Boyd-Franklin, H. (1984). Issues in family therapy with black families. *The Clinical Psychologist*, 37, 54–57.

Burrell, L., & Rayder, N. F. (1971). Black and white students' attitudes toward white counselors. *Journal of Negro Education*, 40, 48–52.

Carkhuff, R. R., & Pierce, R. (1967). Differential effects of therapist race and social class upon patient depth of self-exploration in the initial clinical interview. *Journal of Counsulting Psychology*, 31, 632–634.

Carter, J. H. (1974). Recognizing symptoms in black Americans. *Geriatrics*, 29, 97–99.

Casciani, J. M. (1978). Influence of model's race and sex on interviewers' self-disclosure. *Journal of Counseling Psychology*, 25, 435–440.

Chambers, W. J., Puig-Antich, J., & Tabrizi, M. A. (1978). *The ongoing development of the Kiddie-SADS*. Paper presented at the annual meeting of the American Academy of Child Psychiatry, San Diego.

Endicott, J., & Spitzer, R. L. (1978). A diagnostic interview: The Schedule for Affective Disorders and Schizophrenia. *Archives of General Psychiatry*, 35, 837–844.

Frankl, V. E. (1963). *Man's search for meaning: An introduction to logotherapy*. Boston: Beacon Press

Greenwald, D. P., Kornblith, S. J., Hersen, M., Bellack, A. S., & Himmelhoch, J. M. (1981). Differences between social skill therapists and psychotherapists in treating depression. *Journal of Consulting and Clinical Psychology*, 49, 757–759.

Griffith, M. (1977). The influence of race on the psychotherapeutic relationship. *Psychiatry*, 40, 27–40.

Hamilton, M. (1960). A rating scale for depression. *Journal of Neurology, Neurosurgery and Psychiatry*, 23, 56–61.

Hodges, K., McKnew, D., Cytryn, L., Stern, L., & Klein, J. (1982). The Child Assessment Schedule (CAS) diagnostic interview: A report of reliability and validity. *Journal of the American Academy of Child Psychiatry*, 21, 468–473.

Jenkins, C. D., (1977). Epidemiological studies of the psychosomatic aspects of coronary heart disease: A review. In S. Kasl & F. Reichsman (Eds.), *Advances in Psychosomatic Medicine* (Vol. 9) (pp. 1–19). New York: Karger.

Jones, A., & Seagull, A. (1977). Dimensions of the relationship between the black client and the white therapist: A theoretical overview. *American Psychologist*, 32, 850–855.

Jones, E. E., & Korchin, S. J. (1982). *Minority mental health*. New York: Praeger.

Jones, E. E. (1984). Some reflections on the black patient and psychotherapy. *The Clinical Psychologist*, 37, 62–65.

Jones, J. M., & Block, C. B. (1984). Black cultural perspectives. *The Clinical Psychologist*, 37, 58–62.

Jones, R. L. (Ed.). (1972). *Black psychology*. New York: Harper & Row.

Kovacs, M. (1983). *The Interviewing Schedule for Children (ISC): Form C and the follow-up form*. University of Pittsburgh, unpublished manuscript.

Matarazzo, J. D., & Wiens, A. N. (1972). *The interview: Research on its anatomy and structure*. New York: Aldine-Antherton.

Maultsby, M. C., Jr. (1982). A historical view of blacks' distrust of psychiatry. In S. M.

Turner & R. T. Jones (Eds.), *Behavior modification in black populations: Psychosocial issues and empirical findings* (pp. 39–53). New York: Plenum Press.

Mitchell, A. C. (1978). Barriers to therapeutic communication with black clients. *Nursing Outlook, 6,* 109–112.

Murphy, H. B. M. (1974). Differences between mental disorders of French Canadians and British Canadians. *Canadian Psychiatric Association Journal, 19,* 247–257.

Reik, T. (1948). *Listening with the third ear.* New York: Groner Press.

Schwab, J. J. (1975). Amitriptyline in the management of depression and depression associated with physical illness. *Amitriptyline in the management of depression* (pp. 61–85. Merck.

Singer, B. D. (1977). *Racial factors in psychiatric intervention.* San Francisco: R. E. Research Associates.

Sloane, B. R., Staples, F. R., Cristol, A. H., Yorkston, N. J., & Whipple, K. (1975). *Psychotherapy versus behavior therapy.* Cambridge: Harvard University Press.

Spewack, S., & Spewack, B. (1953). *My three angels.* New York: Random House.

Spitzer, R. L., & Endicott, J. (1975). Assessment of outcome by independent clinical evaluators. In I. E. Waskow & M. B. Parkoff (Eds.), *Psychotherapy change measures* (pp. 222–232). Rockville, MD: National Institute of Mental Health.

Stewart, E. D. (1981). Cultural sensitivities in counseling. In P. P. Pederson, J. C. Draguns, & J. E. Trimble (Eds.), *Counseling across cultures.* Honolulu: University Press of Hawaii.

Thomas, A., & Sillen, S. (1972). *Racism and psychiatry.* New York: Brunner/Mazel.

Thomas, C. S., & Lindenthal, J. J. (1975, Summer). The depression of the oppressed. Mental Health: *A publication of the Mental Health Association,* 13–14.

Turner, S. M., Beidel, D. C., Hersen, M., & Bellack, A. S. (1984). Effects of race on rating of social skill. *Journal of Consulting and Clinical Psychology, 52,* 474–475.

Turner, S. M., & Jones, R. T. (1982). *Behavior modification in black populations: Psychosocial issues and empirical findings.* New York: Plenum Press.

Waterhouse, G. J., & Strupp, H. H. (1984). The patient-therapist relationship: Research from the psychodynamic perspective. *Clinical Psychology Review, 4,* 77–92.

Wing, J. K., Birley, J. T., Cooper, J. E., Graham, P., & Isaacs, A. D. (1967). Reliability of a procedure for measuring and classifying "present psychiatric state." *British Journal of Psychiatry, 13,* 499–515.

Willie, C. V., Kramer, M. B., & Brown, B. S. (1973). *Racism and mental health.* Pittsburgh: University of Pittsburgh Press.

Chapter 2

Mental Status Examination

Renate H. Rosenthal and Hagop S. Akiskal

Introduction

The Mental Status Examination represents the most important step in
the clinical evaluation of individuals suffering from or suspected of having mental disorders. The evaluation is based on observations of a patient's overt and verbal behavior as well as on his or her subjective
experiences. Patients' presenting problems dictate both the types of
questions asked and the depth of inquiry necessary for a coherent and
complete assessment of the mental status. In general, the more deviant
and severely disturbed the patient, the more probing the mental status
examination should be.

Some individuals who present for outpatient psychotherapy or
counseling can be viewed as having "problems of living." In such cases,
the relevant mental status information can be largely gleaned from a
well-conducted history-taking or intake interview. Bizarre ideation, unusual preoccupations, memory or concentration disturbances, and disturbances in mood and perceptions, if any, can be assessed quite readily
in this type of interaction. In the absence of such symptoms, the task
becomes largely a matter of organizing the information gained in the
interview into the structure and terminology used to report a patient's
mental status. On the other hand, if the patient appears to be suffering
from significant disturbance of mood, perception, thinking, or memory,
a formal Mental Status Examination is in order (Kraepelin, 1904). This is

---

RENATE H. ROSENTHAL and HAGOP S. AKISKAL • Department of Psychiatry, University of Tennessee, Memphis, Tennessee 38163.

almost always the case with psychiatric inpatients and with medical patients whose mental functioning is cause for concern. Thus, although much can be learned about a patient's mental status from general observations made during a standard interview, specific probes are often needed to gain essential information about pathology that goes beyond problems of living.

In the past, psychologists tended to be suspicious, if not antagonistic, toward any activities that smack of the "medical model." Psychiatric diagnosis, classification of mental illnesses, and approaches that appeared to sanction the conceptualization of behavioral disturbances as *diseases* were suspect. However, in light of remarkable advances in the fields of genetics, pharamacology, neuroendocrinology, and neurophysiology over the past decade, the idea of underlying physical/biochemical dysfunction in some psychiatric disorders can no longer be disputed. Thus, the *illness* concept has been extended beyond the organic mental disorders (formerly known as organic brain syndromes) to include major "functional" disorders, notably the schizophrenias, the affective disorders, and some anxiety and personality disorders. For patients suspected of suffering from these conditions, a careful Mental Status Examination is mandatory.

Psychologists are often front-line evaluators, particularly in mental health centers where many of these conditions are seen in their milder forms. It is therefore essential to keep in mind that subtle behavioral abnormalities sometimes are the first indicators of underlying medical illness. The Mental Status Examination can provide important data for differential diagnosis. Psychologists are also present in increasing numbers in medical settings, where they are called on to evaluate patients with known medical illnesses and to collaborate with nonpsychiatric physicians in the treatment process. Many medical disorders are accompanied by mental symptoms that may result from the direct impact of illness on the patient's mental functioning (e.g., in metabolic disturbances), from the use of medications that affect mood or cognitive capacity (e.g., antihypertensive drugs or narcotics), or from the personally disabling psychosocial consequences of the illness. Familiarity with mental status terminology enables the psychologist to communicate more effectively with medical specialists, who have been trained to organize their findings in this fashion. Thus, the terminology applied to describe a patient's mental status and the structure used in organizing these findings serve an important communicative function. The structured nature of the Mental Status Examination also forces the examiner to document findings with factual examples and to move from global impressions to specific observations. This, in turn, permits a diagnosis, if indicated, and thereby prepares the ground for a more coherent and focused treatment plan.

Areas Covered in the Mental Status Examination

A systematic examination of the mental status covers several major areas that are outlined in Table 1 and discussed later.

Appearance and Behavior

Although appearance and behavior is the first item in a Mental Status Examination, relevant data on appearance and behavior are gathered throughout the interview. Attire, posture, facial expression, mannerisms, and level of grooming are described in such a way that the person reading or listening to this narration can visualize the patient's physical appearance at the time of the examination, much as if the clinician had taken a photograph. The setting of the interview is also briefly described in this section.

In some cases, little will be revealed about the mental status by these observations, beyond the fact that the patient's physical appearance was unremarkable, failing to distinguish him or her from other people of the same age, educational level, and socioeconomic background. In other instances, this initial section may already give some important clues about the patient's personality, mood, thoughts, awareness of social convention, and ability to function adequately in

Table 1. Outline of Mental Status Examination

Date and time of interview
Appearance and behavior
Attitude toward interviewer
Psychomotor activity
Affect and mood
Speech and thought
Perceptual disturbances
Orientation
Attention, concentration, and memory
Intelligence
Reliability, judgment, and insight

society at the time of the evaluation. Some examples will illustrate the value of this initial paragraph of the Mental Status Examination.

Ms. A., a 20-year-old, single, white student, was interviewed in the Student Counseling Center. She was self-referred. She is a petite, frail-looking woman appearing much younger than her stated age. She wore no makeup, and was dressed in simple attire consisting of a blue button-down boy's shirt, a pair of cutoff blue jeans, woolen knee stockings, and penny loafers. She carried a knapsack full of books which she held closely on her lap. Throughout the interview, her hands were tightly clasped around her knapsack so that her white knuckles showed. Her fingernails were bitten down to the quick.

The description of this patient's appearance gives us clues about a moderate level of anxiety and tension, clues that should be pursued during the remainder of the examination. The next example illustrates a more disturbed patient.

Mrs. B., a divorced white woman, was brought to the mental health center by her distraught son and daughter-in-law because she had become increasingly hostile and combative at home and was staying up all night. She was restless during the interview, rising frequently from her chair, looking at every diploma on the walls, making comments about each of them. She looked her stated age of 53, but her clothes would have been appropriate only for a much younger person: although quite obese, she wore orange "hot pants" and a halter top which showed a bare midriff. Her legs had prominent varicose veins. She wore old wooden beach sandals with spikelike high heels. Her general level of grooming was very poor: her short gray hair was matted on both sides of an irregular part: her fingernails were long and yellowed from nicotine; her toenails were also very long.

The general appearance of this patient suggests a psychotic level of disorder and raises hypotheses of a much different nature from those generated by our first patient, necessitating further inquiry along the lines of a manic or a schizophrenic disorder.

The general appearance of our third patient suggests entirely different diagnostic possibilities:

Mr. Smith, a 25-year-old single, white pharmacy student, was seen in the university health clinic. He was impeccably dressed in a three-piece gray pin-striped suit and matching dress shoes. His hair and mustache were carefully groomed. When he signed his name on the admission form, his hands were visibly tremulous. He generally appeared uneasy, and glanced furtively about the room, paying special attention to electrical outlets, air-conditioning vents, and, most especially to the camera, although he had been assured that it was not in use.

Inquiry along the lines of a delusional illness is suggested by the general appearance of this patient, and differential diagnosis should consider such conditions as amphetamine psychosis and paranoid schizophrenia.

Psychotic patients may display extreme forms of inappropriate behavior (e.g., bare breasts or genitals) or maintain bizarre postures for long periods of time (known as *waxy flexibility*, arising either spontaneously or in response to physical manipulations by the examiner.) All such gross deviations in behavior should be carefully recorded.

Attitude toward the Interviewer

Attitude toward the interviewer is available by observation, without specific inquiry. The patient may relate easily, be cooperative and open, and reveal information freely. Other patients may be suspicious and guarded, requiring frequent reassurance that the content of the session is confidential. Some patients are hostile, engaging in one-upsmanship, and trying to embarrass or humiliate the examiner. This type of patient may make snide remarks about the interviewer's age or credentials: "How old are you, anyway?" "I want to talk to a *real* doctor." In more extreme cases, the patient may refuse to talk altogether. Some patients are manipulative and obsequious, trying to get the interviewer on their side, often by emphasizing how much better and more competent and more likable the examiner is than "all those other doctors who don't seem to care."

Whatever the quality of the interaction, the examiner must document with specific examples how the reported conclusions were reached. For instance, the statement that a patient was "covertly hostile" can be documented by observing that after waiting 15 minutes to be seen, the patient remarked to the examiner, "I thought you had died and . . . gone to hell."

Psychomotor Activity

A patient who displays *psychomotor restlessness or agitation* moves around constantly, appearing to have difficulty sitting still. There may be hand wringing, foot shuffling, crossing and uncrossing of knees, picking on scabs, scratching, nail biting, hair twisting, or even hair pulling. In more severe illness, the patient may get up from the chair or bed, wander around the room, and engage in behaviors inappropriate to the context of the interview, such as trying to make a phone call, combing hair, and the like. Conversely, *psychomotor retardation* is characterized by a general slowing of movement, speech, and thought. The patient will sit quietly, moving very little. Speech is soft and slow, ac-

companied by minimal, if any, gestures. Facial expression can be immo-
bile. Talking seems to be an effort, and there are frequent periods of
silence. Questions are answered after a prolonged latency. In some disorders, such as affective psychoses, psychomotor agitation and retardation may coexist (e.g., the patient may be physically restless and mentally slowed down). Precise description of psychomotor retardation is
now possible through the use of a recently developed scale (Widlöcher,
1983). If neither psychomotor agitation nor retardation is observed, the
patient's psychomotor activity is judged as "normal." This would be the
case in the majority of patients who seek counseling for problems of
living. Abnormal psychomotor activity, observed on repeated examination, tends to be indicative of a major psychiatric disorder.*

Affect and Mood

Affect refers to the prevailing emotional tone during the interview as
observed by the clinician. A "normal" patient will show a range of
affect, laughing when something is funny, and looking somber when
sad or painful issues are discussed. Affect will, in other words, be congruent with the content of the conversation.

Commonly observed disturbances in affect include *hostility* (a predominantly argumentative and antagonistic stance toward the interviewer and others) and *lability* (rapid shifts from happiness to sadness,
often accompanied by giggling and laughing or sobbing and weeping.)
These shifts may cover the whole gamut of feeling states in the course of
an interview.

Inappropriate affect is observed when the patient's feeling state seems
to be incongruent with the content of the conversation (for example,
giggling when the death of a loved one is discussed; weeping while
talking about events which, by objective criteria, should not cause excessive sadness.)

The patient with a *blunted affect* has minimal display of emotion,
with little variation in facial expression. *Emotional flattening* is a more
severe degree of emotional impoverishment and refers to the virtual
absence of all emotional reactivity.

It is important to note that cultural variables play an important part
in the interaction on which the judgment of affect is based. A frightened, insecure patient from a minority background may give the false

*It is beyond the scope of this chapter to provide a detailed description of various motor
disturbances — such as *tics, stereotypies, chorea, ataxia, mitmachen,* and *mitgehen* — seen in
neuropsychiatric disorders. The interested reader is referred to Fish's (1974) *Clinical
Psychopathology.*

impression of emotional flatness because he or she is trying to guard against giving a poor impression by revealing only minimal information with minimal emotional involvement. If the examiner suspects that his or her observations are colored by such contextual variables, definite conclusions should be suspended until there has been an opportunity to observe the patient inobtrusively interacting with peers, family members, nursing staff, or others. Assessment should be carried out to determine if there is an inability to display emotional warmth or if the patient was responding to the social context of a threatening interview with an unfamiliar and inadvertently intimidating professional. Invoking cultural variables to explain abnormal findings requires a thorough knowledge of the culture or subculture in question.

Mood refers to the subjective emotion experienced by the patient over a period of time and therefore is based on self-report. These self-reports do not always coincide with the affect that is observed during the interview. For instance, a patient may look dejected, but vigorously deny a depressed mood; conversely, a patient may interact well and show a good range of affect but report deepening depression over the preceding several weeks. Such incongruities, which are commonplace in the assessment of emotion, should be specifically recorded in the Mental Status Examination. In addition to *depressed* mood (e.g., "I am down in the dumps, and I don't seem to be able to pull myself out of it"), which is probably the most common complaint in a clinical population, one may hear reports of *elated* or *euphoric* mood ("I feel as high as a kite, as if I were on Cloud 9"), *irritability* ("I am short fused, everything seems to bother me; I yell at my kids, at my colleagues. . ."), and *anxiety* or a sense of foreboding ("I feel kind of scared, like something bad is about to happen"). In the absence of specific mood disturbance, the subject is described as *euthymic*.

Speech and Thought

The patient's speech is described with regard to loudness, speed, complexity, usage of words, and ability to come to the point.

Her speech was soft and slow. At times, she was barely audible and had to be asked to repeat what she said. She spoke only in response to specific questions and needed to be asked repeatedly to elaborate on her answers. Her vocabulary was limited, commensurate with her eighth grade education. However, her speech was coherent, and her answers were appropriate.

It is important to document any deviations from what would be considered "normal" by citing relevant examples, using the patient's own words, if possible. Thus, it is not sufficient to summarize one's observations by noting "stilted verbal behavior" or "pressure of speech." Such conclusions must be corroborated by relevant quotes or by a description of the behavior that led the examiner to arrive at them.

His speech was contrived and stilted. He tried hard to convey that he was well-educated, using long words, often inappropriately. For example, when trying to say that things often got hectic at his job as a telephone operator, he stated things got "exuberant."

Thought or *thought process* refers to how ideas are put together, and in what sequence and speed. A patient may exhibit no abnormality. On the other hand, there may be an absence of *coherent thought* that is clear, logical, and easy to follow. *Circumstantiality* is a tendency to answer questions in tedious and unnecessary detail and circumlocution. This is sometimes seen in people from a rural background. Circumstantiality is also frequent in people with extreme obsessional characteristics who want to make sure they include all facts that might be remotely relevant to the point in question. Severe circumstantiality often goes hand in hand with other indications of low intelligence and/or organic mental disturbance. The most severe degree of circumstantiality is known as *tangentiality* (oblique or totally irrelevant responses), often seen in schizophrenic disorders.

In *pressure of speech*, seen in anxiety states and agitated depressions, the patient feels compelled to talk. Patients with flight of ideas, a major diagnostic sign in mania, not only feel pressured to talk, but their thoughts race ahead of their ability to communicate them. The patient will skip from one idea or theme to another. In contrast to *looseness of associations*, the connection between different ideas is not entirely lost, but may be tenuous, consisting of rhymes or puns (*clang associations*).

Her speech was loud and rapid, interspersed with laughter and jokes. At times, she appeared to trip over her words, and her thoughts seemed to be racing ahead of her ability to put them into words. When asked who the president was, she replied: "Johnson, Johnathan, my son, sunshine, Einstein." (This patient entertained the belief that her son was smarter than Einstein and would become the next president.)

In the extreme, it may be difficult to draw the line between flight of ideas and looseness of associations (Andreasen, 1979a). In the latter, the patient's speech loses any meaningful or logical sequence. Patients may actually invent words that have meaning only to them (*neologisms*). Here is an example of severe loosening of associations, interspersed with neologisms. It is the first paragraph of a written statement presented to one of us by a patient who hoped that this would clarify his reasons for coming to the hospital.

Good Day! *Natherath*. In early times man has struggled for the long *surrinel* of the human orator, the inner intestinal cavity, the lungs. It is knowledgeable that the bone structure of man is durable with *tintured* calcium, skin seven epidural thick which replenishes it in the case *endergy* and mental powers.

At times, mild loosening of associations manifests itself in a general vagueness of thinking. However, although not as disjointed as the preceding sample, very little information will be conveyed, even though many words may have been used. This disturbance, known as poverty of thought content, is diagnostic of schizophrenia when known organic mental states are ruled out (Andreasen, 1979a).

In *perseveration*, the patient adheres to the same words or concepts and seems unable to proceed to other topics. For instance, a patient responded to sequential questions as follows: "How many years have you been married?" "Seven." "How many children do you have?" "Seven." "How many weeks have you been out of work?" "Seven." *Echolalia* is the irrelevant echoing or repeating of words used by the interviewer ("Can you tell me what brings you here to the emergency room?" "Room, room, room.") Echolalia is often accompanied by *echopraxia*, which consists of repeating movements initiated by the examiner. These disturbances are often seen in catatonic and organic mental disorders.

Confabulation denotes fabrication of information to fill in memory gaps (seen, for instance, in the Wernicke–Korsakoff syndrome, a complication of chronic alcoholism).

Thought block refers to the sudden stoppage of thought in the middle of a sentence. Sometimes, after a momentary pause, the patient may begin a new and unrelated thought. At other times, the patient may seem perplexed and unable to continue to talk. This experience, when mild, may be due to exhaustion, anxiety, or a retarded depression. More severe thought block is seen in schizophrenia, possibly as the observable counterpart of the subjective experience of thought withdrawal.

Retardation or inhibition of thought processes, characteristic of bipolar depressives, consists of a slowing of thinking — subjectively experienced as poor concentration, indecision, or ruminative thoughts. Such patients may complain of "poor memory" — which, together with poor performance on cognitive tests, may lead to the erroneous diagnosis of dementia in elderly subjects. Such pseudodemented depressions should obviously be distinguished from true dementia, as the former are eminently treatable.

Mutism is the complete loss of speech. The patient cannot be made to talk at all. It is seen in hysteria, catatonia, and with those patients suffering from midline lesions of the brain. Patients who intentionally refuse to speak to certain people display *elective mutism*.

Stupor, which may have its etiology in hysterical, neurologic, depressive, and catatonic disorders, consists of almost total arrest of all motor activity (including speech), with little or no response to external stimuli. Thus, stupor represents an extreme degree of psychomotor retardation and mutism combined. The condition has been observed on the battlefront and in civilian catastrophes as "paralysis by fear," and in catatonic schizophrenia and stuporous depression. However, stupor also can be a sign of severe and life-threatening physical illness, and the first order of business is to rule out medical disease or drug-induced states even if one can find psychologically "plausible" reasons to explain the patient's condition.

Aphonia and *dysphonia*, unless based on laryngeal pathology, are almost always due to hysteria. Here, the patient loses his or her voice and cannot raise it above a whisper. In aphonia — as contrasted with mutism — one observes lip movements or nonverbal attempts to communicate. Aphonia can be an "unconscious" compromise in an inhibited individual who, for example, feels like cursing but is ashamed to do so.

Whereas *thought form* refers to *how* thoughts are communicated, *thought content* refers to what the patient communicates. Much of this information becomes apparent in the course of the interview, but some specific questions may need to be asked. The nature of inquiry into thought content again depends largely on the patient's clinical picture and presenting problem.

Every Mental Status Examination should have an explicit statement about the presence or absence of *suicidal thought content*. Approaching this topic can be difficult for the beginning clinician. There is a popular misconception that one might inadvertently "put ideas into the patient's head" by exploring this issue. In fact, the danger lies in failure to inquire about suicidal ideation, in that the seriousness of suicide risk cannot be properly assessed and appropriate interventions cannot be made. A tactful way to inquire about suicidal ideas is as follows: "You have told me a lot about the painful things that have happened in your life. Have you found yourself thinking that one way to forget it all is to go to sleep and not wake up?" If the answer is affirmative, the next question could be, "Have you had thoughts that you might just want to end it all by taking you own life?" At this point, some patients will vigorously deny that they are considering suicide. Others will admit to suicidal ideas. It is important to find out whether these thoughts have evolved into a specific plan for action and whether there have been suicide attempts in the past. Suicidal risk is greatly increased if the patient feels truly hopeless and helpless.

Homicidal thoughts may emerge during the interview and should be noted; again, direct inquiry may be necessary. *Religiosity* (religious pre-occupation that exceeds culturally accepted standards in the patient's religious denomination) will also probably emerge in the interview. However, *obsessions* (repetitive and irrational ideas that intrude into consciousness and cannot be shaken off) and *phobias* (specific irrational fears) may not emerge spontaneously and should be inquired about. Related symptoms, which may or may not be spontaneously verbalized, include *depersonalization* (the uncanny feeling that one has changed) and *derealization* (the feeling that the environment has changed). Although these two experiences can occur in the normal as isolated events (as in severe exhaustion), they happen most commonly in agoraphobia, (Lader & Marks, 1971) and, less commonly, in depressive illness.*

Delusions are false, unshakeable beliefs that are idiosyncratic to the individual and cannot be explained on a cultural or subcultural basis. For example, the belief that one is possessed by the devil or that one is the victim of a voodoo curse is not necessarily delusional. Neither are beliefs in unusual health practices and folk remedies. However, the judgment that one is dealing with culturally accepted phenomena must be made on the basis of thorough knowledge of the culture. In fact, in cultures where voodoo and witchcraft are still part of daily life, delusions often consist of pathological elaborations of these beliefs that would *not* be endorsed or shared by the patient's kin or associates. The inexperienced examiner may fail to recognize serious pathology by being overly willing to invoke "cultural" phenomena. For this reason, it is often desirable to inquire whether other members of that culture share the beliefs in question.

Delusions should also be distinguished from *overvalued ideas*, which refer to fanatically maintained notions such as the superiority of one sex, nation, race, or of one school of thought, philosophical approach, or artistic endeavor over others. Finally, delusions should be differentiated from *pseudologia fantastica*. This disorder, observed in hysterical psychopaths, consists of fantastic storytelling where the individual eventually loses track of which statements are true and which are false.

Delusions are divided into primary and secondary categories. *Pri-*

---

*A temporal lobe focus is to be suspected if depersonalization and derealization coexist with perceptual disturbances such as *déjà vu* and *déjà vécu* (the feeling that one has seen or experienced a given situation), *micropsia* (objects getting smaller and receding into space) or *macropsia* (getting larger).

mary delusions cannot be understood in terms of other psychological processes (Fish, 1974). They were described by Schneider (1959) as "first-rank symptoms," and they consist of externally imposed influences in the spheres of thought (thought insertion), emotion, and somatic function (passivity feelings) as well as experiences of thought broadcasting (Mellor, 1970). Primary delusions seem to arise out of the context of a "delusional mood" where the patient loses his or her grasp of reality. For example, neutral percepts (such as a black car) may acquire special personal significance of delusional proportion (e.g., the end of the world is imminent). The presence of several of these first-rank symptoms is indicative of schizophrenia, although they can also occur in amphetamine psychosis, temporal lobe epilepsy, and alcoholic hallucinosis. Finally, they can be incidental findings in the affective psychoses (Andreasen & Akiskal, 1983).

Secondary delusions, on the other hand, arise from other psychological experiences (Jaspers, 1962) and are usually explanatory elaborations of other psychological themes. Examples of secondary delusions include:

1. Delusions based upon hallucinations, for example, a patient who hears machinelike noises may be convinced that he or she is being subjected to electrical surveillance.
2. Delusions based on other delusions, for example, a patient who believes that his or her "skin is shrinking" may ascribe it to being slowly poisoned by his or her "enemies."
3. Delusions based on morbid affective states, known as *affective delusions* (Akiskal & Puzantian, 1979). For instance, a manic patient stated that his experience of ecstasy, physical strength, and sharpened thinking was so overwhelming that there was only one explanation, namely that he was chosen by God to serve as the new Messiah.

In terms of content (Wing, Cooper, & Sartorius, 1974), the most common delusions include *delusions of reference* (the idea that one is being observed, talked about, laughed at, etc.); *delusions of persecution* (e.g., that one is the target of malevolent or hostile action); *delusions of misidentification* (the belief that, for example, one's persecutors have been disguised as doctors, nurses, family members); *delusions of jealousy* (false belief in infidelity of the spouse or lover); *delusions of love* (also called *erotomania,* where a public figure is believed to be in love with the patient); *grandiose delusions* (belief in unusual talents or powers, or belief that the patient has the identity of a famous person, living or historical); and *delusions of ill health* (hypochondriacal delusions; the patient pleads for a cure of his or her imaginal and often bizarre "disease"). Others are *delusions of guilt* (the belief that one has committed an unforgivable act);

nihilistic delusions (insistence that body parts are missing); and *delusions of poverty* ("I have squandered all my money; my family will starve").

Perceptual Disturbances

A *hallucination* is a perception without an external stimulus (e.g., hearing voices when no one is around, or seeing things that are not there). Any sensory modality can be involved: hearing, vision, taste, smell, touch, and even the vestibular sense. Certain forms of hallucinations cannot be ascribed to such discrete sensory modalities, however. For instance, patients intoxicated with psychedelic drugs may report that they can "hear colors," "smell music," and the like. This is known as *synaesthesia*.

Illusions are often described by the patient as "hallucinations." However, they are simply misperceptions of actual stimuli, for example, mistaking a clothes tree in a dimly lit room for a person. Such experiences may result from exhaustion, anxiety, altered states of consciousness, delirium, or a functional psychosis.

Perceptual disturbances may occur in individuals who do not suffer from a mental illness. Most of us have had times when, while waiting for an important phone call, we actually "hear" the phone ring; it is not uncommon to "hear" a voice calling one's name when no one is actually there. In normal individuals these experiences are more likely to occur in periods of high emotional arousal or expectancy and tend to be isolated and infrequent events.

Auditory hallucinations are classified as elementary (noises) or complete (voices or words). Both forms are most commonly found in schizophrenic disorders. They may also occur in organic mental disorders and intoxications. For instance, alcoholic patients frequently hear voices (alcoholic hallucinosis). Voices that are continuous, make a running commentary on the patient's behavior, or argue about him or her in the third person are special categories of hallucinatory phenomena included in Schneider's list (1959) of first-rank symptoms. Another Schneiderian first-rank hallucination consists of hearing one's own thoughts spoken aloud (*écho des pensées*). Like primary delusions, these Schneiderian hallucinatory experiences are characteristic of, but not specific to, schizophrenia (Andreasen & Akiskal, 1983).

Auditory hallucinations occur not only in schizophrenic and organic mental disorders but also in depressive and manic psychoses. The term *affective hallucinations* is used to describe hallucinatory experiences based on, or understandable in terms of, a prevailing morbid affective state.

The voice may tell the patient that he or she is "a sinner" or "a mastur-
bator" and should be punished by death. An example of affective hallucinations in mania follows (Akiskal & Puzantian, 1979):

> A 28-year-old black female heard "motors" and believed that this perception
> represented the noise of carriages that were specially sent to transport her,
> her children and the entire household into heaven. (p. 429)

When perceptual disturbances occur in affective illness, they tend
to be transient, usually occurring at the height of mania or the depth of
depression, or during the unstable neurophysiologic transition (mixed
state). They can also appear as organic complications secondary to exhaustion, dehydration, or the superimposed drug or alcohol abuse that
often accompany affective illness.

Visual hallucinations are characteristic of organic mental disorders,
specifically the acute delirious states; they tend to involve figures or
scenes less than life-size ("Lilliputian"), may coexist with auditory hallucinations, and are often frightening in nature. They are common complications of sensory deprivation (e.g., cataract surgery). Psychedelic
experiences with drugs can be pleasant or frightening depending on
mental set. Visual hallucinations are uncommon in schizophrenia but
occur in normal grief (visions of a dead relative), in depressive illness
(e.g., seeing oneself in one's casket) as well as in brief reactive (hysterical) psychoses.

Olfactory hallucinations are difficult to distinguish from illusions of
smell. (The same is true for *hallucinations of taste*.) Some delusional
female patients, for instance, are always conscious of their vaginal odor
and tend to misinterpret neutral gestures made by other people as indicative of olfactory disgust. In temporal lobe epilepsy, hallucinations of
burning paint or rubber present as auras.

Hallucinations of touch, or *haptic hallucinations,* usually take the
form of insects crawling upon one's skin and characteristically occur in
cocaine intoxication, amphetamine psychosis, and delirium tremens.
When they occur in a schizophrenic disorder, they may take such
bizarre forms as orgasms imposed by an imaginary phallus.

Vestibular hallucinations (e.g., those of flying) are most commonly
seen in organic states such as delirium tremens and LSD psychosis.
Patients with such misperceptions have been known to sustain serious
injuries or even death by trying to fly out of windows.

In *hallucinations of presence,* experienced by schizophrenic, histrionic,
and delirious patients, the presence of another individual is somehow
sensed. In *extracampine hallucinations,* the patient visualizes objects outside his or her sensory field (e.g., seeing the devil standing behind him
or her when he or she is looking straight ahead). In *autoscopy* the patient

sees himself or herself in full figure without the benefit of a mirror; this experience that can occur in organic, hysterical, depressive, and schizophrenic conditions is also known as *doppelgänger,* or seeing one's double. It is skillfully portrayed in Dostoevski's novel *The Double.*

Other varieties of hallucinations include visual experiences that occur in the twilight state between wakefulness and sleep (*hypnagogic*) or sleep and awakening (*hypnopompic*). Although their occasional occurrence is normal, repeated experiences suggest narcolepsy. Some narcoleptic subjects may actually have difficulty distinguishing vivid dreams from reality. It must be kept in mind, however, that patients with histrionic personalities may also give flamboyant accounts of hallucinations: they may actually "perceive" objects or events that fit their fantasies, and they may, in addition, dramatize the occurrence of normal hallucinatory experiences such as dreams in an attention-seeking manner.

Orientation

Orientation is conceptualized in four spheres: orientation to *time* (day, week, month, and year), *place* (location of interview, name of city), *person* (identity of self and interviewer), and *situation* (interview as opposed to, for example, inquisition or trial). A patient who is oriented in all spheres is noted to have a *clear sensorium.*

Patients with signs and symptoms of psychosis may or may not be oriented in all spheres. Those with affective and schizophrenic psychoses are not typically disoriented, whereas patients suffering from organic brain syndromes are characteristically disoriented. In an acute brain syndrome, the mental status tends to fluctuate; in a hospital setting, these patients often show remarkable changes depending on time of day, with worsening orientation at night (known as *sundown syndrome*). The symptomatic picture of acute organic brain syndromes (e.g., drug intoxication) often closely resembles acute psychoses of "functional" origin (schizophreniform and manic disorders). Whether the patient is disoriented and whether his or her mental status fluctuates are therefore important diagnostic clues. For this reason, the examiner must state the time of day of his or her interview on the report to permit serial assessments.

Some specific questions that should be asked are as follows: *Orientation to time:* Can you tell me what day of the week it is today? Do you know what day of the month it is? And what month? What year is it? *Orientation to place:* Can you tell me the name of this place? What is the name of our city? What is the name of the state? *Orientation to person:* Tell me your name. Do you know who I am? (If the patient cannot be expected to know your name, let him or her look at your name tag.) Can you tell me what I am doing here? *Orientation to situation:* Tell me what this is all about. Why are we talking to you? What is the purpose of this visit to the clinic? If the patient is not able to answer these questions, the examiner should, in a reassuring and supportive manner, provide answers and clarification. At a later point, the patient can be asked the same questions again. Whether he or she is able to retain this information will give important clues regarding short-term memory.

Obviously, it is not necessary to inquire formally about orientation items in every patient. A student with the chief complaint of fear of public speaking need not be examined in depth about his or her orientation; this will be evident from his or her general demeanor and life situation.

Attention, Concentration, and Memory

Much can be learned from careful observation of the patient during the interview. A patient with deficits in *attention* has trouble achieving the appropriate set that would permit the interview to proceed: he or she may fall asleep as you talk; he or she may practically ignore you, being distracted by television, telephone, and other irrelevant stimuli. He or she cannot filter relevant from irrelevant stimuli as they pertain to the interview situation. Care must be taken to distinguish between *deficits in attention,* which are involuntary, and *lack of cooperation* or oppositional behavior, which is a purposeful attempt to obstruct the interview process. An example of the latter would be a patient who pointedly leafs through a magazine while you are trying to talk to him.

A patient with deficits in *concentration* may be able to achieve the set required for a successful interview, but has trouble maintaining it. Thoughts are easily distracted, questions will have to be repeated, and complaints like "my mind is not working" are common. If the patient shows deficits in attention and/or concentration, a more formal inquiry into these areas is indicated.

Deficits in *memory* can be of four types: *immediate* (the patient cannot recall things he or she has just been told); *short term* (the patient cannot retain information for 5 minutes or so); *long term* (the patient is unable to remember the events of the past months or years); and *remote* (concerning events many years in the past).

Impairment in immediate and short-term memory may actually reflect inability to concentrate, a distinction that is not always easy to make. The patient whose deficits arise from difficulty concentrating will appear preoccupied, anxious,and will have problems following the clinician's instructions. On the other hand, the patient with memory deficits will try his or her best and will understand what he or she is supposed to do but be unable to perform. Anxiety may also be present, but this will be more of a response to the patient's realization that his or her mind is not functioning properly. A supportive and reassuring stance on the part of the examiner is essential.

Sometimes the examiner may actually decide to "coach" a patient with memory deficits: severely depressed patients often display concentration disturbances that result in poor performance on cognitive tests (*depressive pseudodementia*). With encouragement and reassurance, these patients often find the correct answers. However, such coaching does not work in true dementia.

Some specific tasks that can be used in assessing memory and concentration are as follows:

Street address: "Now I am going to give you an address that I want you to remember for me. I will ask you again in about 5 minutes what this address is, and you tell me. The address is 1625 Poplar Avenue. Can you repeat this for me? (Let the patient repeat the address.) O.K. I'll ask you about it in 5 minutes. Now let's go on and talk some more about the other things we were discussing." After 5 minutes, most patients without organic impairments will be able to recall the address correctly, or almost correctly.

Digits forward and digits backward: "Now I am going to ask you to repeat some numbers for me. I say the numbers, and when I am done, you say them after me. Now I start: 1-4-5. Can you repeat these for me?" One then goes on to increasing numbers of digits. When the patient has reached the maximum number of digits he or she can recall, the process can be repeated with the instruction to recall digits backward, starting with two numbers, and going on to longer strings. Most patients with normal intelligence and without organic impairment can repeat six digits forward and at least five in reverse. For this exercise to be useful, the clinician should *not* try to make up the numbers but should read them off a table, in an even cadence.

Memory for three objects: "Now I am going to ask you to remember three things for me. I will ask you again in about 5 minutes, and you tell me what they are. Here are the three things: The color *red*; the word *pencil*, and the number 17. Repeat these for me. O.K., try to hang on to these three things, and I'll ask you again, in about 5 minutes."

Serial subtraction: This is more specifically a test of concentration. Ask the patient to subtract 3 from 100, then 3 from that number (hopefully, 97), then 3 again, and so forth. If this poses no problem for a few rounds, ask him or her to subtract 7 from 100, from 93, and so forth. Educational level and calculating ability must be taken into consideration.

Recall of recent events: By asking a patient about verifiable events that transpired in the past days, one can assess mental functioning in an unobtrusive way. These questions can include what the patient ate for lunch, the current issues in the TV news (if the patient reports having watched the news), and the like. It is important that the answers can be verified, because patients with organic brain dysfunction often *confabulate* their answers (e.g., they invent plausible responses in order to avoid the painful realization that they cannot remember). Intellectual functioning can also be unobtrusively assessed in this way, by asking the patient about current events and his or her understanding of their implications.

Remote memory: Such memory function is often well preserved, even in patients who suffer from significant organic impairment. It can be checked by getting patients to talk about their childhood and adolescence, places where they have lived, military service, occupations, and (most verifiably) by assessing recollections of important historical events and their impact (e.g., Pearl Harbor, the Great Depression, who was president during those times, etc.) Some specific questions may include "Who was John F. Kennedy and what happened to him?" "What is the Berlin Wall?" "What was Sputnik?" "What was Watergate?"

Intelligence

One can get a general estimate of a patient's intelligence simply by talking to him or her. Specifically, the patient's *vocabulary* will give clues about intelligence, especially if considered in view of educational level. A college graduate can be expected to have a good vocabulary, but if a laborer with a third grade education shows evidence of a rich vocabulary, one may conclude that his intelligence is much above his level of scholastic achievement.

Abstraction ability is another indicator of intellectual functioning. Some specific questions will help in this assessment: the "similarities" section of the Wechsler Adult Intelligence Scale lends itself to use in a Mental Status Examination. One may wish to set the stage for this line of questioning by giving an example.

> Now I am going to ask you a few more questions. They have to do with how some things are like other things. Here is an example. A hammer and a screwdriver are like each other in that they both are tools. Now, can you tell me how an apple and an orange are like each other? A table and a chair? A coat and a dress?

Concrete answers are more likely to reflect lack of education than intellectual impairment. However, the answers to these questions can be revealing at both ends of the spectrum. A patient with minimal schooling who shows a high level of abstraction ability can be assumed to have good intelligence. A patient with a college degree whose answers are concrete (an apple and an orange both have peels; a table you eat at and a chair you sit on. . .) shows significant intellectual deterioration.

Another way to test abstraction ability is by asking the patient to interpret proverbs. However, knowledge of the patient's sociocultural background is essential because one cannot assume that the patient has ever heard or understood the proverbs that we take for granted. Proverb interpretation can be approached as follows: "Now I am going to give you a few sayings, and I want you to tell me what they mean. Have you ever heard the saying, 'Don't cry over spilt milk'?" If the patient says yes, ask him or her to interpret. If he or she says no, interpret it for him or her. ("It means that there is no use worrying about something bad that has happened and that can't be fixed.") "Now let's try another one: can you tell me what could be meant by 'a stitch in time saves nine'?" Concrete interpretations should be evaluated in the same way as concreteness in "similarities."

Reliability, Judgment, and Insight

The interviewer must decide whether the patient can be deemed to be a *reliable* informant. This will largely depend on an estimate of the patient's intellectual functioning and on the clinician's impression about the patient's honesty, attention to detail, and motivation. For example, a patient who comes to treatment under family duress may give a very self-serving story that cannot be judged as reliable. A very histrionic patient may believe his or her own reports, but they may be colored by exaggeration, retrospective falsification, and wishful thinking. A patient with antisocial traits may tell bold-faced lies to get out of legal trouble, and a patient with limited intelligence may simply make up facts to avoid embarrassment and to get the doctor "off his back." Psychotic patients and patients with organic mental disorders are often unreliable informants. Whether or not the patient is deemed reliable must be stated explicitly.

Unreliability due to carelessness, poor memory, or psychosis should not be confused with *talking past the point* or *vorbeireden*. First described in prisoners (and labeled *Ganser syndrome* after the psychiatrist who observed it), it consists of giving deliberately wrong answers in a fashion that indicates that the question was understood. Like, "Who is the president?" "Jimmy Reagan." "Who was president before him?" "Ronald Carter." Such patients, typically sociopathic, are either malingering to appear insane or, in the case of schizophrenic individuals, are simply amused by the question–answer sequence. Because in most instances the impression given is one of dementia, the condition is also described as *hysterical pseudodementia* (Fish, 1974).

Judgment must be evaluated clinically in light of the entire history. Many patients who have normal intellectual functioning suffer from notoriously poor judgment in organizing their personal lives. This information can be gleaned from the facts obtained during the interview; evidence of poor judgment should, again, be documented with specific examples. For instance, walking around city streets wearing a bikini is poor judgment, as are a history of repeated suicidal gestures or of impulsive job changes. Judgment can, if necessary, be assessed more specifically by using items from the Wechsler Adult Intelligence Scale, such as the well-known "What would you do if you were the first one in a movie house to see smoke and fire? What would you do if you found a sealed letter which has an address and a stamp on it?"

The clinician has to assess whether the patient has adequate awareness that he or she has a problem, and if so, of possible causes and reasonable solutions. This is known an *insight* and can be poor or absent (as in a psychotic illness), partial (some cognizance of the emotional nature of the problem), or good (understanding of the emotional roots of the problems). Insight usually depends on adequate intellectual functioning, but the converse is not true, that is, many highly intelligent people may be sorely lacking in insight.

Commonly Misused Terms and Their Diagnostic Significance

Beginning clinicians often find it difficult to distinguish between *apathetic, depressed,* and *flat* affect (Andreasen, 1979b). Apathy can sometimes be due to severe physical illness wherein the patient simply feels too ill and too weak to engage in a conversation. Apathy can, however, also be encountered in chronic schizophrenia and organic mental states.

A patient with *depressed* affect is best described as being in a state in which he or she experiences mental anguish, or is unable to experience joy or pleasure (James, 1903). He or she will not be cheered up by reassurance or jokes; he or she cannot imagine a time when he or she will not be suffering the pain of depression. This is typically a phasic disturbance and tends to fluctuate with episodes of the disorder.

On the other hand, a patient with *blunted* or *flat* affect shows emotional impoverishment. He or she not only fails to experience joy but cannot feel sadness, anger, desperation, or any other emotion. Such emotional impoverishment, which is characteristic of schizophrenia, tends to go hand in hand with formal thought disorder and is often present throughout the course of the illness, not just during florid psychotic flare-ups (Andreasen, 1979b).

Apart from using the patient's history, differentiation of depression and emotional flatness on a Mental Status Examination can be accomplished as follows. The facial expression of the chronic schizophrenic is typically vacant; that of the depressed patient is one of gloom, pain, and dejection. The interviewer usually has difficulty empathizing with the schizophrenic (known as *praecox feeling*) except on an intellectual level ("How this person must suffer inside!"), but the depressed person's dejection and pain tends to be communicated to the clinician and elicits emotional as well as intellectual empathy. Admittedly, this is a subjective criterion, but it is valuable in the hands of experienced clinicians.

Another difficult distinction is that between a *labile* affect (which changes quickly, often from one extreme to the other) and *incongruent* affect (which is inappropriate to the thought content or the context). Both labile and incongruent affect should be differentiated from *affective incontinence*, where the patient laughs or cries for extended periods with little or no provocation (i.e., the patient loses control over emotional expression). Lability may be encountered in character disorders such as histrionic personalities; in mixed states of manic-depressive illness where there is rapid shift from elation to irritability to depression; and in acute organic mental disorders, where the affect can quickly change from anxiety to terror to panic. By contrast, incongruent affect (e.g., laughing while relating the gory details of a fatal accident) should raise the suspicion of schizophrenia. Emotional incontinence occurs most commonly in organic mental states such as arteriosclerotic dementia and multiple sclerosis.

Euphoria and *elation*, although characteristic of manic states, can also occur in organic mental disorders such as those resulting from systemic lupus erythematosus and multiple sclerosis. The euphoria seen in mania has warmth that is communicated to the observer, although, in the extreme, the manic patient can be irritable, cantankerous, obnoxious, and alienating. A silly kind of euphoria occurs in chronic schizophrenia and frontal lobe lesions; this sign is known as *Witzelsucht* and consists of the patient's relating patently silly jokes. Manic euphoria tends to be contagious or infectious—the clinician cannot help but enjoy the patient and laugh along with him or her. This is not the case with the silly euphoria found in schizophrenic and organic states. Again, these are not entirely reliable judgments but seem to carry diagnostic weight in the hands of experienced clinicians.

The term *paranoid* refers to psychotic conditions where delusions predominate (e.g., paranoid schizophrenia and paranoid disorder). Thus, the term *paranoid delusion* is redundant and should be replaced in the psychiatric vocabulary by more precise phrases such as *persecutory delusions, delusions of reference,* or *delusions of jealousy.*

Thought disorder is a rather nebulous term and should not be used without qualification. One should always distinguish between *formal thought disorder* and *disorder of content.* Thus, the presence of delusions is not necessarily indicative of formal thought disorder. As already discussed, delusions can arise from affective and memory disturbances. Furthermore, in paranoid schizophrenia, delusions can exist in the absence of gross disturbances in the formal aspects of thought.

Formal thought disorder is a disorder in associations whereby thoughts are dissociated, disconnected, or rambling. It is also known as *derailment* (thoughts that are off the track). If mild, it leaves the impression of "vagueness"; if extremely severe, the patient makes no sense at all and is often said to exhibit *word salad.* The phrase *loose associations* is used for an intermediate degree of severity whereby one finds fragments of thoughts that seem totally illogical. Nevertheless, such thinking may have some symbolic significance — a highly personalized meaning that derives from "primary process" or "unconscious" associations; for that reason it is referred to as *autistic thinking,* that is, entirely related to the self, the inner world, and divorced from reality (Bleuler, 1950). Autistic patients invent neologisms to convey highly personalized concepts or meanings for which they find conventional language inadequate. The incoherence that one observes in the thinking of organic patients is qualitatively different from formal thought disorder in that it lacks symbolism and the autistic quality. It is sometimes difficult to assess whether a patient whose answers are vague and rambling is intellectually dull or has trouble focusing ideas: that is, has a mild thought disorder. In the absence of intellectual impairment (e.g., if the patient has completed college), the hypothesis of a thought disorder should be entertained. Beginning clinicians may be overly eager to give such patients the benefit of the doubt, supplying in their interview accounts connections and logical transitions that the patient has failed to produce. This is especially likely when the patient is intelligent and shares other characteristics of the examiner, thereby making it threatening for the examiner to recognize the patient's pathology.

The converse can also occur. Some clinicians tend to diagnose schizophrenia with minimal evidence. This is often based on proverb interpretation. Andreasen's work (1977) has shown proverbs to be generally unreliable in diagnosing schizophrenia. Yet it is often erroneously assumed that inability to abstract on proverbs or similarities (i.e., *concrete thinking*) carries major diagnostic weight for schizophrenia. If a patient does not exhibit gross loosening of associations and displays concreteness on proverbs, he or she is said to have a *subtle thinking disorder.* There is little scientific rationale for this type of practice, because concreteness correlates best with poor intellectual endowment, cultural impoverishment, and organic mental disorders. All three frequently coexist with schizophrenia, and to this extent schizophrenics will have impaired ability in abstraction. Schizophrenic patients are often annoyed by proverbs. In our opinion, it is best to avoid direct testing of abstracting ability, unless one suspects organicity or mental retardation. The main value of the proverbs test in schizophrenia lies not in the degree of concreteness of responses (which may be due to low intelligence and social restriction) but in the patient's tendency to give bizarre and idiosyncratic responses.

In its severe manifestations, hysteria may mimic major affective illness, schizophrenia, and even organic mental disorders. The histrionic patient may transiently display (or *report* to have experienced) a plethora of severe symptoms suggestive of a major psychotic disorder. There can be repeated, bizarre, and florid symptoms; such symptomatology is often reported with an affect known as *la belle indifference*, (i.e., a remarkable lack of concern for what to others would seem heart-rending problems). This attitude is often mistaken for flat affect, and the flighty and disorganized verbal accounts for formal thought disorder. In these situations, it is of the utmost importance to see the patient more than once, preferably after the emotional turmoil that provoked the clinical picture has had a chance to abate.

Some Illustrative Case Reports

In this section we will provide samples of Mental Status Examinations performed in different settings.

Case 1.

Ms. A. was a 38-year-old black woman, married, mother of three teenagers. She was referred by her gynecologist because gynecologic examination had failed to elucidate the cause of her decline in sexual interest. Her Mental Status Examination was as follows:

She was a tall, slender woman, impeccably dressed and groomed. Her hair was carefully styled. She wore makeup, conscientiously applied, and expensive-looking jewelry. She sat at the front of her armchair, appearing very "edgy." Her facial expression was one of worry. She was oriented in all spheres. She engaged in considerable hand wringing when she talked about her troubles and often picked nervously on her clothes, removing tiny specks of lint. She was cooperative and appeared to answer all questions to the best of her ability. Her affect showed a good range and was generally appropriate; she also exhibited several instances of nervous laughter when relating painful events. She described her mood as dysphoric and worried, "like I feel something bad is going to happen, and I have no control in the matter." She wept at times but always managed to pull herself back together. No history of discrete panic attacks was elicited, nor did she have specific obsessions or compulsions. She admitted to feelings of extreme irritability and frustration because she was unable to cope with the "teenage problems" of her kids. While discussing these, she stated that she felt worse in the mornings, which was the time her husband wanted to engage in sex. She said she could be more receptive sexually at night, though she was anorgasmic then as well. There had been no change in appetite, but she had difficulty falling asleep. Her attention appeared good, but she had trouble concentrating and often had to be brought "back on track"; she had a tendency to get lost in the details of her complicated story. She asked several times "What was it we were talking about?" Her memory for events appeared normal, but she complained that she had "trouble remembering things." For example, she almost had a fire at home last week because she forgot to unplug her iron; she often came home from the store without items she had intended to buy. She said this was not like her; she always prided herself in being conscientious and well organized. She stated, "I guess I just have too much on my mind." Her intelligence was above average, commensurate with her education (a Master's degree in education). She expressed herself well and stated the nature of her problems in sophisticated language. Her report is considered reliable. There was no abnormality in her thought form or content. She stated she was worried that she was about to "really lose it" when, a few days ago, she heard the doorbell ring, and nobody was there. She described no other instances of perceptual disturbances. She vigorously denied suicidal thoughts, stating her faith (Catholic) would keep her from even considering such acts because she feared eternal damnation. Although she freely verbalized anger toward her husband, children, and friends who had sometimes "let her down," there was no evidence of homicidal ideation. She expressed guilt for feeling angry. Her judgment and insight were good, as she realized the emotional nature of her presenting problem. She felt her main problem was her inability to communicate it properly to her husband.

This mental status is compatible with a generalized anxiety disorder, major depression, or both, a differential diagnosis that should be resolved on the basis of present illness, past psychiatric and medical history, and family history.

Case 2

Mr. B. was a 21-year-old white male who was brought into the emergency room by the police after he had disrupted a funeral at a local cemetery.

He was pale and disheveled. His clothes were dirty. Although it was summer, he wore two woolen hats and a long muffler. He was oriented to time and place. However, he stated with a silly grin he was the "Antichrist" and the examiner was "the Virgin Mary." He was restless during the interview and often stood up from his chair. He seemed bewildered and was reluctant to talk. When asked who had brought him to the hospital, he stated: "The police! Inquisition! Ha! Ha! Armageddon!" He was reluctantly and superficially cooperative, asking repeatedly "Done now? Let me go!" His affect was silly. He giggled inappropriately, often after saying "quiet!" at which time he seemed to be listening to voices. When asked about them, he said he received instructions from "above," but refused to elaborate. He denied other Schneiderian first-rank symptoms. He stated his mood was "wonderful." His attention and concentration were impaired, possibly by distraction from inner stimuli or thoughts. He refused to try serial subtractions and cursed at the examiner, stating, "Don't you ever mess with the Antichrist no more." His intelligence could not be assessed. His educational level is unknown. He claims he has a "PhD and an EdD and an MD degree also." When asked about what it meant to be the Antichrist he said, "If you don't know that by now, you never will." After this, he refused to communicate any further and stared quietly into space for the remainder of the session. For this reason, suicidal or homicidal thoughts, or specific delusions, could not be assessed. His judgment and insight are considered to be nil.

This mental status raises differential diagnostic possibilities ranging from schizophrenic to manic and drug-induced psychoses. Historical, familial, and laboratory (e.g. urinary drug screen) evaluations are necessary to differentiate between these alternatives.

Case 3

Ms. C. was seen for consultation on the Medicine Service where she was hospitalized following a large overdose of diazepam, which she had stolen from her mother's medicine cabinet.

She sat propped up in her bed, dressed in a hospital gown. She looked younger than her stated age of 24. Her hair was braided in corn rows and slightly disheveled, but she was otherwise neat and clean. She stated with a smile that she knew the examiner thought she was a "real mental case" but that she had taken the pills following an argument with her fiance and had had no intention to die. She just thought he "needed to be taught a lesson." Her psychomotor activity was normal, and she was oriented in all spheres. Her affect appeared shallow. She denied depression and stated that "all is well now": the boyfriend had "come around" to her way of thinking, and there were not going to be "any more problems." When asked how the future looked to her, she said "perfect." Her attention, concentration, and memory appeared normal. Her intelligence and vocabulary seemed commensurate with her educational level (10th grade). Her account of what led up to her overdose seemed reliable, but her judgment was immature. There was no evidence of formal thought disorder, and her speech was normal in flow and content. She denied any hallucinations, stating "You really think I'm a nut!" Her insight is deemed to be poor, but she has no suicidal or homicidal ideas at the present time.

This mental status, which fails to reveal the presence of a major Axis I disorder, is indicative of a personality disorder, the nature of which should be explored in future sessions of individual or preferably, group therapy (assuming, of course, that the patient is willing to follow through).

Case 4

Mrs. D., a 57-year-old widowed former schoolteacher, was seen in consultation on the medical service. She was hospitalized for observation and diagnostic work-up of gastric complaints.

According to the referring physician, her mental status on admission was "unremarkable." On the fifth day in the hospital, she became visibly anxious, and her condition worsened during the night. The night shift reported she refused to stay in her room and was found wandering the halls in the nude on two occasions. The nurse on the morning shift described the patient as "a sweet lady who has gone bonkers on us!" In retrospect, the nurse recalled that the patient had complained of insomnia and nightmares beginning with the second night of hospitalization. However, her request for a hypnotic had not been granted by her physician. When Mrs. D. was seen by the consultant the following morning, she wore only her pajama bottoms and had a towel twisted around her head like a turban. She mumbled to herself and displayed considerable restlessness, getting up and wandering around her room, picking invisible objects off her chest and arms. Her hands showed a coarse, irregular tremor. She was marginally cooperative, agreeing to put on her pajama top and following simple directions such as "stick out your tongue," "turn your head to the left," and the like. However, her attention span appeared very impaired, and she seemed to be distracted by visual and auditory hallucinations. She stated, with irritation, that she could not sleep because "these Jehovah's Witnesses were singing hymns in my room all night long." She also complained that the nurses had put a half gallon of vanilla ice cream on her night table where it was "melting and dripping away." (There had never been any ice cream.) Her affect was labile, alternating from pleasant cooperation to irritability. Her orientation was marginal. She stated she was in a hospital but seemed genuinely puzzled about why she was there. She knew her name and home address. She was disoriented to time. There was no gross loosening of associations; rather, she proved to be extremely distractible and often drifted off the subject, mumbling to herself. At one point, she announced she needed to go now because she was tired of hearing "Big Mama" call her for a "bologna sandwich." Her memory and concentration were extremely poor. She was unable to perform any of the relevant tasks (serial sevens, three objects, digits forward and backward). There was no evidence of systematized delusions. Her insight and judgment were nil.

This patient exemplifies an acute organic brain syndrome. Further history revealed that she had been taking various types of minor tranquilizers since her husband's death a year ago to help her sleep. Enforced abstinence in the hospital had resulted in drug-withdrawal delirium, similar to that seen in alcohol withdrawal states, but occurring much later than the two- to three-day latency from abstinence typical for delirium tremens. This is due to the longer half-life of minor tranquilizers.

Summary

Current evidence indicates that, despite overlapping manifestations, discrete categories of mental disorders do exist. The diagnosis of these disorders requires systematic history taking and interviewing. Eliciting the various signs and symptoms described in this chapter is not only necessary to support differential diagnostic decisions, but it also serves the important task of communication with other colleagues and objective documentation of current difficulties for future reference.

A carefully conducted mental status is the cornerstone of good clinical work and research in psychopathology (Fish, 1974). In addition to presenting a general psychopathologic framework pertinent to all professionals who come into contact with the mentally ill, this chapter has emphasized situations and concerns particularly relevant to psychologists.

References

Akiskal, H. S., & Puzantian, V. R. (1979). Psychotic forms of depression and mania. *Psychiatric Clinics of North America, 2,* 419–439.

Andreasen, N. C. (1977). Reliability and validity of proverb interpretation to assess mental status. *Comprehensive Psychiatry, 18,* 465–472.

Andreasen, N. C. (1979). The clinical assessment of thought, language and communication disorders. *Archives of General Psychiatry, 36,* 1315–1330.(a)

Andreasen, N. C. (1979) . Affective flattening and the criteria for schizophrenia. *American Journal of Psychiatry, 136,* 944–947.(b)

Andreasen, N. C., & Akiskal H. S. (1983). The specificity of Bleulerian and Schneiderian symptoms: A critical re-evaluation. *Psychiatric Clinics of North America, 6,* 41–54.

Bleuler, E. (1950). *Dementia praecox, or the group of schizophrenias.* (J. Zinkin Trans.) New York: International Universities Press.

Fish, F. (1974). Clinical psychopathology: Signs and symptoms in psychiatry In M. Hamilton (Ed.). Bristol: John Wright & Sons.

James, W. (1903). *Varieties of religious experience.* Glasgow: William Collins & Sons, 1982.

Jaspers, K. (1962). *General psychopathology* (M. W. Hamilton & J. Hoenig, Trans.) Manchester: Manchester University Press.

Kraepelin, E. (1904). *Lectures on clinical psychiatry.* London: Balliére, Tindall, and Cox.

Lader, M., & Marks, I. M. (1971). *Clinical anxiety.* New York: Grune & Stratton.

Mellor, C. S. (1970). First rank symptoms of schizophrenia. *British Journal of Psychiatry, 117,* 15–23.

Schneider, K. (1959). *Clinical psychopathology* (M. W. Hamilton, Trans.) New York: Grune & Stratton.

Widlöcher, D. J. (1983). Psychomotor retardation: (clinical, theoretical and psychometric aspects. *Psychiatric Clinics of North America, 6,* 27–40.

Wing, J. K., Cooper, J. E., & Sartorius, N. (1974). *The measurement and classification of psychiatric symptoms.* Cambridge: Cambridge University Press.

Part II

Psychiatric Disorders

Chapter 3

Anxiety-Based Disorders

H. E. Barbaree and W. L. Marshall

Introduction

This chapter presents a general approach and method for the conduct of interviews with the anxiety-disordered patient. The chapter does not present a structured approach to the derivation of differential diagnoses according to decision rules in any single diagnostic system. Rather, it presents a more general approach to the gathering of data in the interview, which results in a useful understanding of the patient's fears. The general approach we propose is based on the scientific method (hypothesis testing) in which the interviewer constructs a theory of the patient's fear, derives hypotheses from the theory, and subjects these to empirical validation in the interview.

A Method for Gathering Data in the Interview

Kozak and Miller (1982) make an important distinction between fear as an intervening variable and as a hypothetical construct. For clinicians who want to come to a good understanding of their patients' fears, the distinction is important. As an intervening variable, *fear* is nothing more than a label that serves to summarize the collection of empirical facts concerning the fearful behavior. According to MacCorquodale and

H. E. BARBAREE and W. L. MARSHALL • Department of Psychology, Queen's University, Kingston, Ontario, Canada K7L 3N6.

Meehl (1948), these variables offer no hypotheses concerning the existence of unobserved entities or processes and contain no words in their
definition that cannot themselves be defined in terms of the observed
facts.

On the other hand, fear as a hypothetical construct is less restricted
in scope by the empirical facts. This concept of fear makes predictions
concerning its generality in time and place and postulates variables that
may serve to increase or reduce it. Kozak and Miller (1982) argue that
without guidance from a theory of fear, we would not know which
combination of measures to use to appropriately collect the "facts" concerning fear.

> One can only attribute factual status to an observation if a theory is
> available to determine that it is indeed significant, i.e. a fact. Facts are *the-*
> *oretically* significant observations, not neutral or "hard" data. (Weimer, 1976,
> pp. 18–19, italics added)

When diagnostic labels are applied to patients according to modern
diagnostic systems, as for example, the *Diagnostic and Statistical Manual
of Mental Disorders*, third edition (DSM-III), the resultant label is in the
form of an intervening variable. These are labels for sets of "facts" or
criterion levels of observable behavior. Nothing in the way of inferences
or hypotheses enter into the process by which these labels are applied.
The modern diagnostics are in contrast to earlier systems (e.g., DSM-II)
that depended heavily on inferences concerning etiology and mechanisms of the disordered behavior. Unreliability of the diagnosis and
conflicts over the etiology and mechanisms have forced the development of the modern inference-free systems. The modern diagnostics
show a distinctly improved reliability of diagnosis and lend themselves
well to hospital record keeping, experimental and statistical sampling,
epidemiology, and the like. However, for the working clinician, labels
for patients that simply summarize the empirical facts in the case are not
particularly helpful. Clinicians need to construct theories of their patients' fear to guide their choice of treatments and to predict outcome in
therapy. In this sense, clinical practice ought to be indistinguishable
from the guiding principles of research, and both may be seen as ver-
sions of the scientific method (Marshall, 1982). Indeed, Yates (1975) has
argued that this approach is the distinguishing feature of behavior
therapy.

In arguing for the necessity of inference in clinical practice and
scientific enquiry regarding fear, Kozak and Miller (1982) do not argue
for a return to the inferentially based diagnostic systems. It is important
here to distinguish between appropriate and inappropriate inferences in
this regard. In the earlier diagnostics, inferences were frequently stated
in terms that could not be operationally defined nor empirically validated. For example, distinctions between diagnostic categories on the

basis of etiology could not be verified in individual cases. However, that is not to say that all inferences need be so ill defined or unverifiable. Inferences can be stated in hypothetical (testable) terms and later subjected to empirical validation.

> Ideally theory and data advance through a process of mutual feedback as each changes to accommodate the developments in the other. This would seem to be the proper relationship of data and construct: theory suggests a crucial test, data provide the test, and theory must then evolve to accommodate that data. Data are uninterpretable, however, in a theoretical vacuum. (Kozak & Miller, 1982, p. 351)

When a clinician sits down with a patient in an interview and tries to come to some useful understanding of the patient's fear or anxiety, he or she does not simply record the facts in the case, nor does he or she use labels or jargon to code summaries of the facts and relationships among the facts. Rather, the clinician constructs a theory of the patient's fears not just on the basis of information provided by the patient, but also on the basis of knowledge derived from the clinician's general background and training and the current scientific understanding of fear and anxiety.

The better interviewer forms a series of hypotheses about the patient's fear early in the interview, and the interview proceeds as a continuous stream of hypothesis formation, hypothesis test, and theory modification or reconstruction. A good theory of the patient's fear will allow the clinician to

1. Outline the important cognitive, motoric, social, and physiologic processes that contribute to or determine the patient's fear.
2. Highlight aspects of the clinician's understanding of the fear that do not place undue reliance on the patient's self-reports. Hypotheses based on self-reports at the interview will be open to subsequent examination by objective testing or behavioral assessment.
3. Caution the patient concerning situations or circumstances in which he or she may be at high risk for failure.
4. Facilitate choice of treatment strategies in general terms and subsequently quide the clinician in planning the details of treatment strategies. The application of the interventions in turn serve to further evaluate the hypotheses.
5. Determine a set of dependent measures and assessment procedures with which to monitor the patient's fear throughout therapy.

The questioning in interviews is designed to gather response data in each of three separate modes or channels (Cone, 1978; Lang, 1968, 1971,

1977), including physiologic, motoric, and verbal response modes. Of course, although these response modes function somewhat independently in some circumstances (Rachman & Hodgson, 1974), they usually interact and often serve to augment one another. Physiologic responses in anxiety are those associated with hyperventilation, sympathetic over-arousal, and with skeletal muscular tension. These responses include palpitations, chest pains, difficulty in breathing, dizziness, peripheral tingling sensations, sweating, faintness, and trembling. These physiologic reactions may escalate to extreme levels, and when they do the patient is said to experience a panic attack. The most obvious motor or gross behavioral responses in anxiety are escape or avoidance behaviors, but also anxiety may be observed as behavioral signs (e.g., trembling, speech dysfluencies, etc.). These responses may be directed by stimulus location, as in animal or height phobias, or may seemingly be generalized to all location stimuli as in agoraphobia. The content of verbal responses in anxiety usually connote some expectation of harm or threat of harm, including dread and apprehension. Also, persons may experience a change in their sense of themselves (depersonalization) or in their sense of their reality (derealization).

General Description of Anxiety Patients

The DSM-III groups several disorders under the heading "Anxiety Disorders," including Phobic Disorders and Anxiety States. Included in this last category are Obsessive-Compulsive Disorder and Posttraumatic Stress Disorder. We will not address these latter disorders in this chapter but rather restrict our discussion to maladaptive behaviors that involve direct manifestations of anxiety or fear as their defining feature.

Anxiety disorders are classified in DSM-III in terms of the predominant symptoms from among the three response modes. Phobic Disorders are primarily characterized as combinations of motor and verbal anxiety responses. Anxiety States are primarily characterized as combinations of physiologic and verbal anxiety responses. Agoraphobia with Panic Attacks is described as a combination of all three anxiety responses in the one disorder. Although the DSM-III encourages a clear-cut distinction among these various disorders, the evidence is not as compellingly supportive of the distinctions as would appear to be implied. For example, Emmelkamp (1982) has argued that we should not consider anxieties and phobias as distinct diagnostic categories but rather as displays of fearful symptoms lying along the three dimensions of responding described previously (which are common to all forms of anxiety and fear). On the other hand, Klein and his co-workers (Klein, 1980; Zitrin, Klein, Lindemann, Toback, Rick, Kaplan, & Ganz, 1976; Zitrin, Klein, & Woerner, 1980) have found that panics occur in a wide range of phobic and anxiety states, and they consider the presence or absence of panics to be of greater importance than the object or range of fear. Other authors, for example Hallam (1978) and Marks (1969), have reviewed evidence that they take to mean there is little or no difference between generalized anxiety and agoraphobia; certainly, diagnosticians have difficulty reliably distinguishing these disorders (Gorman, et al., 1981).

Although this diagnostic issue remains problematic, Klein (e.g., Mendel & Klein, 1969) has for many years maintained that these two disorders (generalized anxiety and agoraphobia) are distinguishable on the basis of the presence or absence of panics. Klein (1980) claims there is a group of patients who suffer from generalized anxiety and yet do not have panics. These patients, so Klein says, have a high level of chronic anxiety reflected in muscular tension, hyperactivity in various autonomic indexes (e.g., excessive sweating, digestive distress, cardiac acceleration, increased blood pressure, elevated respiration rates, genitourinary problems, etc.), hypervigiliance, and apprehension and dread. Klein considers these individuals to be characterized by a pervasive demoralization, vulnerability to criticism and rejection, and a general inability to deal with life's problems. They do not, however, develop phobic avoidance. These descriptions fit the DSM-III criteria. As Klein notes, this group of patients has been inadequately studied but appears to include a heterogenous group of individuals who may or may not be readily distinguishable from those diagnosed as having other anxiety disorders. Recent research reported by Hoehn-Saric (1981) indicates that patients having generalized anxiety without panics differ from patients having panics primarily in terms of the type and severity of particular somatic symptoms. Panic patients have more severe respiratory distress, a greater incidence of palpitations, hot and cold flashes, and more severe headaches. However, these two groups do not differ in reports of tiredness and sleep disturbances nor in the frequency of gastrointestinal or genitourinary symptoms. Although this study offers support for Klein's position in terms of the relevance of panics (note that the somatic features that distinguished the disorders are primarily those manifest in panics), it does not support a single-minded distinction among the anxiety disorders in terms of the predominance of somatic symptoms in general.

From Hoehn-Saric's study and other research, the two features that may most readily distinguish generalized anxiety from both panic disorder and agoraphobia are the presence or absence of both panics and specific, or generalized, phobic avoidance. In the latter respect, patients with generalized anxiety disorder appear to restrict their activities somewhat but do not consistently avoid any specific object or situation. Further, they do not become as excessively restricted as do agoraphobics.

Panic-disordered patients are so diagnosed if they experience recurrent panics that are not in response to some specific, readily identifiable stimulus and that appear in the absence of clear agoraphobic symptoms. Although these patients usually develop some degree of anticipatory fear of panics and may be reluctant to enter situations in which they previously experienced panic, their lives are not as circumscribed as are those of agoraphobics, nor are their anticipatory fears attached to a particular setting but rather to the possibility of experiencing a panic. In this latter respect their fears are similar to those of agoraphobics who experience panics; that is, they are afraid of fear. The panic attack itself involves discrete periods of extreme anxiety manifested by difficulties in breathing and associated feelings of choking or smothering, radical fluctuations in heart rate, severe chest pain, faintness and dizziness, and experiences of depersonalization and derealization. During these panics the patient believes he or she will die, go crazy, or lose control.

A substantial number of these panic-disordered patients suffer from mitral valve prolapse (Crowe, Pauls, Kerber, & Noyes, 1981), as do a number of agoraphobics who experience panics (Kantor, Zitrin, & Zeldis, 1980). For patients in whom panics have been identified, therefore, it may be prudent to make a referral to a cardiologist as part of the diagnostic investigation.

Although by far the majority of agoraphobics appear to experience panics, according to DSM-III not all do. The presence of panics may very well be quite important not only for theories of the etiology of these disorders but most importantly for treatment decisions. Klein and his colleagues (Klein, 1967, 1980; Zitrin, Klein, & Woerner, 1978, 1980) have found that antidepressants (imiprimine in particular but also the MAO inhibitors) suppress panics but fail to affect anticipatory anxiety or avoidance behavior. Anxiolytics and behavioral treatments, on the other hand, appear to attenuate anxiety but have no affect on panics. However, the latter conclusion by Klein and his co-workers concerning the value of behavioral treatments has been criticized (Marshall & Segal, 1984). Chambless and Goldstein (1981) have offered an alternative perspective that suggests that it is countertherapeutic to pharmacologically suppress panics in treatment. Whatever the empirical outcome of this debate, it will remain important to identify panics and to distinguish them from anticipatory fear and avoidance.

Agoraphobics experience fear in situations which they define as "lacking safety," by which they mean those situations that do not offer ready help should they have a panic or become distressed. Thus, situations where they are isolated or from which escape is difficult are typically avoided by agoraphobics. Because this encompasses an evergrowing range of situations, as the agoraphobic becomes increasingly sensitized to fear (i.e., develops a "fear of fear" as Goldstein & Chambless, 1978, call it), the agoraphobic becomes increasingly constricted in movement and frequently ends up housebound. It is important to note that for agoraphobics, being alone is one of the most dreaded situations, and consequently they quickly develop dependent relationships. Indeed, an important aspect of this problem and possibly of other anxiety or phobic disorders concerns a variety of relationship difficulties. For example, agoraphobics often display a persistently dependent interpersonal style (Andrews, 1966; Fodor, 1974), although the evidence on this is equivocal (Buglass, Clarke, Henderson, Kreitman, & Presley, 1977). Similarly, agoraphobics are frequently passive, unassertive individuals (Chambless & Goldstein, 1981), who are involved in dysfunctional relationships (Kleiner & Marshall, 1984). In addition, agoraphobics in particular but also other anxiety and phobic patients are characteristically depressed (Bowen & Kohout, 1979; Gardos, 1981). Marks (1982) provides evidence suggesting that the beneficial effects of antidepressants with phobics may be due to their pretreatment level of dysphoric mood. Because none of these features (dependency, passivity, poor relationships, and depression) occurs in all agoraphobics, it will be necessary, in a proper analysis of the presenting problem, to identify the magnitude of these defects in each patient in order to define assessment strategies in addition to ascertaining treatment goals and procedures.

Social phobias are common after the onset of adolescence (Abe & Masui, 1981; Agras, Chapin, & Oliveau, 1972) and involve primarily a fear of scrutiny by others. The DSM-III takes much fear of scrutiny to be the defining characteristic of social phobia, although it also notes that these patients are afraid of behaving in a way that may humiliate or embarrass them. Included among the social phobics are people who are afraid of public speaking, who are beset by anxiety about eating in public, working in front of others, conversing with others, crossing a crowded room, or using public lavatories. The social phobic, therefore, can identify situational features that elicit anxiety, and he or she takes care to avoid these if at all possible.

Perhaps the easiest diagnostic task of all in this area is to identify the simple phobic. This person, who, it might be said, rather rarely appears in clinical practice, is afraid of some specific, readily identifiable stimulus. These problems may involve fear of closed spaces (claustrophobia), of heights (acrophobia), of flying, of animals or insects, of death or illness, of storms or the dark, or indeed fear of any other

circumscribed situation or object. Although the majority of these patients do not experience spontaneous panics, they do experience situational panic in response to exposure to their feared stimulus. Also Zitrin,
Woerner, and Klein (1981) have found that some phobics, usually claus-
trophobics, do have spontaneous panics, and they refer to these patients
as *mixed phobics*. Again, the presence or absence of these panics is important in designing treatment.

Case Interview

This patient was a 34-year-old self-referred male. When he called to
make an appointment he described himself as *agoraphobic*, a problem he
said he had read about in the local newspaper and realized that the
description fitted him. He expressed much apprehension about the trip
from his home to our office. On the day before his appointment he
called to outline a contingency plan should it snow the next day. He
explained that he was afraid of riding in a car during a snowfall. Because
it was a warm and sunny day in late March, the probability of a snowfall
seemed extremely remote. This concern revealed the extent of his restricted movement and suggested that his self-diagnosis was probably
accurate. He arrived well ahead of time for his interview, and he seemed
unable to await for the appointed hour, so we commenced immediately.
The following is an abbreviated, edited transcript of the first three interviews. We have dispensed with introductory exchanges and start at the
point where information gathering began. We first investigated the role
of panics in the problem. Given the literature on agoraphobia, it was
reasonable to suppose that panics were a central problem for this man.

T: You mentioned on the telephone that you were quite concerned about a
   variety of possible problems you might have encountered on your way to this
   appointment. Perhaps you could begin by telling me what some of these
   possible problems might have been and what difficulties they might present
   for you.
P: Well, I told you how I can't ride in a car when it's snowing.
T: Yes you did, but why is that a problem?
P: Well, I think the car will slide off the road.
T: I see. You think you might be injured in an accident.
P: Not really. Of course I don't want to get hurt, but I am more afraid that if we
   had an accident I might have an attack and I wouldn't be able to get help.
   That's what I am really scared of.

As we suspected, panics were a key feature of this man's problem.
We then proceeded to determine the nature of these attacks.

T: Oh, I see. Perhaps you could tell me what you mean by an "attack."

P: Well, I guess it's called a *panic attack*. I read that in the newspaper article.

T: Alright. Tell me, do you have many panic attacks?

P: Oh yes. I have them all the time.

T: How often?

P: Probably two or three times a week.

T: How long have you been having these attacks? Has the frequency changed over time?

P: I've been having them for about 6 or 7 years. They started a bit before I was married and that's been about 6 years. At first, I had them only occasionally, but not long after I was married they increased to about the same rate as now.

T: That must be very upsetting. What happens to you when you have an attack? Take the last time you had an attack and try to remember what it felt like.

P: Oh it's terrifying really. I am certain I am going to die when it happens. I know you're going to say I won't die. That's what my family doctor says, and that's what a psychiatrist I saw 2 years ago said. And probably it's true; at least that's what I think sitting here talking to you. You see I don't feel too bad sitting here; after all, you're a doctor; you'd know what to do if I had an attack. You could get me to emergency or give me a pill or an injection to make me OK.

T: I'm glad you feel OK here, but tell me, you said you thought you were going to die when you had an attack. Is that still true? If you had an attack later today, for example, do you think you would feel the same, feel you are going to die?

P: Definitely. I tell you it's so frightening, I can't breathe properly; my heart pounds like its going to burst. I know I'm dying, but no one ever believes me. I guess they're right, but I wish they'd take me more seriously at the time. I remember once when I was at the psychiatrist's office. While I was waiting I felt an attack coming on; all those other patients were looking at me, and I began to get nervous, and I knew I was going to have an attack. I told the secretary, but she told me I'd have to wait, but I couldn't, so I pushed past her into the doctor's office and pleaded for help. He made me go back to the waiting room, and I ran outside terrified. The doctor came after me along with my wife, and again I pleaded for an injection or something to stop me from dying. Jeez, I'm getting upset just talking about it. Can we stop for a while and talk about something else.

T: Sure. Don't worry, you're safe here. I'll believe you if you tell me you are terrified and think you are going to die. You won't, of course, but I promise to look after you and take your concerns seriously.

At this point a shift in topic seemed appropriate in order to calm the patient. Because we also needed more information about the general effects of his problem on his life we pursued those issues.

T: Maybe you can tell me a bit about your present circumstances, your marriage, where you are living, your job, that kind of thing. Why don't you start wherever you feel comfortable.

P: Well, I am not working and haven't been for the past 6 years. In fact, I gave up work about 6 months after we married.

T: So you've been married for about 6 years. Why did you give up work?

P: Well, I began to have attacks at work. At first, I just went to emergency and then took the rest of the day off, but after, I think, the third attack, which was very embarrassing to me. I'm sure the other staff thought I was silly and weak. Anyway, after this third attack, I just couldn't go back; everytime I tried I'd start to panic and have to give it up. I've never been back since.

T: Have you tried to get another job?

P: No. My wife and I agreed that it would be better for my health if I stayed at home until these panics went away. In fact, it was her idea that I give up work for a while. I'm not so sure she still thinks it was a good idea since we have had to live off her limited income and we have had to shift into a basement apartment in my parents' house. We all get along OK, in fact my mother in particular loves having us there, but I guess it's not how married people are supposed to live.

T: Has it placed a strain on your marriage, the fact that you are not working and bringing home some money or the fact that you are living with your parents?

P: No, not at all, really. My wife says she likes looking after me, and her and my mother get along real well.

T: It must be nice for you to have their support. I see your address is in the country. How do you feel being left alone during the day while your wife is at work? Are you not afraid of having an attack?

P: Not really. First of all, I rarely have an attack at home, and if I do it usually passes before it gets too bad. Then, of course, my mother is always there. She doesn't go out unless my wife is home and [my wife] always gets home from work by five o'clock.

These remarks about the support offered by his wife and mother suggested several possible hypotheses having to do with his dependency upon them and their possible need for him to continue to be dependent.

T: Every night your wife comes directly home from work, and every day your mother stays at home with you?

P: My mother is not actually with me. She is upstairs, and I am in the apartment, but yes she does always stay home until my wife gets back. She [mother] doesn't think I should be left alone, and she's right; I'd be terrified if I was alone.

T: And your wife, she always comes straight home from work?

P: Yes. Always. They both realize, you see, how bad my problem is.

T: That's interesting. We might come back to this later. But for now let's turn to something else. Can you remember when all this started? When did you have your first panic?

P: It was years ago. I think I said earlier they began about 7 years ago. Actually, the first one was earlier than that, but they began to occur regularly about 7 years ago. About 9 years I'd guess was when I had the first one. It happened one night when we were coming home from doing a show. I used to be in a country and western band, and we'd played in [a small town some 10 miles from his home] until about 1 A.M. On the way home in the van the drummer gave me a hit of acid [LSD]. I'd done acid before and enjoyed it, but for some reason I had a bad time that night. I didn't know it at the time, but what I had was a panic. I was scared to death. In fact, I thought I would die for sure. They took me to emergency where they gave me something; I don't know what it was, some kind of injection. Anyway I felt OK after a bit.

T: That sounds awful. So that's when they began. Can you remember the next time? Was it soon after or what?

P: No, it didn't happen again for about 3 years. Of course, I never took acid again or dope [marijuana]. Too scared.

T: Tell me about the time it happened again. What was going on at the time? Where were you? Tell me as much about the circumstances as you can remember.

Here we were interested in the possibility that stress was a precipitant. If so, we may need to do stress management training as part of treatment.

P: Oh I remember it very clearly. In fact I've never got over it. I was engaged and we were to be married in 3 weeks.

T: You and your wife?

P: No. She was before I met my wife. In fact, I married my wife on the rebound, you might say.

T: Go on.

P: Well, we'd been going out for about 4 years and had been engaged for about 5 months. We were always planning things for the marriage and after. Anyway, I went over to her place one night after [band] practice. We'd finished early, and she didn't expect me, but I'd often gone without her expecting me. Mind you, she sometimes got annoyed if I arrived unexpectedly, but I was always so eager to see her I'd put up with her annoyance. Anyway, I let myself in her apartment — I had a key — and found her in bed with a friend of ours. Christ, it killed me really. I didn't know what to do. I started to get upset and she got angry; told me to get out and pushed me out the door. I banged on it, but they wouldn't let me in. God, I felt terrible, my world was turned upside down. I got in my car and drove away. Didn't know where I was going. I got just a bit outside [the town where she lived some 15 miles from his home], when I felt this panic coming over me. It was like the bad acid trip over again. That's all I could think of; it's a flashback. I'd heard of them. I stopped the car. It was dark, and I was all alone way out in the country; didn't know where I was; couldn't get help. It was awful. I was sure I was going to die way out there all alone. Of course I didn't but I was scared for days; couldn't think about [his fiancée]. Everytime I started to think of her I'd start to panic again. I never saw her again or spoke to her. Never. My mother looked after getting my things back and giving [his fiancée] her things back. I've never even gone back to [the town where his fiancée lived]; can't bear the thought even now, of going into the town. That's when it all started really. I've had panics ever since.

T: At the present rate? Two or three times a week?

P: Yeah, pretty much the same as now, although they were probably more severe when I was still going out to work and so on.

Because he had mentioned marrying "on the rebound," we wished to explore the possibility that his attachment to his present wife was not as deeply felt as it might be. Also, lingering affection for his former girlfriend might be relevant to his failure to have made a serious attempt to overcome his agoraphobia.

T: You said you married on the rebound. When?

P: Well, I already knew my wife, and my mother liked her so she invited her over a couple of weeks later after the nightmare with [his fiancée]. She was nice; we got along well. She looked after me; was really kind. We got married within 2 months. Silly, really, I suppose. I didn't give it enough thought. I didn't really love her then.

T: Well, if you're happy now, I guess it doesn't matter what the circumstances of your marriage were. Are you happy now?

P: Yeah, I guess so.

T: You guess so? Are you really happy? If you had your choice in an ideal world would you be married to [his wife]?

P: I'm not sure. I think I really still. . . [He began to cry].

T: It's OK to cry. Go ahead. [Crying subsides].

T: Tell me, what you were going to say?

P: It's silly really. You'll think I'm a fool and a jerk.

T: I doubt it, but tell me anyway.

P: I still love [his former fiancée; cries again].

T: I see. Does your wife know this?

P: No. [Still crying].

T: Well that's obviously a distressing subject. Let's get back to that later. You said your wife "looked after you" after the awful news about your fiancée. You said she was kind and nice. Does she still look after you, would you say?

Some agoraphobics tend to be rather dependent, and some of his remarks suggested that he might be.

P: Yes, I guess so. She does everything except the housework. I suppose our roles are reversed. I'm the scared one who needs looking after. She goes out to work, earns the money, drives me around when I can go out, does the shopping.

T: Does it bother you that you are not fulfilling the usual male role?

P: No, not really. I do my bit around the house as far as I am capable. My wife and my mother and father realize my problem and don't expect me to do anymore than I do.

T: I see. So they are all supportive. Did they also encourage you to get help?

P: Yes. My sister told my mother about you, and it was her that called.

T: Oh, I thought it was your wife that called, but it was your mother, eh? Is your wife supporting your efforts to get treatment?

P: Oh yes. She drove me here.

We try not to concentrate too fully on any one aspect of a patient's problems for a prolonged period but rather to shift back and forth from topic to topic in an attempt to keep the interview alive and also to avoid the development of defensiveness arising from pressing the patient too hard on a specific topic. We were interested in how he had responded to earlier treatment and particularly how cooperative he was and what support he got from his family for attempts to change.

T: You said you saw a psychiatrist sometime ago. Did he or she help you?

P: Not much. He gave me Valium, which I still take.

T: How much?

P: Ten milligrams a day. It helps with my anxiety a bit, but it doesn't stop the panics. You know it makes me feel like I can get through. Maybe, I don't need it, but I'm too scared to stop. Matter of fact, I went to see another psychologist about a year ago, and he said I would have to give up the Valium if he was to treat me. I didn't go back. I was too scared to stop. He doesn't know what it's like. Nobody does really except probably my wife and my mother.

T: When you went to see this psychiatrist or the psychologist, did either of them urge you to get out of your home a bit? I get the impression you spend most of your time at home. Is that true?

P: Definitely. In fact, pretty well the only time I leave is on Saturdays; I go shopping with my wife. Well, I don't always make it. Sometimes I start to panic, and my wife has to take me back home.

T: If you make it to the shopping center do you go in with your wife?

P: Very occasionally. The crowds are too much. Usually, I sit in the car and she checks on me about every 15 minutes or so. It's just a chance to get out.

T: I was asking you before if the psychiatrist had ever suggested that you go out more, perhaps even try doing so on your own?

P: Yes he did, and I started to do it too, but I got really upset once, and my wife and mother got very annoyed with the doctor and said I shouldn't go to see him anymore because he was making me worse.

T: Was he? Do you really think it was making you worse?

P: Probably not, but I did start to have more panics and [his wife] was really angry so I just stopped going.

T: How does your wife feel about you coming here?

P: Oh, she thinks it's a good idea.

T: So she'll be supportive. What if I ask you to try to go out on your own? Will your wife and mother support that, or do you think they will get angry again especially if you get upset?

P: Oh yes. I don't think they liked Doctor. . . . They thought he was pushing me too hard. He wasn't very understanding really. He told me I had to get off my ass and conquer my fear as if it was easy to do.

T: Well, I am sympathetic, and I realize it's not easy for you to go out alone, but I do want you to understand that an important part of treatment will require you to get out and about on your own. We'll do it slowly and proceed at a pace that suits you, and initially I will accompany you. But sooner or later you will have to go it alone, and you will always have to make the effort to go a bit further than you might be prepared to go; that's how you overcome these things. Anyway, more of that later. I wanted to ask you a bit more about your relationships and what you were like before this problem developed.

Again, we are interested in exploring the extent of his dependence on others and the likely associated unassertiveness.

T: Perhaps you could start by telling me about your friends at school. Did you have many friends?

P: No. Only one really. The other kids always picked on me for some reason, and my friend had a couple fights over it.

T: He fought other boys because they were nasty to you?

P: Yeah. I don't know what I'd have done without him.

T: You're a reasonable-sized fellow; how come you didn't fight for yourself?

P: I'm not a good fighter. I don't like fighting. It scares me; always did.

T: Me too; so I understand what you mean. Fighting is no way to solve problems anyway. Did you say anything to these other kids when they were nasty to you?

P: No. I'd run away if I could.

T: What if you couldn't?

P: Usually I'd do what they told me. God, I used to even agree with whatever they said about me. But I used to imagine what I'd do to them. I used to pretend to myself that I was superstrong and in my daydreams I'd beat them up and they'd all be scared of me. Of course, I never did any of that stuff. Once I did get angry and started screaming at them, but I got so upset that I made a fool of myself, and they all laughed. That made everything worse; they never left me alone after that so I never did that again.

T: How about with other people, when you were older, say in your teens?

P: What do you mean?

T: Well, I understand why you didn't stand up to these nasty kids at school, but I'm just wondering if you learned from that to let others push you around. What do you think?

P: I don't think so. I guess I've always been a bit shy, and I like doing things for people. I enjoy helping people out.

T: Could you give me an example?

P: Well, when I was in the band I'd always do most of the organizing and loading and unloading the van. It relieved the other guys, and anyway they didn't like doing it. They thought I was great.

T: I see. Well, we'll get back to that later. I'd also like to know a bit about how others helped you out. You sound like someone who enjoys doing things for other people. Did other people do things for you?

P: Well, actually I don't always enjoy doing things for others. Even in the band I used to get annoyed sometimes because the other guys were a bit lazy, and I'd have to do everything. On the other hand, as I said, I was shy and too scared to do any singing or announcing, so the other three would do all that. That was a great relief to me, I can tell you; it was bad enough to have to stand up on stage in front of all those people.

T: That was nice of them. What about your girlfriend? The one you found in bed with your friend. What was she like to you? Was that the first time she had been unkind or unfaithful?

P: I'm not sure, but I think she might have been unfaithful before. She used to go off for weekends to Toronto and wouldn't let me go with her. I often thought that maybe she was meeting someone, but I never said anything.

T: Why didn't you say anything?

P: She would have just got angry. It might have made her annoyed enough to tell me to hit the road; leave and not come back. I don't know, I never felt like I could tell her what I was thinking. She'd get pissed off at the simplest things.

T: What about the time you spent together. Who decided where to go, what to do? You or her?

P: Oh, she did. Mind you, I didn't mind. I was just happy to be with her. She was great, really. I still love her. I think I told you that already.

T: In what way was she so great?

P: I don't know. She was so capable; such a strong personality. She would arrange everything we did. I didn't have to worry about anything. She was so different from my wife. She [his wife] wants me to decide everything all the time. What we eat. What TV show we watch. God, it gets me down. I wish she was more like [his former girlfriend].

T: But your wife does the shopping. She goes out to work. So she does contribute something.

P: Oh, yeah. Actually, I usually end up getting her to decide on dinner and the TV, for that matter.

T: What about going out? I know you don't go out often, but when you do who decides?

P: Well, the only places we go are shopping and to visit her parents, and she plans those, although I often can't go, so we cancel out.

T: What about if you have to go to the doctor or the dentist?

P: I'm too afraid of dentists, although I badly need work on my teeth. If I have to go to a doctor my wife makes the appointment and takes time off work to take me.

Obviously, this man was very dependent and had managed to manipulate things so that others took care of him. Clearly, his agoraphobia was maintained by factors in addition to fear, and these other factors could be understood as secondary benefits that may have become more important than the fears and panics. At this point, we clearly needed a better picture of the anxieties associated with his problems.

T: I need to know a bit more about your panics and what you think causes them. Tell me, what goes through your mind when you have an attack? What do you think about?

P: Well, I think I'm going to die.

T: Yes, you mentioned that before. What else do you think?

P: I don't know. What do you mean?

T: Well, I guess you feel frightened, and I know you feel as if you're going to die, but is there anything else you think might happen?

P: Maybe I'll go mad, and I always make a fool of myself. I mean, other people think I'm foolish because they don't understand what I'm going through. My father-in-law thinks I'm weak. He says I'm afraid of everything. He calls me a "suck" and a "wimp."

T: Do you actually think about this when you have a panic? I mean, do you think about behaving foolishly?

P: Oh, yeah. When I start to panic, the first thing I think is "Christ I'm going to look like a goof again." I'm tired of being a goof. I wish I could be like everyone else. I'm sure this is caused by some physical problem. Jeez, I'd love to find out it is caused by a heart problem or something. I'd love to have a doctor's certificate to show my father-in-law and all those other jerks who laugh and sneer at me.

T: Do you ever think that something dreadful will happen? I mean other than that you will die or go mad or look foolish. You know you mentioned that you are afraid to be in a car in winter in case it slides off the road. Do you ever think something terrible like that will happen either before or during a panic?

P: I don't think so. I'm just afraid I will have a panic. That's on my mind most of the time.

T: Are there times when you think panics are more likely? Places or times actually?

P: Oh, definitely. That's the reason I never go out. Panics are always more likely when I'm away from home.

T: Why do you think that's true?

P: Everything is more uncontrolled. You don't know what might happen. At home I feel in control, and in any case I can get help from people who understand. Also, there's no one around who will think I'm silly if I get afraid.

T: That's very interesting. You are doing a great job; being very helpful. We'll get back to that in a bit. What do you feel when you panic? I mean as far as your body is concerned. You said earlier that your heart pounds, and I think you said your breathing was upset. Tell me more about this and about anything else your body does.

P: It's mainly because of my heart and the fact that I can hardly breathe that I think I'll die. Even if there's nothing wrong with my heart, I'm sure that all the strain on it during my panics will eventually cause it to give out. I'm also sure that one day my breathing will get so tight that I will stop [breathing] altogether and just die.

T: Do you have any other body symptoms?

P: Not that I can remember. The heart and breathing problems are overwhelming. I probably wouldn't notice anything else.

T: Perhaps we'll come back to this again leter. Maybe you can tell me what you do when you either have a panic or feel one coming on.

P: I try to get help. If I'm in a car, I get out; ask the driver to stop and get out. I don't really know why since all I really want to do is get home or get to emergency [hospital].

T: What if you're in a crowd?

P: I don't go where it's crowded. I used to, but after having a panic in a crowd I've always avoided them. Since then I wouldn't even talk to more than three or four people. That's too many for me.

T: So you avoid situations that might be unsafe in the sense that help may not be readily available and people who don't understand might laugh at you.

P: Yes; that's it. I'm like a hermit, really.

T: You said earlier that you have about three or so panics a week. Has that been consistent over the past few years?

P: Yeah; pretty much so.

T: Are they just as intense as always?

P: No. But that's cause they usually happen at home where I'm safe so they don't get worse. They would get worse if I was out somewhere.

T: If you're safe at home how come you have panics?

P: Well, my mom doesn't hear too well and sometimes she's out back or doing the laundry or mowing the lawn, and she can't hear the phone so I have to answer it and that always makes me anxious until I find out who it is.

T: I see. When you find out who it is you're OK.

P: No; not always. If it's someone I know, except my father-in-law, it's OK, but if it's a stranger, that will start a panic especially if they won't let me get off the phone.

This man is obviously afraid of interpersonal interactions as well as being agoraphobic. Subsequent interviews supported this. By the time we had completed four interviews, we had formulated several hypotheses about his problem that we had repeatedly tested throughout the interviews, and they were sufficiently strongly supported to justify additional examination by psychological and behavior testing. These test procedures further strengthened our hypotheses that this man was agoraphobic; panicked readily when stressed or when in an "unsafe" situation; was markedly upset by looking foolish; was very anxious interpersonally; was excessively dependent and unassertive; and harbored some degree of resentment toward those upon whom he was, or had been, dependent (his family and the band members, for example). We were also convinced that he had not resolved his feelings for his former girlfriend and that these feelings were contributing to both his housebound behavior (he was afraid he would come in contact with reminders of her) and his resentment toward his wife. On this latter issue, he told in an interview that he felt his wife had taken advantage of his vulnerability to get him to marry her. These hypotheses were then subjected to a somewhat more rigorous test by implementing specific treatment strategies to deal with each problem in a somewhat sequential manner. Although these strategies did not represent the rigorous single-case approach typical of the best examples of behavior therapy (Hersen & Barlow, 1976), they nevertheless were characterized by repeated probe assessments that tended to confirm all our hypotheses. We also thought it possible that he might have genuine heart problems; particularly, we were concerned over the possibility of mitral valve prolapse (see Marshall & Segal, 1984, for a consideration of this issue). However, thorough evaluations, including echo-cardiogram, revealed nothing in the way of supporting evidence.

In addition, we hypothesized that his wife and mother might become resentful when he made progress in treatment. This was a rather weak notion based on the few remarks about their anger over the previous therapist's attempts to have him do self-managed *in vivo* exposure. When he began treatment, his wife and mother were supportive and encouraging. However, once he made progress both these women began to undermine his efforts, urging him to give it up. At a meeting with the family, it became clear that his wife was afraid he would become independent of her and find himself another woman, whereas his mother was afraid that if he was cured, both he and his wife would move out and not visit her anymore. An open discussion of these issues resolved the problem, and progress thereafter was rapid. This man remains somewhat shy, somewhat anxious, and rather restricted in his social activities. However, he is no longer housebound, and he has a responsible, well-paying job. Despite her worst fears, his relationship with his wife is now excellent. He has put his former girlfriend in the past and now declares his love for his wife. Moreover, this couple has maintained affectionate and constant relations with his parents even though they have found themselves independent accommodation. Finally, even his father-in-law seems to have warmed toward him.

Summary and Some Cautionary Notes

Tables 1 and 2 detail the information that should be collected in an interview with respect to the anxiety response in particular (Table 1) and

Table 1. Information Specific to Anxiety Disorder

1. Behavioral topography of anxiety
   (a) Cognitive/verbal
      —Self-statements
      —Expectations, evaluations, attributions
      —Apprehension and dread or threat
   (b) Physiologic/somatic
      —Autonomic arousal such as accelerated HR, sweating, etc.
      —Muscular tension
   (c) Motor/behavioral
      —Escape or avoidance behavior
      —Trembling or fidgeting
      —Approach behavior
2. Severity and generality of component behaviors
3. Antecedents—Investigate through patient's detailed description of at least two illustrative actual events—preferably recent events
   —Conditions or events which intensify anxiety
4. Consequences—How do spouse and friends respond to the anxiety?
5. History
   (a) First occurrence—when and how did first anxiety response occur?
   (b) Family history—other members of family who have experienced similar difficulties
6. Other fears—number and specify, e.g., animals; high, closed, open or dark places; anger or emotions that might result in homicide or uncontrolled sexual behaviors; dentists; speaking in public; social behaviors; illness; storms; being alone; being somewhere unsafe; death; surgery; and injections.
7. Current and anticipated stress
8. Previous attempts at control of anxiety
   (a) By others, including treatment history related to anxiety.
   (b) By self

extraneous variables that might influence the anxiety or its treatment (Table 2). It may be difficult to investigate each of the issues specified in one interview. Two or three interviews may be required to come to an adequate understanding of the patient's fear.

The primary purpose of the interview we have described is to develop a treatment strategy that will be most likely to succeed for the individual patient. Most often, the treatment strategy must include a combination of individual treatments (i.e., desensitization, flooding, social skills training) that is idiosyncratic to the individual patient and that depends on the details of the patient's anxiety response and life circumstances. The clinician cannot arrive at an overall treatment strategy without a good understanding of the patient's fear. The primary source of information that contributes to the understanding is the interview described previously.

Table 2. General Information Pertinent to Anxiety Disorder

1. Marital relationship
   (a) Satisfaction
   (b) Dominance/submission
   (c) Who does housework
   (d) Leisure—conjoint or separate
                —extent
   (e) Amount of time spent in house/alone
2. Work
   (a) Satisfaction
   (b) Effectiveness
   (c) Easy/difficult
3. Education
   (a) Level up to, above, or below competence
   (b) Any training would like to pursue?—why not?
4. Interpersonal effectiveness
   (a) Range of friends
   (b) Frequency of social contacts
   (c) Quality of social contacts
   (d) Confidence in social interactions
   (e) Assertiveness
5. Sexual functioning—satisfaction of both patient and partner
6. Positive experiences
   (a) Frequency of pleasure/enjoyment
   (b) Leisure time and activities
7. Attributions for behavior control and belief in personal competencies
8. Dependence/independence—including need for approval and attention
9. Health
   (a) Sleep
   (b) Appetite
   (c) Somatic complaints
   (d) Psychiatric history (not related to anxiety)

The theory of a patient's fear that will be most helpful in developing effective treatment strategies is constructed by the clinician through a specification of both empirical and theoretical functional relationships between antecedents and the patient's fear and between related behaviors and the patient's fear. Taken together, these functional relationships have been referred to as a *functional analysis of fear* (Goldfried & D'Zurilla, 1969; Kanfer & Saslow, 1965). As we have illustrated in the case history, the theory is developed through a process of hypothesis testing. Once an hypothesized relationship has been formulated, information is sought to verify the relationship. Hypothesized functional relations that are supported by empirical evidence remain in the theory. Those that are contrary to, or incompatible with, evidence are excluded or modified. Through a continuous process of hypothesis testing, a theory of the patient's fear will evolve, one that will form a good foundation for developing an effective treatment strategy.

Hypothesis testing does not end with diagnostics or with the last introductory interview. Treatment is properly applied as a test of an hypothesis, and unsuccessful treatment calls the therapist's theory of his or her patient's fear into question. Further revision of the clinician's theory will involve further interviews and new proposals for treatment.

Two cautionary notes are in order here. We have noticed in teaching this approach to interviewing that novice clinicians concentrate on a single topic for too long, repeatedly testing a single hypothesis by asking the patient many questions concerning what seems to him or her to be a very small aspect of his or her fear. Patients react to this prolonged focus with boredom, frustration, and confusion, and questions as to why the minute details are so important. The case illustration provides the reader with strategies for switching focus in the interview. The clinician will have to rely on her or his own sensitivity as to when a switch in topics is appropriate.

A second common error is to conduct interviews that are too long. It is true that patients are more comfortable ending the interview after they are satisfied that clinicians have achieved a good understanding of their fears and that a reasonable hope for effective treatment and relief of their suffering has been achieved. Clinicians should communicate a good understanding of the patient's fear and an optimism for treatment early in the interview. This should be done before they are certain of the details of their patients' fears or life circumstances and before they have worked out the details of a treatment strategy. In this way, the initial interview can be terminated before either the patient or clinician becomes fatigued or inattentive. The details of the clinician's understanding and the treatment strategy obviously can be worked out in subsequent interviews.

References

Abe, K., & Masui, T. (1981). Age–sex trends of phobic and anxiety symptoms in adolescents. *British Journal of Psychiatry, 138,* 297–302.

Agras, W. S., Chapin, H. N., & Oliveau, D. C. (1972). The natural history of phobia: Course and prognosis. *Archives of General Psychiatry, 26,* 315–317.

Andrews, J. D. W. (1966). Psychotherapy of phobias. *Psychological Bulletin, 66,* 455–480.

Bowen, R. C., & Kohout, J. (1979). The relationship between agoraphobia and primary affective disorders. *Canadian Journal of Psychiatry, 24,* 317–322.

Buglass, D., Clarke, J. Henderson, A. S., Kreitman, N., & Presley, A. S. (1977). A study of agoraphobic housewives. *Psychological Medicine, 7,* 73–86.

Chambless, D. L., & Goldstein, A. J. (1981). Clinical treatment of agoraphobia. In M.

Mavissakalian & D. H. Barlow (Eds.), *Phobia: Psychological and pharmacological treatment*. New York: Guilford Press.

Cone, J. D. (1978). The behavioral assessment grid (BAG): A conceptual framework and a taxonomy. *Behavior Therapy, 9*, 882–888.

Crowe, R. R., Pauls, D. L., Kerber, R. E., & Noyes, R. (1981). Panic disorder and mitral valve prolapse. In D. F. Klein & J. G. Rabkin (Eds.), *Anxiety: New research and changing concepts* (pp. 103–116). New York: Raven Press.

Fodor, I. G. (1974). The phobic syndrome in women. In V. Franks & V. Burtle (Eds.), *Women in therapy*. New York: Brunner/Mazel.

Gardos, G. (1981). Is agoraphobia a psychosomatic form of depression. In D. F. Klein & J. G. Rabkin (Eds.), *Anxiety: New research and changing concepts*. (pp. 367–379). New York: Raven Press.

Goldfried, M. R., & D'Zurilla, T. J. (1969). A behavioral-analytic model for assessing competence. In C. D. Speilberger (Ed.), *Current topics in clinical and community psychology* (Vol. 1). New York: Academic Press.

Goldstein, A. J., & Chambless, D. L. (1978). A reanalysis of agoraphobia. *Behavior Therapy, 9*, 47–59.

Gorman, J. M., Fyer, A. F., Glicklich, J., King, D. L. & Klein, D. F. (1981). Mitral valve prolapse and panic disorders: Effects of imipramine. In D. F. Klein & J. G. Rabkin (Eds.), *Anxiety: New research and changing concepts*. (pp. 317–326). New York: Raven Press.

Hallam, R. S. (1978). Agoraphobia: A critical review of the concept. *British Journal of Psychiatry, 133*, 314–319.

Hersen, M., & Barlow, D. H. (1976). *Single-case experimental designs: Strategies for studying behavior change*. New York: Pergamon Press.

Hoen-Saric, R. (1981). Characteristics of chronic anxiety patients. In D. F. Klein & J. G. Rabkin (Eds.), *Anxiety: New research and changing concepts*. (pp. 399–409). New York: Raven Press.

Kanfer, F. H., & Saslow, G. (1965). Behavioral analysis: An alternative to diagnostic classification. *Archives of General Psychiatry, 12*, 529–538.

Kantor, J. Zitrin, C., & Zeldis, S. (1980). Mitral valve prolapse syndrome in agoraphobic patients. *American Journal of Psychiatry, 137*, 467–469.

Kleiner, L., & Marshall, W. L. (1984). *Marital conflict and agoraphobia*. Unpublished Manuscript, Queen's University.

Klein, D. F. (1967). Importance of psychiatric diagnosis in prediction of clinical drug effects. *Archives of General Psychiatry, 16*, 118–126.

Klein, D. F. (1980). Anxiety reconceptualized. *Comprehensive Psychiatry, 21*, 411–427.

Kozak, M. J., & Miller, G. H. (1982). Hypothetical constructs versus intervening variables: A reappraisal of the three-systems model of anxiety assessment. *Behavioral Assessment, 4*, 347–358.

Lang, P. J. (1968). Fear reduction and fear behavior: Problems in treating a construct. In J. M. Shlien (Ed.), *Research in psychotherapy* (Vol. 3). Washington, DC: American Psychological Association.

Lang, P. J. (1971). The application of psychophysiological methods to the study of psychotherapy and behavior modification. In A. E. Bergin & S. L. Garfield (Eds.), *Handbook of psychotherapy and behavior change*. New York: Wiley.

Lang, P. J. (1977). The psychophysiology of anxiety. In J. Akiskal (Ed.), *Psychiatric diagnosis: Exploration of biological criteria*. New York: Spectrum.

MacCorquodale, K., & Meehl, P. E. (1948). On a distinction between hypothetical constructs and intervening varibles. *Psychological Review, 55*, 95–107.

Marks, I. M. (1969). *Fears and phobias*. London: Heinemann.

Marks, I. M. (1982). Drugs combined with behavioral psychotherapy. In A. S. Bellack, M. Hersen, & A. E. Kazdin (Eds.), *International handbook of behavior modification and therapy* (pp. 319–345). New York: Plenum Press.

Marshall, W. L. (1982). A model of dysfunctional behavior. In A. S. Bellack, M. Hersen, & A. E. Kazdin (Eds.), *International handbook of behavior modification and therapy* (pp. 57–78). New York: Plenum Press.

Marshall, W. L., & Segal, Z. (1984). The role of drug therapies in the behavioral treatment of phobias and anxieties. In M. Hersen & S. E. Breuning (Eds.), *Pharmacological and behavioral treatment: An integrative approach*. New York: Wiley.

Mendel, J. G. C., & Klein, D. F. (1969). Anxiety attacks with subsequent agoraphobia. *Comprehensive Psychiatry, 10*, 190–195.

Rachman, S., & Hodgson, R. (1974). I. Synchrony and desynchrony in fear and avoidance. *Behaviour Research and Therapy, 12*, 311–318.

Weimer, W. B. (1976). Manifestations of mind: Some conceptual and empirical issues. In G. G. Glorbus, B. Maxwell, & I. Savodnik (Eds.), *Consciousness and the brain: A scientific and philosophical inquiry*. New York: Plenum Press.

Zitrin, C. M., Klein, D. F., Lindemann, C. G., Toback, P., Rock, M., Kaplan, J. H., & Ganz, V. H. (1976). Comparison of short-term treatment regimens of phobic patients: A preliminary report. In R. L. Spitzer & D. F. Klein (Eds.), *Evaluation of psychological therapies*. Baltimore: Johns Hopkins University Press.

Zitrin, C. M., Klein, D. F., & Woerner, M. G. (1978). Behavior therapy, supportive psychotherapy, imipramine, and phobias. *Archives of General Psychiatry, 35*, 307–316.

Zitrin, C. M., Klein, D. F., & Woerner, M. G. (1980). Treatment of agoraphobia with group exposure *in vivo* and imipramine. *Archives of General Psychiatry, 37*, 63–72.

Zitrin C. M., Woerner, M. G., & Klein, D. F. (1981). Differentiation of panic anxiety from anticipatory anxiety and avoidance behavior. In D. F. Klein & J. G. Rabkin (Eds.), *Anxiety: New research and changing concepts* (pp. 27–46). New York: Raven Press.

Chapter 4

Affective Disorders

Charles VanValkenburg and Hagop S. Akiskal

Conceptual, Terminologic, and Nosologic Aspects

Transient feelings of depression are a universal experience, and depressed mood is easy to recognize. The outward expression or *affect of depression* is on a continuum with normal experience, and even when a depressive state has a known organic precipitant (e.g., reserpine toxicity), the observable change in affect is usually more one of degree than of quality.

Numerous common and uncommon stimuli can precipitate depression. A partial list includes failure or defeat, unemployment, bereavement, other losses, anemia, low thyroid function, seasonal variation in daylight, brain tumor, Parkinson's disease, subacute viral infections, antihypertensive medication, and numerous other chemicals. Because only a small proportion (typically not more than 10%) of people exposed to such stressors develops depression, they cannot be considered to be truly causative; familial-hereditary and developmental-characterologic predisposition appear to be necessary substrates (Akiskal & McKinney, 1975; Akiskal & Tashjian, 1983).

No matter what the provoking factors, the constellation of signs and symptoms associated with depressed mood—the depressive syndrome—is remarkably consistent. There is often a pervasive loss of

CHARLES VANVALKENBURG • Department of Psychiatry, University of Minnesota, School of Medicine, Minneapolis, Minnesota 55455.   HAGOP S. AKISKAL • Department of Psychiatry, University of Tennessee, Memphis, Tennessee 38163.

interest and the ability to experience pleasure; appetite and sleep are usually diminished, although sometimes increased; energy is impaired, and mental and physical functioning is slowed, although there is often agitated purposeless movement; ability to concentrate or remember is impaired; self-esteem is lowered, and feelings of guilt and worthlessness become painful preoccupations; and, finally, there may be thoughts of death or suicide, or actual suicide attempts. Clinical depression is diagnosed when mood change is accompanied by several of these symptoms. According to the third edition (1980) of the American Psychiatric Association's *Diagnostic and Statistical Manual of Mental Disorders* (DSM-III), *major depressive disorder* refers to an illness of acute onset over a period of days to a week, a syndromal depression with a minimum of four signs and symptoms, and sustained duration for at least 2 weeks. The diagnosis of *dysthymic disorder* is based on insidious onset over many months, subsyndromal level of illness with a minimum of two symptoms, and chronic or intermittent duration for at least 2 years. Dysthymia can precede or predispose to major depression, or it can be a sequel to it.

As a deviation from normal mood, depression may be compared to fever, which is a deviation from normal body temperature. Like depression, fever is a syndrome with numerous associated symptoms, including chills, shivering and muscular rigor, malaise, headache, and sometimes photophobia, delirium, shock, convulsions, and death. In antiquity, fever was itself considered an illness. Later fevers became a class of illnesses, and now, except in the case of "fever of unknown origin," the syndrome is not considered a diagnosis but rather a manifestation of such diseases as influenza, malaria, or pneumonia, collagen disease, or spreading cancer.

The diagnosis of depression is generally reserved for cases where the cause of the syndrome is unknown, like the "fever of unknown origin." This is the position taken by DSM-III, which excludes normal bereavement (caused by death of a loved one) and organic affective syndromes (caused by a known physical illness or medication) from the rubric of major affective disorders. However, as pointed out previously, organic causes of depression, like psychosocial stressors, are often insufficient explanations for the occurrence of depression. Accordingly, we prefer (see Akiskal, 1984), a modification of the DSM-III schema for depression whereby phenomenologic affective diagnoses—irrespective of causative factors—are noted on Axis I, personality factors on Axis II, organic contributions on Axis III, and relevant psychosocial stressors on Axis IV. This multifactorial approach, in which depression is viewed as the final common pathway of many etiologies, both psychologic and biologic (Akiskal & McKinney, 1975), appears most consistent with current data. However, as in the case of fever, future research may demonstrate many discrete etiologies.

From a clinical standpoint, the most meaningful distinction within the class of affective disorders is that between bipolar disorder and depressions pursuing a unipolar course. *Bipolar disorder* in its "classical" form (also known as *Bipolar I*) is characterized by syndromal episodes of depression and mania. Mania is the hallmark of bipolar illness and is characterized by euphoric, irritable, or hostile mood; decreased need for sleep; psychomotor excitement; pressured speech and flight of ideas; inflated self-esteem; expansive and grandiose ideation; and poor judgment, especially with regard to excessive involvement in social, sexual, or business activities with little insight of painful consequences. Mania is typically of psychotic proportions and often leads to hospitalization. A milder degree of illness is known as *hypomania*. In *cyclothymic disorder*, depressive and hypomanic manifestations alternate on an attenuated (subsyndromal) plane and tend to pursue a lifelong course. Major depressive or manic syndromes often complicate the course of cyclothymia; the reverse—that is, cyclothymia appearing for the first time after a major bipolar breakdown—is rarely if ever seen clinically. Bipolar I and cyclothymic conditions appear to be phenomenologically bridged by Bipolar II disorder that refers to recurrent major depressions and infrequent and short-lived hypomanic periods. Related to this disorder are Bipolar III or "pseudounipolar," typically recurrent, depressions with bipolar family history; here, hypomania does not occur spontaneously but appears on pharmacologic challenge with tricyclic antidepressants (Akiskal, 1983c).

Another widely accepted distinction within the class of affective disorders is based on the presence or absence of melancholic or psychotic features, as such features usually dictate vigorous somatic interventions, with psychosocial modalities viewed as ancillary (Klerman, 1983). This is not to say that other major depressions would not respond to somatic interventions; indeed, longitudinal prospective follow-up of nonmelancholic depressions has shown melancholic, psychotic, or even bipolar outcome in at least 40% of cases (Akiskal, Bitar, Puzantian, Rosenthal, & Walker, 1978). Such findings suggest that melancholic, psychotic, and bipolar depressions often arise from the background of milder depressive reactions, although it is not always easy to prospectively define which of these milder expressions will show such denouement (Akiskal *et al.*, 1979b).

Investigators from Washington University have proposed that, in research studies where homogeneous samples are needed, affective disorders occurring in the setting of preexisting psychiatric disorders must

be distinguished from primary affective disorders without such antecedents (Robins & Guze, 1972). The psychiatric disorders that are commonly complicated by depression include anxiety disorders, somatization and antisocial personality disorders, alcoholism and substance
abuse, ego-dystonic homosexuality, schizophrenia, and early dementia.
Although mania can be secondary to medical disease or drugs, bipolar
illness is almost never secondary to another disorder. When alcohol and
substance abuse precede the onset of overt bipolar manifestations, such
abuse is probably best explained as an early manifestation of cyclothymic mood swings leading to self-treatment with drugs. Thus, the rubric
secondary affective disorder almost always refers to dysphoric states, either
dysthymic or major depressive. Although the primary/secondary distinction is not made in DSM-III, we find it useful in view of the differences in course dictated by the underlying psychiatric illness (Goodwin & Guze, 1984). As the underlying disorders are usually chronic,
superimposed depressive conditions tend to run an intermittently or
continuously chronic course. Furthermore, the primary/secondary distinction carries treatment implications. For instance, dysphoric states
(dysthymic or major depressive) superimposed on panic disorder tend
to respond better to monoamine oxidase inhibitors than to tricyclic antidepressants, and those complicating the course of somatization, antisocial, and related personality disorders generally do not respond well
to most forms of somatic therapy.

Description of Subtypes

The different subtypes of affective illness are distributed on a continuum of signs and symptoms and can be reliably distinguished only in
the most extreme cases. When interviewing a patient, the clinician must
evaluate each new bit of information that is reported or observed and
must consider how this information pertains to each of the possible
subtypes. In many cases, a preponderance of information will eventually point to one subtype; in others, it will not be possible to establish the
classification with much certainty. The most important clinical differential diagnostic problems involve:

1. deciding whether an underlying and treatable medical cause
   exists;
2. depressive versus anxiety disorders;
3. unipolar versus bipolar conditions; and
4. character-based dysphorias versus cyclothymic and related dysthymic disorders.

Affective Syndromes in the Setting of Medical-Neurologic Disease

It is not always easy to decide if affective symptoms represent understandable psychologic reactions to concurrent medical-neurologic disorders or whether they are caused by the physiochemical impact of these disorders. However, it is the obligation of the clinician to first rule out such contributions that are potentially reversible. In general, there are no distinctive clinical features that distinguish these medical-neurologic affective states from their primary counterparts. Their detection depends heavily on the clinician's index of suspicion. It is wise to insist that all affectively ill patients—especially those with first breakdowns after age 40—undergo physical evaluation. Table 1 lists medical-neurologic conditions most commonly associated with depressive and manic disorders. Especially treacherous are occult malignancies—whether systemic or involving the brain—as well as endocrine and subictal (temporal lobe) disorders; these conditions should in particular be suspected

Table 1. Common Medical Causes of Depressive and Manic States

Type of cause	Depression	Mania
Pharmacologic	Steroidal contraceptive	Corticosteroids
	Antihypertensive drugs	Levodopa
	Alcohol and other sedatives	Stimulants
	Cholinesterase inhibitor insecticides	Monoamine oxidase inhibitors
	Amphetamine withdrawal	Tricyclic antidepressants
Infectious	Influenza	Influenza
	Infectious mononucleosis	St. Louis encephalitis
	TB	Q fever
	General paresis (tertiary syphilis)	General paresis (tertiary syphilis)
Endocrine	Hypothyroidism	Thyrotoxicosis
	Cushing's disease	
	Addison's disease	
Collagen	Systemic lupus erythematosus	Systemic Lupus erythematosus
	Rheumatoid arthritis	Rheumatic chorea
Neurologic	Stroke	Stroke
	Multiple sclerosis	Multiple sclerosis
	Cerebral tumors	Diencephalic and 3rd ventricle tumors
	Parkinson's disease	
	Sleep apnea	
	Dementing diseases in early stages	

Note. Reproduced with modification from *The Merck Manual of Diagnosis and Therapy,* 14th ed., pp. 1448–1462, edited by R. Berkow. Copyright 1982 by Merck & Co., Inc. Used with permission.

when psychologic and pharmacologic interventions do not yield expected positive results within a few weeks. Unfortunately, this may sometimes be too late as is described next.

Case 1

A 46-year-old woman presented to a mental health center with the chief complaint of lassitude, irritability, hostile outbursts, insomnia, low self-confidence, and poor concentration of insidious onset over a period of 8 weeks. It was felt at the time that this was a "reaction" to her hysterectomy (for benign fibroid tumors) a year before and the fact that her husband had been neglecting her romantically since then and was increasingly immersed in his job. Their two children were attending college in another city, and the patient had no other relatives close by. Although she had always been a rather anxious person, past psychiatric history was negative for major psychopathology. She was treated with individual psychotherapy with a cognitive-behavioral focus and having made no progress within 6 weeks, she was referred for psychiatric evaluation. Mental status revealed a woman who looked exhausted, having lost 20 lb in a few weeks, and who complained of inability to think. There was no evidence for memory and cognitive deficits; however, systems review indicated that she had had mild diarrhea for 8 weeks. Laboratory studies were ordered at this time. Thyroid indexes were normal, CBC revealed a mild anemic state, and blood chemistry revealed abnormalities in protein levels. Internal medicine consultation led to referral to a surgeon who performed a laparotomy, revealing an intestinal malignancy (lymphoma). The patient died 6 months later.

Major (Melancholic) Depression

The syndrome of depression can occur for no apparent reason in a previously well person. Major depression in its full-blown melancholic form typically appears in the 40s and 50s, which explains the former label *involutional melancholia*. The depression often begins insidiously with irritability and minor mood changes; as it gradually worsens, it is accompanied by insomnia, agitation manifested in pacing and hand wringing, self-reproach, fearfulness and, sometimes, panic attacks. When depression reaches psychotic severity, it is characterized by delusions of guilt, persecution, or ill health. In some cases, impairment of memory and orientation in elderly melancholics may give the false impression of a primary dementia. Premorbidly, melancholics tend to be conscientious, perfectionistic, meticulous, self-sacrificing, scrupulously honest, rigid, and frugal. Before electroconvulsive and antidepressant medication therapies became available, recovery was slow, and psychiatric wards were filled with these patients. With the advent of early diagnosis and effective treatment, this extreme form of melancholia has become relatively uncommon. Much of the distinctive quality of the syndrome can be attributed to its severity and the pathoplastic effects of aging itself.

Melancholia has, in the DSM-III classification, replaced the term *endogenous* (i.e., unprecipitated) depression because current evidence indicates that the presence of precipitants carries no diagnostic specificity (Akiskal *et al.*, 1978). The syndrome is currently defined by anhedonia, pathologic guilt, marked psychomotor disturbance, middle and late insomnia, and weight loss that occur in an autonomous fashion.*

Whether precipitated or not, these manifestations pursue a course of their own that is minimally affected by psychosocial contingencies. Untreated episodes, if not ended by suicide, may continue unabated for many months—even several years—and there are records of patients who have been ill for a decade or longer. This autonomy of the morbid process imparts to the syndrome of melancholia the attributes of a medical disease. The patient is unable to sit still or concentrate well enough to answer questions and cannot be distracted from perseverative expressions of guilt, persecution, and woe. Memory or attention may be so poor that little or no information can be elicited about the circumstances or symptoms of the illness. In these "pseudodemented depressions" the initial difficulty is distinguishing the illness from a primary degenerative dementia. In cases where paranoid symptoms predominate, the illness can resemble late-onset schizophrenia.

Although both the dexamethasone suppression test (Carroll, 1982) and rapid eye movement (REM) latency test findings (Kupfer & Thase, 1983) tend to be most deviant in severe melancholic illness, the clinical picture may be dominated by somatic complaints to such an extent that a definitive diagnosis can be established only by a therapeutic trial of antidepressant medication or of electroconvulsive therapy (Akiskal & Cassano, 1983). Such cases are subsumed under the rubic of *masked depression* because of the patient's denial of subjective depression. In milder cases, or those seen early in the course of the illness, the patient will report irritability, anxiety, and insomnia. The following case illustrates a full-blown form of melancholia.

A 60-year-old widow was brought to the psychiatric hospital by her children, who had obtained a court commitment order. She had been admitted to the hospital several times in previous years and had always been treated with electroconvulsive therapy (ECT). On admission, the patient was grossly agi-

---

*As described later in this chapter, the endogenous pattern in bipolar depressions may manifest with hypersomnia and weight gain.

tated, seemed unable to sit or stand still to answer questions about herself, and walked away from anyone who tried to talk to her. When alone, she often walked in circles. In bed, she thrashed around or kicked her legs. Her appearance was one of anguish. At times she would admit that she felt depressed but said that she believed that nothing could be done for her and that she should be allowed to leave or to die. At other times, she asked members of the hospital staff to poison her, to put an end to her misery. The nurses confirmed that the patient stayed awake much of the night, especially after 2:00 A.M. She believed that her bowels had completely stopped working and sometimes said that her brain was dead and not working anymore. At other times she would speak of having cancer. When given medication, she often expressed the concern that somebody might be poisoning her for past sins. She said that she had done horrible things (which she never specified) that had ruined the lives of her family members. Interviewing her proved difficult because she generally would not answer questions about herself and would not cooperate with the cognitive portion of the mental status examination. She did try to name the past presidents of the United States and was able to name only three since Franklin Roosevelt and did not name the current or immediate past presidents.

It was not possible to learn much from her about the past course of her illness. Most of the information in her medical record had been obtained from her family. She had had an episode of depression when she was 38, following the birth of her youngest son. Otherwise, she had apparently been well until her late 50s, when she had gradually become depressed, agitated, and delusional, a description very similar to the current illness. She had been hospitalized four times and had never recovered without ECT. She had generally returned to her normal self for periods of up to 5 years, although recently she had had a tendency toward quick relapses. Outside of her episodes of depression she had always been an extremely religious person, conscientious and self-sacrificing, caring for disabled members of her family at considerable inconvenience to herself, and exerting a strong role in maintaining family traditions. She had never abused alcohol or other substances. Her father had suffered from repeated bouts of the same illness and had committed suicide on his 49th birthday.

Her physician prescribed antidepressant medication, but she would not take the pills with any regularity. Antipsychotic medication diminished her agitation but did not resolve the melancholic syndrome, necessitating the use of ECT.

Anxious Depression

Anxiety and depression are often associated. The agitation of typical melancholia is not always easily distinguished from physically expressed anxiety. Psychic anxiety is also frequently a part of depression. Patients with anxiety disorders are often troubled by some degree of depressed mood, and many even develop episodes of major depression. Those anxiety disorders that eventually lead to depression tend to be the most severe, chronic, and disabling variants. Depressions that are accompanied by severe anxiety are similarly likely to become chronic and to respond poorly to the usual treatments (VanValkenburg, Akiskal, Puzantian, & Rosenthal, 1984).

The most reliable indicator of anxiety disorder is the spontaneous panic attack, that is, an episode of intense anxiety that is usually unprovoked and lasts a few minutes to an hour. Associated physical symptoms include shortness of breath, hyperventilation, palpitations, chest pain or discomfort, numbness or tingling, and a feeling or fear of physical or mental loss of control or impending death. Between the attacks, the patient may manifest or experience nervousness and tension, worrying, apprehensiveness, overactivity of the autonomic nervous system resulting in flushed or pale skin, excessive perspiration and rapid pulse, and overarousal, with vigilant scanning of surroundings for possible danger.

To evaluate whether a depressed patient is suffering from an anxious depression, the clinician must document history of panic attacks and other anxiety symptoms such as excessive worrying, tension, depersonalization, and derealization. If these are present, it is important to learn whether they are part of a long-standing anxiety disorder or whether they have been limited to the period of the depressive episodes. Clues to differential diagnosis follow:

1. If the patient is older, the anxiety and agitation are more severe, and there were no previous neurotic or unstable personality manifestations, the illness might be melancholia in an early stage (Akiskal & Cassano, 1983).

2. If the anxiety and tension had their onset with or after the depression, then according to DSM-III (1983), major depression is the most appropriate diagnosis. However, current evidence from family (Leckman, Weissman, Merikangas, Paula, & Prusoff, 1983), follow-up (VanValkenburg et al., 1984), and sleep EEG studies (Akiskal, Lemmi, Dickson, King, Yerevanian, & VanValkenburg, 1984) indicates that depression with concurrent anxiety states may be more like panic disorders than primary depressive disorders. Further, monoamine oxidase inhibitors like phenelzine appear to be the treatment of choice for both panic disorder and anxious depression (Davidson, Miller, Turnbull, & Sullivan, 1982). In Great Britain these patients with anxiety/depression have been subclassified as *atypical depressions* by the occurence of reverse diurnal variation (feeling worse in the evening) and reverse vegetative signs (hypersomnia and hyperphagia). Why some anxious depressives complain of insomnia and others of hypersomnia is not known with certainty. However, in many anxious patients, excessive daytime fatigue and somnolence appear secondary to multiple awakenings at night (Akiskal & Lemmi, unpublished date).

3. If there has been a long history beginning at an early age of unexplainable physical symptoms, associated with self-dramatization, hostility, flamboyance, manipulativeness, and less objective evidence of depression, the most likely diagnosis is depression associated with somatization disorder or related personality disorder.

Anxious depressions are best conceptualized as secondary depressions—either major or dysthymic—superimposed on anxiety (usually panic) disorders. An illustrative case follows:

Case 3

A 33-year-old single woman was referred to a psychiatric clinic by her psychotherapist, who thought medication might help her increasingly severe and uncontrollable depressions. She had been in psychotherapy for several years, working on problems of generalized anxiety and tension, unhappiness, and dissatisfactions with career and relationships. She reported history of anxiety and tension since her late teenage years. She was also able to identify fluctuating depression, which she could not clearly distinguish from her more frequent periods of anxious brooding, but stated that the dysphoric mood and pessimism had been constant and incapacitating over the past 6 weeks. Panic attacks, which had begun in the past year, were not brought on by any specific stimuli, although she felt that she was under considerable stress at these times. She reported difficulty falling asleep and feeling inadequately rested in the mornings, getting out of bed with great difficulty. Appetite and weight were not changed. She stated that her concentration was not as good as it had been, although she could not think of definitive examples of this. She volunteered that her ambition and energy level were diminished. She denied feeling guilty but said that her chronic problems with low self-esteem and self-confidence had worsened recently. Her interest in sex was reportedly quite low, and self-confidence had recently been extremely low. She admitted recent thoughts of suicide but had not made any serious plans or attempted suicide. On specific questioning, she said that she had been feeling more angry and hostile toward others recently. She had also had some episodes of tearfulness associated with unpleasant memories, and she became briefly tearful as she reported this. At the time of interview she appeared only slightly tense and agitated. She reported she had been having two to three panic attacks in each of the past several weeks. A few of these had been extremely severe and had caused her to leave the public places in which they occurred. Most of her panic attacks began very suddenly with feelings of intense fear, shortness of breath and smothering sensations, heart palpitations, mild chest discomfort, numbness and tingling, and a subjective feeling that her skin was flushing and that she was losing control of herself and attracting the attention of others (which was not the case). In her most severe attacks, she reported a very unsettling feeling that things around her seemed to have changed and taken on an "unreal" or "eerie" quality. She stated that during the more serious attacks she became afraid that she would die, even though she was able to tell herself on a rational level that she would not. She was treated with alprazolam and phenelzine and continued her psychotherapy. Her panic attacks ceased soon after she began these medications. Although the level of depression was bearable now, low-grade depressive symptoms persisted and self-esteem remained low.

Recurrent Major Depression, "Pseudounipolar" Type

Many otherwise normal persons are subject to bouts of depression, typically beginning in the second or third decade of life, which last a few months and then resolve spontaneously. Mood, energy, and interest in life decrease, there may be a tendency to oversleep, thought processes and activities become slowed, self-esteem diminishes, and self-doubts multiply, concentration and memory are less than normal, tranquility is lost, appetite becomes disturbed, and the value of continued existence is increasingly questioned. In these early-onset retarded depressions, in contrast with the agitated depressions described earlier, family history is often positive for manic-depressive illness, and many of these patients tend to respond to tricyclic antidepressants with mild and short-lived hypomanic periods. Most of these depressions turn out to be prodromal or mild manifestations of manic-depressive disorder, in that long-term prospective follow-up often shows evidence for spontaneous hypomanic and manic episodes (Akiskal, Walker, Puzantian, King, Rosenthal, & Dranon, 1983). DSM-III subsumes these patients under *major depression* because evidence for bipolarity cannot be readily evaluated on a cross-sectional basis. We prefer the designation *major depression, pseudounipolar type*, because this illness is phenomenologically distinct from other depressions (Akiskal, 1983c) and has clear treatment implications. These patients respond poorly on tricyclic antidepressants but well to lithium carbonate (Kupfer, Pickar, Himmelhoch, & Detre, 1975).

Case 4

A 42-year-old college professor was seen in consultation on the surgical service. He had shot himself through his calf muscles and reluctantly admitted having done this "to have a legitimate excuse to be in the hospital." He felt his colleagues would not understand that depression could be an incapacitating illness. Since his late teens, he had had "paralyzing depressions" every 2 to 3 years, lasting 3 to 4 months at a time and characterized by hopeless despair, inability to face students in the classroom, excessive sleep, preoccupation with death, and a sense of failure. These were initially ascribed to romantic disappointment or job stress, but both he and his wife now recognized that no adequate explanations for these episodes could be found in recent years. His father, a successful physician, had committed suicide in his early 40s. A paternal uncle was a diagnosed manic-depressive who had been placed on lithium after he ruined the family business during a manic episode.

Although no discrete periods of hypomania could be elicited, after 8 days of desipramine he began feeling "unusually lucid," corrected in one evening 70 exam papers that had previously seemed like an onerous task, made love to his surprised wife six times during the weekend pass, and refused to come back to the hospital, stating that a poet who was as good as "Lowell, Berryman, and Delmore Schwartz combined need not stay under some shrink's care." Fortunately, he also stopped the desipramine, and his wife reported that his pharmacologic hypomania abated over a week's period.

Bipolar Disorder

The large subgroup of recurrent major depressives who experience spontaneous but infrequent and mild periods of elevated mood without meeting the full criteria for full-blown mania have been classified as Bipolar II (Fieve & Dunner, 1975). In DSM-III, these patients are referred to as *atypical*, partly because of difficulties involved in ascertainment of the elevated periods. Yet, current evidence indicates that these conditions are as common as more classical bipolar disorders (Akiskal, 1981, 1983c; Weissman & Myers, 1978). Patients with these conditions have retarded depressions very similar to pseudounipolars; the major difference is that hypomanic periods can occur spontaneously as well as on pharmacologic challenge. Hypomanic episodes are thus of considerable diagnostic importance here and must be specifically inquired about in the diagnostic interview of all depressives. The pertinent point is a history of abnormally elevated mood, a clear departure from ordinary experience. Typical symptoms might include a degree of optimistic enthusiasm that does not seem justified by the situation, little need for sleep, sexual risktaking that is out of character, exuberant spending sprees or drinking bouts, or energetic overachievement that might be cut short by the consequences of faulty judgment. To be classified as hypomania, there should be several symptoms at the same time, all of them plausibly attributable to elevated mood, lasting at least a few days. As these sorts of behaviors are common in individuals with personality disorders, hypomania should not be considered unless the symptoms represent a clear break from the habitual self and are preceded or followed by retarded depression. A certain degree of such uninhibited behavior can be dismissed in sociopathic individuals as not indicative of manic-depressive disorder, whereas in patients with episodic depressions it may be necessary to discount denials of such past episodes. For example,

Bipolar II patients, when depressed, have difficulty remembering that they have ever felt otherwise.

Case 5

The patient was a 46-year-old divorced woman, previously hospitalized for a retarded depression. Her medical records indicated that she had had an almost stuporous depression, with hypersomnia and psychomotor retardation; she had been treated with electroconvulsive therapy. Her main symptoms at this time were "dragging" in the morning, some pessimism, and hostility toward her former husband. She had been taking an antipsychotic-tricyclic combination without interruption for 12 years. These drugs had been prescribed by her GP because of a history of "lazy depressions" lasting 6 to 8 weeks at a time in early fall and midwinter months. She resisted all attempts to change her medication regimen, insisting that she always had relapsed in the past when any other medications were used. Because her relapses were so very bad—"life coming to a screeching halt"—she did not want to do anything that might bring another one on. After a television feature on tardive dyskinesia she finally agreed to have her antipsychotics stopped. Following several dramatic episodes of physical symptoms, insomnia, and of restarting the pills on her own, she finally managed to stop using them. About this time her moods began to become more labile. For several weeks she was easily excitable and had restless energy. She became involved in an affair with a man she met at a singles party, marveling in her clinic visits about how wonderfully sexually compatible they were. She then broke off with him abruptly and flew to California for a weekend with a boyfriend from high school whom she had not seen for 30 years. This was followed by another retarded depression, less severe than the previous one. She was successfully managed with lithium carbonate. When fully euthymic,* she recalled that the "lazy periods" in her 20s had been on few occasions followed by episodes when she felt so energetic that she could go for 48 hours without sleep and during which she wrote passionate love letters.

The full-blown form of manic-depressive illness is known as *Bipolar I disorder* (Fieve & Dunner, 1975). This is more severe than Bipolar II disorder in that the excited periods in Bipolar patients develop into full syndromal height. Thus, manic psychosis is the hallmark of the disorder. However, the distinction between hypomania and mania is more one of degree than of quality. Elevated periods become classified as *manic* when they last more than a week and are of such intensity that they result in disruption of the patient's social standing or employment or in serious financial or legal difficulties to such an extent that the patient's friends and family act in concert to get him or her into a psychi-

---

Euthymic: In a state of normally elevated mood, as distinguished from *dysthymic* and *manic.*

atric hospital. The excessive energy of these patients cannot be contained or tolerated by relatives and associates. Their grandiose ideas and plans strike those around them as not merely unrealistic but distinctly pathological. Most episodes of mania lead to hospitalization, making a past history of manic disorder relatively easy to document.

As the severity of manic disorder increases, the mood of euphoria typically gives way to one of irritable dysphoria. The manic energy may increasingly come to resemble purposeless psychomotor agitation and may alternate with or give way to periods of profound depression and psychomotor retardation or catatonic immobility (mixed state). The flight of ideas typical of mania may become so severe that speech appears disorganized or incoherent. Whereas a euphoric manic might cheerfully entertain thoughts of personal divinity, the paranoid manic might be more inclined to be belligerent toward any unbelieving infidel. As delusional and hallucinatory, even mood incongruent experiences are not uncommon in these patients, they can be misdiagnosed as schizophrenics. Younger, acutely psychotic, assaultive, and combative patients who give evidence for a biphasic course are likely to be manic (Akiskal & Puzantian, 1979). They often can be identified by a history of more typical manic and depressive symptoms. They are less likely than other manic depressives to have had periods of normal functioning, tend to be noncompliant with treatment, and often have poor prognosis (Jamison & Akiskal, 1983). By contrast, the response of compliant Bipolar patients to lithium carbonate is one of the most dramatic and professionally gratifying experiences in all of medicine.

Case 6

A 35-year-old male was referred by the psychiatric nurse of a mental health center because he suspected manic-depressive illness despite the fact that all past records described him as an acute paranoid schizophrenic. He had more recently been seen in the hospital because of accelerated speech, extreme irritability, insomnia, weight loss, crying spells alternating with euphoria, religious ideation followed by sexual advances toward the nurses, and fleeting visual hallucinations of "Jesus in the sky." This psychotic state had been attenuated with a neuroleptic, and he had been sent to the mental health clinic for aftercare.

Past history revealed that the first episode requiring psychiatric hospitalization had occurred when the patient was 25; records indicated poor sleep, physical hyperactivity, singing on the streets, disturbing the peace, and euphoria. The second episode requiring hospitalization, at age 31, involved similar behavior plus preaching the Bible and having "visions" of God. This was followed by a protracted depressive episode characterized by psychomotor retardation, lack of energy, lack of social initiative, feelings of being unloved, staying in bed, gloomy thoughts, and decreased sexual drive. Between these episodes, the patient described himself as "neither depressive nor optimistic" but nervous and irritable with occasional periods of insomnia. However, at age 18, he had had a 3-month period characterized by hypersomnolence, thoughts of death, irritability, and hopelessness; at the time, a general practitioner had treated him with "vitamin shots." As a result of this illness, he had graduated 1 year late from high school. The patient had not been able to maintain jobs between episodes and hoped to find a job in the near future. Family history revealed that his father, who was a "wild man" and drank heavily, had spent 2 years in a state psychiatric hospital and had committed suicide at the age of 43.

Mental status revealed the patient to be oriented in three spheres. He was pleasant and cooperative, with somewhat slow thought progression. Content of thought did not reveal delusions; he avoided talking about religion. Affect was slightly depressed; cognitive functions were intact.

The patient was advised to have a lithium work-up in view of psychotic manic, retarded depressive, and mixed (the most current) episodes.

Cyclothymic Disorder and Subaffective Dysthymic Variants

The bipolar swings in these patients are of subsyndromal intensity. Thus, cyclothymic individuals seem vivacious and energetic at times, dull and neurasthenic at others. They might report periods of enthusiasm, decreased need for sleep, and high productivity alternating with periods of "laziness" and eating and sleeping too much. As cyclothymia has its onset by adolescence or early adulthood, it can initially be mistaken for a personality disorder. Many of these patients describe their mood as "always either up or down." Counting up every symptom of elevated or depressed mood they have ever had, each part of the full syndrome of manic-depressive disease might have been present at one time or another—albeit for short periods (see Table 2). These mood swings often lead to serious personal complications such as episodic promiscuous behavior, repeated conjugal failure, dilettantism, and geographic instability (Akiskal, Djenderedjian, Rosenthal, & Khani, 1977). Compared with antisocial personalities, they have fewer antisocial behaviors, fewer problems with drugs or alcohol, and a mood disorder that is more phasic than continuous, with normal periods being more likely than in pure characterologic disorders. A therapeutic trial of lithium carbonate might also help distinguish cyclothymia from mood swings associated with primary characterologic disorder. However, many of these individuals neither need nor want help, perhaps because they are reluctant to jeopardize the creative talent that has been described in some cyclothymics (Andreasen & Canter, 1974).

Case 7

This 31-year-old architect presented for outpatient care with the chief complaint of having been a "moody person" since his midteens. He had been

Table 2. University of Tennessee Criteria for Cyclothymic Disorders

I. General characteristics
   A. Onset < age 21 years
   B. Short cycles (days), which are recurrent in an irregular fashion, with infrequent euthymia
   C. May not attain full syndrome for depression & hypomania during any one cycle, but entire range of affective symptoms occur at various times
   D. Abrupt and unpredictable mood change, often unrelated to external circumstances
II. Biphasic course
   A. Pessimism and brooding alternating with optimism and care-free attitudes
   B. Unexplained tearfulness alternating with excessive punning and joking
   C. Lethargy and decreased verbal output alternating with eutonia and talkativeness
   D. Hypersomnia alternating with decreased need for sleep
   E. Introverted self-absorption alternating with uninhibited people-seeking
   F. Mental confusion and apathy, alternating with sharpened and creative thinking
   G. Shaky self-esteem alternating with low self-confidence and grandiose overconfidence
   H. Marked unevenness in quantity of productivity (unusual working hours)

Note: Modified from Akiskal *et al.* (1979a).

divorced twice and was separated from his third wife, who accompanied him to the clinic to make sure he would receive appropriate care. She described the marriage as "living on a roller coaster"; having attended lectures on manic-depressive psychosis, she felt her husband had a "miniature" form of the illness. She also said "all his family is extremely temperamental—even wild—yet charming and talented" but that she could no longer live with him unless he received psychiatric treatment. The patient admitted to periods of low mood during which he would oversleep, lack energy and motivation, and "vegetate." These periods were followed, often with a switch in the morning upon waking, by high periods of 2 to 3 days when he would be energetic, overconfident, sexually active, witty, sleepless, often carrying out in one day "all the backlog of postponed activity accumulated from the 'down' days." Such periods were often followed by 1 to 2 days of irritable and hostile mood, heralding the transition back to depression. Thus, he typically had few euthymic periods. He admitted to the frequent use of alcohol during "up" moods to help him sleep and to occasional cocaine use during the "down" periods. Medical history was unremarkable. The patient's mother was diagnosed *paranoid schizophrenic*, but history obtained from the patient was more compatible with bipolar illness with recurrent manic episodes. For example, she had been married six times!

As exemplified by this case, relatives of manic-depressives may suffer from attenuated intermittent cyclothymic disorders (Akiskal *et al.*, 1977, 1979a). Other relatives of bipolar patients suffer from mild and intermittent depressions (Akiskal, Rosenthal, Haykal, Lemmi, & Rosenthal, 1980; Rosenthal, Akiskal, Scott-Strauss, Rosenthal, & David, 1981). This illness has an early onset and is present enough of the time that it can seem to be a part of the personality. As is typical of manic-depressive disease, sleep and appetite disturbances are more likely to take the form of overeating and oversleeping. This has led some to call these depressions *atypical*, whereas others reserve this term for depressions of the more anxious and hysteroid type (Davidson *et al.*, 1982). Chronic antisocial and drug abuse problems are less likely in these patients than in primary personality disorders, but this difference is usually not sufficiently dramatic to classify individual patients. When bipolar family history has been obtained, these patients can sometimes be identified with a trial of a noradrenergic tricyclic antidepressant, which often precipitates a hypomanic state, thereby establishing the primacy of the dysthymic disorder.

Case 8

A 24-year-old divorced female presented with the chief complaint of "I have been depressed as long as I remember." Upon further questioning, she dated this back to age 9, when she took an overdose of aspirin "because I was disappointed in myself—I did not make straight A's." She had always been nonassertive, introverted, and self-denigrating. Other current manifestations included hypersomnolence, decreased energy, poor concentration, inability to comprehend her low moods, and death thoughts (but no suicidal wishes). Mornings were especially difficult, as she felt "gloomy much of the time." Upon further probing, it was apparent that her dysphoria was not continuous but manifested in periods lasting 7 to 10 days, with intervening 2 to 3-day periods of feeling "just OK." She stated that at times she would "gradually sink into deeper states of suicidal despair." Her husband had divorced her because he could not live with her "pervasive gloominess." Her father was a known manic-depressive responding to lithium carbonate. Accordingly, she was placed on desipramine (a tricyclic antidepressant) 50 mg twice a day and on the eighth day she began to wake up early in the morning (5 A.M. versus her usual rising hour of 11 A.M.), feeling an overabundance of energy, increased sexual urges, and an unexplainable feeling of well-being unknown to her. After proper medical evaluation, lithium carbonate was substituted. With lithium levels of 0.7 mEq/L, much of her gloominess was gone, and she and her ex-husband remarried.

Such patients are not easily distinguished from the chronic dysphoric conditions seen in primary characterologic disorders to be described next. Accordingly, in Table 3, we are providing proposed operational criteria for their identification (Akiskal, 1983b).

Table 3. Proposed Criteria for Subaffective Dysthymic Disorder

---

A. Not due to a nonaffective condition
B. Early indeterminate onset (< age 21 years)
C. Intermittent subsyndromal depressive features with infrequent euthymia
D. Introverted, self-denigrating, and masochistic
E. Habitual
   (1) Brooding
   (2) Anhedonia   Worse in
   (3) Hypersomnolence   A.M.
   (4) Psychomotor inertia

Note: Modified from Akiskal (1983b).

"Characterologic Dysphorias"

Personality disorders are often associated with intermittent dys-regulation of mood, predominantly manifested in depression, irri-tability, and poor anxiety tolerance. A dysthymic level of disturbance is more common than sustained major depression. Although DSM-III lists numerous types of personality disorders, they seem to conform to three broad categories: (a) a withdrawn, reclusive, or suspicious type, referred to as *schizoid* or *paranoid-schizotypal*, which in some cases may represent mild forms of schizophrenia; (b) a histrionic-somatizing type; and (c) an aggressive, antisocial type. Mood disturbances are common presenting symptoms in the last two groups. *We shall detail the description of these disorders not because they are representative of affective disorders but because they are often confused with them.* Case Histories 9 and 10 that depict, respectively, the unstable mood of antisocial and histrionic character disorders should be contrasted with those depicting primary mood disorders.

Antisocial personalities are a risk-taking, sensation-seeking preda-tory group of individuals who, in their full-blown form, seem to cause trouble at every opportunity. As children, they disrupt classes and get in trouble with authorities, whereas at home, as adolescents, they fight, steal, vandalize, and overindulge in drugs and sex. As adults, they have unstable work histories, break laws and get arrested, abuse marital part-ners and children, fail to pay their bills, and are given to wanderlust. Many of these individuals have an almost "maniclike" level of energy and self-esteem, and on psychological tests like the MMPI, they show the same personality profile (4–9; acting-out psychopath) as manic pa-tients. But in most cases, the predominant mood is one of dysphoria. The mood disturbance may be due to the constant level of trouble and turmoil in their lives or may result from their frequent abuse of alcohol and other substances. Such abuse may also give rise to elation and psychomotor excitement, leading to difficult clinical differentiation from the chronic mild variants of manic-depressive disease. The hallmark of character-disorder-based dysphorias is the associated unremitting personality disorder, which seems quite clearly to be a different illness from manic-depressive disease. Although a minority of aggressive psychopaths—possibly misdiagnosed cyclothymics—may respond to lithium carbonate (Sheard & Marini, 1978), there is effective treatment neither for the personality disorder nor for the associated dysphoria in the majority of cases. An illustrative case follows

Case 9

A 38-year-old divorced man was seen in a public mental health clinic for a renewal of his prescription for "depression." He had been taking amitriptyline at bedtime for sleep and during the day to calm his "nerves." He made it quite clear that he would prefer a medication that would better relieve his general nervousness and muscle tension and named several benezodiazepines and other sedatives. His medical record indicated that he had abused and probably been physically dependent on at least two of these in the past. When specifically asked, he admitted this, although he denied that he had ever had a problem with alcohol or with other types of drugs. He had taken amphetamines before and said that they helped him when he drove trucks (which is how he supported himself intermittently). He said that he had been depressed all of his life, particularly since his early teenage years and that he was "not fit to work." When asked specifically, he reported that he had had occasional panic attacks in the past but that they were no longer a problem. He also reported fears of animals, particularly police dogs. He thought that a lot of his dysphoria had to do with his frequently unfavorable life circumstances. He had been in prison after having been apprehended in what was, by his account, the only major crime he ever committed (selling drugs). However, past records indicated that he had, on numerous occasions, falsified signatures of his sisters and girlfriends on checks. He said that prison had been particularly depressing. His medical records indicated that while in prison he had received negative medical work-ups for headaches, a buzzing sensation in one ear, spells of unconsciousness associated with urinary and fecal incontinence but without seizurelike shaking, abdominal gas pains associated with nausea and numerous food intolerances, chronic low-back pain and pains in the hips and knees, and that he had sought treatment or had been prescribed medication for many other minor ailments. He had been briefly married four times and had two children from different marriages, but he had never supported his children financially and did not wish to visit them. Although he denied that he had ever been aggressive or violent and said that he had never physically harmed anyone, past records indicated he had physically abused each one of the women he had married.

Although somatization is not uncommon in those with antisocial life-styles—as seen in this case—it is most characteristic of histrionic individuals. The hallmark of the latter personality disorder is a lifelong tendency to develop physical or mental symptoms that bring them special favors from others. In some cases, particularly in men, the goal may be obvious—to obtain money or free services, to escape legal judgments or incarceration, or to avoid military service. In others, the "secondary gains" may be less obvious—perhaps increased attention and consideration from a spouse or an excuse to avoid usual obligations. The natural tendency to accord preferential "sick-role" status to those who are disabled by illness may be regarded by manipulative or predatory individuals as a natural resource to be exploited. As clinicians, we cannot reliably determine the somatizing individual's true motivation; therefore, somatization is identified not by its presumed etiology but by its pattern of symptoms. The somatizers we can identify with a fair degree of certainty are those who have had so many physical and emotional symptoms over the years that no other diagnosis or combination of diagnoses can plausibly account for them all. DSM-III requires a total of 14 different symptoms affecting several systems (neurologic, digestive, menstrual, sexual, pain, and cardiopulmonary) as well as a lifelong pattern of sickliness. Antisocial behavior is also common in these patients, as is depressed mood. It should be noted that patients with "true" depression also often become hypochondriacal but typically lack such preoccupation before the onset of depression. Because they may not remember this when they are depressed, the past history should be obtained from a reliable informant. Some somatizers will give themselves away by admitting to multiple past pseudoneurologic conversion symptoms, but many have become too smart for that. Some will still show *la belle indifference* toward their symptoms or seem to be enjoying themselves too much for their reported symptoms to be credible. A history of juvenile or adult antisocial symptoms also tips the diagnosis toward somatization disorder. Because of their tempestuous life histories and rapid mood swings, this group can be easily confused with cyclothymic conditions. But a detailed history, as exemplified in the next case, would suggest otherwise.

Case 10

The patient, a 31-year-old divorced woman, was admitted through the emergency room at night because of urges to kill herself. She reported she had been feeling depressed and suicidal for 2 weeks because of conflicts at work. Upon questioning, she said her energy had been low and she had lost a few pounds, that she had lost all interest in sex but not in social activities, that she was feeling very guilty and worthless but that her sleep had not been disturbed. She said that she had been feeling hopeless, pessimistic, worried, irritable, hostile, and suspicious. She had been worrying about her health and reported nausea and vomiting and a general increase in aches and panic and "bad sensations" in her body.

Her medical records indicated that she had recently had an extensive evaluation for "intractable seizures"; no evidence of seizure disorder had been found, and a diagnosis of conversion hysteria had been made. When asked about other neurologic symptoms, she said that she had at various times had loss of all sensation in parts of her body, had lost her voice, and had experienced difficulty walking, paralysis, loss of consciousness, and double vision. She denied episodes of blindness or deafness. She reported past serious problems with dysmenorrhea. She said she had never climaxed during sex with men. She reported having heard voices occasionally, most recently of a man's voice telling her to kill herself. She had also been bothered by visual hallucinations—typically of insects crawling on her. When asked, she said she had felt that others were talking about her and harassing her. However, her hallucinatory behavior and other evidence of psychosis were not observed. She denied sustained periods of elevated mood but did report short periods (4 to 5 hours at a time) of unusually irritable and dysphoric mood, associated with hyperactivity, pressured speech, distractability and buying sprees, reckless, uninhibited behavior, increased meddling in others' affairs, and angry, hostile, and abusive behaviors. In response to specific questions, she said she had been having panic attacks for the past 6 months. The symptoms had been intense anxiety, hyperventilation, heart palpitations, dizziness, faintness, shakiness, restlessness, and hot flashes. She also reported general anxiety for the past 2 months and long-standing fear of crowds with some avoidance, which she said had not particularly interferred with her functioning.

She admitted past problems with alcohol, including memory blackouts, and objections of friends to her drinking. Her heavy drinking had begun at age 17 and ended by her mid-20s. She said she had not abused street drugs but had once been addicted to oxazepam, which had been prescribed for her. When specifically asked, she reported that she had several juvenile antisocial problems, beginning at age 10 or 12, including truancy, running away from home, chronic violations of the rules at school and at home, and shoplifting. She was specifically asked about each adult antisocial symptom in DSM-III and denied them all. She had been divorced twice and said she had had pelvic inflammatory disease once, though she said this could not have been sexually transmitted as she had never had any sexual contact before its onset. Despite the extreme number of symptoms she reported, she did not look particularly disturbed; one could describe her as "drowsy" and "dissatisfied." In the hospital, she twice signed requests for discharge against medical advice but withdrew them after long talks with a doctor. She also requested and received several hours of supportive psychotherapy from various nurses. In spite of her threats to leave the hospital and kill herself, she resisted transfer to an unlocked ward. Within the next few days, she told another of her doctors that she had just remembered that she had been raped when she was 14. She said she had previously totally suppressed this, but the questions regarding her gynecologic history (which included pelvic inflammatory disease) brought it all back.

At this stage, both her family and employer had telephoned to warn that she was "an extremely convincing and shameless liar." She had worked for a medical clinic and had just been fired for stealing confidential patient records, tranquilizers, uniforms, and equipment. Her family said that she had been writing many bad checks that they could not afford to make good "this time." She had been receiving rape-victim counseling and seemed to respond well, although her family was certain that she had neither been raped nor had pelvic inflammatory disease. She had been a very troublesome child and had been taken to various specialists for "incorrigibility" since before age 10 and had been hospitalized for a year as a juvenile because of these behaviors. She was an avid reader of psychology and medical texts, and tended to "catch" diseases she read about, most recently bulimia and premenstrual tension. She also wondered if she was a "lesbian" as she believed the female psychiatric resident entrusted to her care was "making passes" at her. After her negative seizure evaluation, she had told this psychiatrist that the exam had in fact been positive for four different kinds of "amnesic seizures" that were all very rare in that there was no electroencephalographic evidence of seizures except during the actual seizures. She had vaguely indicated that during her periods of amnesia she did bad things—such as "lesbian acts"—that others later told her about. She had also begun to talk about there being two people in her, a good one and a bad one, who were fighting. Her mother said that when told of things she had done, she very convincingly denied all memory of them, but when pressed with evidence would give good indications that she actually did remember and would then lose her temper, "go hysterical," or run away.

This extensive case is presented to illustrate the fact that affective dysregulation does not necessarily constitute a primary mood disorder.*

Diagnostic Interviewing

Reliability and Validity

Structured interview schedules for affective disorders—of which the best known is the Schedule for the Affective Disorders and Schizo-

*Some dysphoric patients display labile mood that is highly reactive to environmental support or adversity. This is considered by Klein's group to suggest "hysteroid dysphoria" (Liebowitz & Klein, 1979). A severe depressive "crash," with oversleeping, overeating, and a leaden inertia will follow any personal rejection, whereas acceptance and approval by others will bring back the usual personality, likely to be histrionic, flamboyant, intrusive, seductive, self-centered, demanding, preoccupied with physical attractiveness. If a patient shows these "reactive" mood changes, the interviewer should ascertain whether the patient has consistently become depressed upon interpersonal rejection. Many of these patients probably represent variants of characterologic dysphorias, though a subgroup might be related to subaffective dysthymic and cyclothymic disorders.

phrenia (Spitzer, Endicott, & Robins, 1979)—were designed to provide instruments for investigating the phenomenology and nosology of affective disorders and their differentiation from boundary conditions. Such instruments have achieved acceptable reliability in the hands of relatively inexperienced clinicians who have undergone training in their rigorous application, making them suitable for use in clinical research. However, at this writing, these instruments are best regarded as exploratory tools. Their main limitations are as follows:

1. The validity of the nosologic concepts that they embody is uncertain.
2. Questions are asked in a more or less "standard" manner, which would preclude delving into phenomenologic subtleties.
3. They do not incorporate—or are not sufficiently detailed regarding—many phenomenologic categories commonly encountered in clinical work, for example, anxious depressions, chronic affective disorder subtypes, and milder forms in the bipolar spectrum.
4. Rare but treatable forms of affective disorder—that is, those due to a specific toxin or medical disease—are not specifically inquired about.
5. Such an interview cannot be conducted in severe forms of affective disorders, or when the patient is uncooperative.

For these reasons, we prefer semistructured interviews, in which there is adherence to rigorous diagnostic criteria but greater freedom for the patient and the interviewer to express or inquire about subtleties of affective experience and behavior. The senior author has developed such a schedule—the Mood Clinic Data Questionnaire (MCDQ)—that is particularly suitable for ambulatory affective disorders. The use of this instrument requires phenomenologic sophistication and should be administered by the psychiatrist, clinical psychologist, or social worker with considerable clinical experience.

The beginning clinician must remember that an affective diagnosis—or *any* diagnosis—is not just a collection of signs and symptoms that have reached a certain threshold of severity and duration. If this were the case, self-rating instruments that assess severity of depression, like the Beck Depression Inventory (Beck, 1967) or the Hamilton Rating Scale for Depression (Hamilton, 1960) would suffice, and there would be no need for diagnostic interviewing. (These instruments merely measure the *severity* of the depressive syndrome in an individual who is known to be suffering from an affective disorder.) Clinical judgment is required in assessing whether (a) individual signs and symptoms are present; (b) whether, *taken together*, they constitute a coherent affective disorder; and (c) whether appropriate exclusion criteria are met. Finally, the presence of an affective disorder must be validated by certain external validating strategies such as familial aggregational illness, laboratory indexes, treatment response, and course (Feighner, Robins, Guze, Woodruff, Winokur, & Munoz, 1972). For the clinician, the most important validation is the ability of a diagnosis to predict treatment response and course (or prognosis). For the researcher, familial and laboratory markers are often more significant because they are potentially useful in construct validity. It must also be kept in mind, however, that indexes that help in construct validation may also prove useful in predicting treatment response. Further discussion of these issues is beyond the scope of this chapter, and the interested reader is referred to reviews on the subject (Akiskal, 1983a; Akiskal & Webb, 1978; Carroll, 1982: Kupfer & Thase, 1983).

Context Areas

Diagnostic interviewing should not be overly directive to avoid projecting symptoms onto a suggestible individual. The questions should be asked neutrally, without obvious response expectation. For instance, one should not phrase questions in a judgmental or leading manner, for example, "You're not an alcoholic, are you?" The far more common problem is, unfortunately, not asking about such important matters at all.

Diagnosis is based on what we observe to be wrong (signs) and what patients tell us is wrong (symptoms). Most, though not all, persons who are depressed will look depressed. In some cases sad facial expression, downcast gaze, and stooped posture might be accompanied by very slow speech and movement, or there might be a long pause between questions and responses. This mental and physical slowing (psychomotor retardation), when present to an obvious degree, is suggestive of a *retarded depression*. Retarded depressions are more likely to be accompanied by "endogenous" features, so if retardation is observed, the interviewer should ask about pervasive loss of interest in usual activities and sex, early morning awakening (though hypersomnia may predominate in some patients), fatigue and low energy, increased feelings of guilt and self-reproach, and diurnal variation (feeling worse in the morning). The depressed phase of bipolar disorder is likely to be a retarded type of depression, especially if the patient is a young adult, so it is particularly important to ask about past episodes of manic or hypomanic symptoms.

In older depressed patients, anxiety and motor agitation are more common. These patients should be observed for restlessness, fidgeting, squirming, wringing their hands or pulling their hair, or feeling compelled to get up and pace around. The clinical picture is termed *agitated depression*. Although physically overactive, such patients often show slowed mental processes in performing specified cognitive tasks. Cognitive functions should be tested to distinguish depressive pseudodementia from dementing diseases. They should also be asked about reduced appetite or weight loss, sleep trouble, especially early morning awakening, feelings of guilt and hypochondriasis. These depressions are not only melancholic but are often of psychotic severity, and, therefore, one should directly inquire to learn whether there are the delusions of guilt or of physical illness, or hallucinations that typically occur in more severe forms which tend to have hypochondriacal, self-denigrating, or persecutory content. As is the case with retarded depressions, these patients are relatively unlikely to have shown traits of generalized anxiety or personality disorder before they became depressed. On the contrary, they are more likely to have been hard working, self-sacrificing, scrupulously honest, or perfectionistic—what is often termed *stable premorbid personality*.

If the dominant affect is one of milder depression mixed with anxiety, muscle tension, tremulousness, blushing or pallor, perspiration, mental overarousal, jumpiness, a tendency to startle easily, and fearfulness and if frank psychomotor agitation is not evident, an anxious depression (major depression or dysthymia with panic disorder) is more likely. These patients should be asked about panic attacks, obsessive thoughts and compulsions, and whether these began to occur during the depression or predated it. These patients are more likely to report chronic and unremitting anxiety and depressed mood, trouble falling asleep and poor quality of sleep, poor appetite or weight loss, and hypochondriacal preoccupations with their health—but not to delusional proportion. These patients often display "reverse" vegetative signs—such as early insomnia, daytime or morning hypersomnolence, hyperphagia, and feeling worse in the evening—and are contrasted to those with retarded or agitated melancholia. Panic attacks with onset during the period of depression seem to be the best single indicator of anxious depression, but a combination of other anxiety symptoms may also help in pointing to this subtype.

Other patients complain of depression and anxiety but do not look particularly anxious nor depressed. Some will report profound depression for brief periods (hours or days), but this can rapidly give way to a normal or even cheerful mood. This inconsistent affect suggests a personality disorder such as somatization disorder. This disorder—which can mimic every other mental and physical illness—also gives rise to depressive symptoms, though rarely of convincing syndromal depth.

These patients should be asked about a variety of past physical symptoms: lifelong sickliness, neurologic symptoms such as past episodes of blindness, paralysis, amnesia, or seizures, abdominal pains and vomiting, menstrual symptoms, lifelong sexual dysfunction, bodily pains (particularly burning pains in the mouth, anus, or genitalia), headaches, and heart or breathing symptoms. They should also be asked about symptoms of other psychiatric illnesses. In some cases they will also report fleeting hallucinations, panic attacks, binge eating followed by vomiting, drug or alcohol abuse, and antisocial symptoms. What is diagnostic is a collection of ominous-sounding symptoms without the signs that would normally accompany them if a known medical disease were present. Checking old medical records might reveal a history of many more unremembered symptoms. Usually these patients will report "continuous" anxiety and depression, but collateral information will reveal that these symptoms come and go. Those who tend to be vivacious, theatrical, flamboyant, and energetic might complain of lower energy and increased need for sleep when they are depressed. They should be asked about their relationships, which are likely to have been troubled and marked by overdependence, manipulativeness, and hostility. Dysphoric states that could be of either dysthymic or major depressive proportions are also commonly seen in antisocial personalities. Rather than concentrating on manipulativeness, one should ask about overtly abusive and predatory behavior such as physical assaultiveness, thefts, arrests, rights, unstable employment, vagrancy and wanderlust, and irresponsible financial and sexual behaviors. Depressed mood is likely to be described as absolutely unremitting—although this is rarely borne out by objective evidence—and although superimposed episodes of major depression may also occur. In interview, this type of dysphoria is best identified by asking about drinking, drug use, the symptoms of the antisocial personality disorder and symptoms that might be summarized as indicative of a sociopathic character. The number of antisocial symptoms will often fall below the DSM-III criterion for antisocial personality disorder, which is based on the extreme stereotype of this disorder.

The major differential diagnosis of depressions that are character based is from anxious depressions, subaffective dysthymic disorder, and cyclothymia. Often individuals with severe personality disorder abuse substances that can, during withdrawal, produce a mixture of anxiety and depressive symptoms. In addition, they invite life situations that can augment their dysphoric states. By contrast, in cyclothymic and subaffective dysthymic disorders, the personality disturbances are secondary to subsyndromal affective instability (Akiskal et al., 1977, 1983b). A careful longitudinal history will reveal that mood swings began a few years earlier than the personality difficulties. Some of these patients actually meet the DSM-III criteria for borderline personality disorder, which further clouds differential diagnosis. However, current data indicate that many of these patients represent a variant of affective disorder, most commonly subaffective dysthymic, cyclothymic, and Bipolar II disorders (Akiskal, 1981; Akiskal, Yerevanian, Davis, King, & Lemmi, 1985; Stone, 1984). Diagnostic criteria for subaffective dysthymia and cyclothymia developed at the University of Tennessee (Akiskal, 1979a, 1983b) have already been summarized in Tables 2 and 3. The most important distinctions from primary characterologic disorders include (a) course, that is, the fact that the affective manifestations preceded the personality difficulties, though this is not always easy to document; (b) affective manifestations are sustained from a few days to a week, rather than just hours; (c) affective symptoms often come "out of the blue," cannot be accounted for by substance abuse, and do not disappear when social rewards are provided; (d) the subsyndromal patterns are biphasic; and (e) they appear spontaneously in cyclothymia but require pharmacologic challenge in subaffective dysthymia. The interview schedule by Depue, Slater, Wolfsetter-Kaush, Klein, Coplerud, and Farr, (1981) has been used in research studies for identifying cyclothymic individuals but remains largely untested in a clinic patient population.

Related to cyclothymia—and likewise confused with personality disorder—are patients with Bipolar II disorder (Akiskal, 1981). The tempestuous biographies of these individuals are superimposed on recurrent retarded depressive episodes, typically of relatively short duration (4 to 12 weeks), and infrequent and mild hypomanic periods of very brief duration (1 to 3 days). In other words, these patients resemble cyclothymics except that the depressive episodes are of longer duration and hypomania is infrequent. Because hypomania in these patients is often pleasant and adaptive, they do not complain about it or seek help during such times. Thus, the presence of hypomania is only ascertained by history and requires skilled interviewing. Table 4 summarizes the

Table 4. Setting the Threshold for Clinical Hypomania

1. It is often dysphoric in its drivenness
2. Tends to be labile
3. May lead to substance abuse
4. Impairs social judgment
5. It is often preceded or followed by retarded depression
6. Typically springs from positive familial background for classical bipolar disorder

Note: Summarized from Akiskal (1983a).

University of Tennessee criteria for distinguishing clinical hypomania from normal happiness (Akiskal, 1983a). Treatment with antidepressants will sometimes mobilize a hypomanic state in these patients, thereby serving as an external validator. This is also how the diagnosis of pseudounipolar depressions (Bipolar III/Unipolar II) is suggested. Family history for bipolar illness is helpful in this regard.

Because bipolar patients often deny past psychopathology, the history of past retarded depression or excited periods is best obtained from someone who has known the patient for a long time. Regarding current mania and hypomania, it is useful to ask about sleep, that is, whether there has been a recent change, and less sleep than usual is needed. Expansive grandiosity is best assessed by asking questions about indirect indicators—whether there has been a recent increase in spending, recently developed great plans for the future, a recent dramatic improvement in sexual interest and prowess, or a recent increase in heroic drinking without the usual degree of impairment. Again, most reliable information regarding such behavior comes from significant others. The affect of frank mania is easy to recognize. The infectious exuberant energy of these patients is qualitatively different from anything seen in ordinary human beings or those with primary characterologic disorders. Mania is more difficult to recognize when it progresses to a psychotic stage or a mixed episode where irritability, dysphoria, and hostility may replace euphoria. Delusions, hallucinations, and thinking disturbances are likely to be observed (Akiskal & Puzantian, 1979). These patients can be very difficult to differentiate from those with schizophrenia. Their frenzied activity actually makes them seem more psychotic than patients with schizophrenia (Carlson & Goodwin, 1978). These paranoid or delusional manics can become assaultive with minimal provocation and are best interviewed briefly and in the company of assistants trained in physical restraint of the mentally ill. Therefore, the definitive diagnosis of primary bipolar affective disorder is established by obtaining an outside history—from family, friends, or old psychiatric records—for an episodic course of illness with periods of recovery from psychotic symptoms, by a past history of more typical episodes of mania and depression, and by a lack of psychotic symptoms during periods when neither mania nor depression were present.

Summary

Although recent approaches using psychometric, family history, pharmacologic response, neuroendocrine, and neurophysiologic techniques have provided new and provocative ways to assist in the diagnostic process, phenomenologic diagnosis remains the solid foundation of the clinical and research endeavor. Diagnosis of depression and mania and their subtypes is based on observed signs and reported symptoms. The core signs and symptoms of depression are depressed mood, appetite and sleep changes, loss of interest, energy, self-esteem, memory and concentration, thoughts of death or suicide, and psychomotor agitation or retardation. Additional features or a preponderance of certain features will suggest a particular subtype of depression. Anxiety often coexists with depression and creates problems in differential diagnosis. Mania is characterized by euphoric or irritable mood, increased energy, hyperactivity, racing thoughts, pressured speech, flight of ideas, grandiosity, decreased need for sleep, and disinhibited behavior. Subtypes of bipolar disorder—where depression and mania coexist— are identified by severity and by associated psychotic symptoms. As personality disturbances commonly occur in the setting of depressive and bipolar disorders, their differentiation from primary characterologic disorders is often problematic.

In this chapter we have elaborated on the distinction between primary affective disorders and dysphoric states that are secondary to, or represent complications of, anxiety and personality disorders. Such differentiation of true affective illness and its subtypes from overlapping mental disorders is important for reasons of predictive and construct validity. In brief, the clinician must distinguish between affective subtypes because of differential treatment implications, whereas the clinical investigator must specify the subtype that he or she wishes to examine for hypothesis testing. Unfortunately, many researchers testing etiologic hypotheses or the efficacy of various treatment approaches in depression fail to specify whether their study populations conform to primary affective disorder or represent dysphoric states in the setting of non-affective disorders. We hope that future work in affective disorders will make increasing use of rigorous principles necessary for proper diagnostic subtyping of these disorders.

References

Akiskal, H. S. (1981). Subaffective disorders: Dysthymic, cyclothymic, and Bipolar II disorders in the "borderline" realm. *Psychiatric Clinics of North America, 4*, 25–46.

Akiskal, H. S. (1982). Affective disorders. In R. Berkow (Ed.), *Merck manual of diagnosis and therapy* (pp. 1448–1462). New Jersey: Merck, Sharp, and Dohme Research Laboratories.

Akiskal, H. S. (1983). Diagnosis and classification of affective disorders: New insights from clinical and laboratory approaches. *Psychiatric Developments, 1*, 123–160. (a)

Akiskal, H. S. (1983). Dysthymic disorder: Psychopathology of proposed chronic depressive subtypes. *American Journal of Psychiatry, 140,* 11–20. (b)

Akiskal, H. S. (1983). The bipolar spectrum: New concepts in classification and diagnosis. In L. Grinspoon (Ed.), *Psychiatry update: The American Psychiatric Association annual review, II,* Washington, DC: American Psychiatric Association. (c)

Akiskal, H. S. (1984). The boundaries of affective disorders: Implications for defining temperamental variants, atypical subtypes, and schizoaffective disorders. In G. Tischler (Ed.), *DSM-III: An interim appraisal.* Washington, DC: American Psychiatric Association.

Akiskal, H. S., & Cassano, G. B. (1983). The impact of therapeutic advances in widening the nosologic boundaries of affective disorders: Clinical and research implications. *Pharmacopsychiatria, 16,* 111–118.

Akiskal, H. S., & McKinney, W. T. (1975). Overview of recent research in depression: Integration of ten conceptual models into a comprehensive clinical frame. *Archives of General Psychiatry, 32,* 285–305.

Akiskal, H. S., & Puzantian, V. R. (1979). Psychotic forms of depression and mania. *Psychiatric Clinics of North America, 2,* 419–439.

Akiskal, H. S., & Tashjian, R. (1983). Affective disorders: Part II. Recent advances in laboratory and pathogenetic approaches. *Hospital and Community Psychiatry, 34,* 822–830.

Akiskal, H. S., & Webb, W. L. (Eds.). (1978). *Psychiatric diagnosis: Exploration of biological predictors.* New York: Spectrum Publications.

Akiskal, H. S., Djenderedjian, A. H., Rosenthal, R. H., & Khani, M. K. (1977). Cyclothymic disorder: Validating criteria for inclusion in the bipolar affective group. *American Journal of Psychiatry, 134,* 1227–1233.

Akiskal, H. S., Bitar, A. H., Puzantian, V. R., Rosenthal, T. L., & Walker, P. W. (1978). The nosological status of neurotic depression: A prospective three-to-four year examination in light of the primary-secondary and unipolar-bipolar dichotomies. *Archives of General Psychiatry, 35,* 756–766.

Akiskal, H. S., Khani, M. K., & Scott-Strauss, A. (1979). Cyclothymic temperamental disorders. *Psychiatric Clinics of North America, 2,* 527–554.

Akiskal, H. S., Rosenthal, R. H., Rosenthal, T. L., Kashgarian, M., Khani, M. K., & Puzantian, V. R. (1979). Differentiation of primary affective illness from situational symptomatic and secondary depressions. *Archives of General Psychiatry, 36,* 635–643.

Akiskal, H. S., Rosenthal, T. L., Haykal, R. F., Lemmi, H., Rosenthal, R. H., & Scott-Strauss, A. (1980). Characterological depressions: Clinical and sleep EEG findings separating "subaffective dysthymias" from "character-spectrum" disorders. *Archives of General Psychiatry, 37,* 777–783.

Akiskal, H. S., Walker, P. W., Puzantian, V. R., King, D., Rosenthal, T. L., & Dranon, M. (1983). Bipolar outcome in the course of depressive illness: Phenomenologic, familial and pharmacologic predictors. *Journal of Affective Disorders, 5,* 115–128.

Akiskal, H. S., Lemmi, H., Dickson, H., King, D., Yerevanian, B. I., & VanValkenburg, C. (1984). Chronic depressions: Part 2. Sleep EEG differentiation of primary dysthymic disorders from anxious depressions. *Journal of Affective Disorders, 6,* 287–295.

Akiskal, H. S., Yerevanian, B. I., Davis, G. C., King, D., & Lemmi, H. (1985). The nosologic status of borderline personality: Clinical and polysomnographic study. *American Journal of Psychiatry.*

American Psychiatric Association. (1980). *Diagnostic and statistical Manual of Mental disorders* (3d ed.) Washington, DC: Author.

Andreasen, N. C., & Canter, A. (1974) The creative writer: Psychiatric symptoms and family history. *Comprehensive Psychiatry, 15,* 123–131.

Beck, A. (1967), *Depression: Clinical, experimental and theoretical aspects.* New York: Harper & Row.

Carlson, G. A., & Goodwin, F. K. (1978). The stages of mania: A longitudinal analysis of the manic episode. *Archives of General Psychiatry, 28,* 221–228.

Carroll, B. J. (1982). Clinical applications of the dexamenthasone suppression test for endogenous depression. *Pharmacopsychiatria, 15,* 12–24.

Davidson, J. R. T., Miller, R. D., Turnbull, C. D., & Sullivan, J. L. (1982). Atypical depression. *Archives of General Psychiatry, 39,* 527–534.

Depue, R. A., Slater, J. R., Wolfsetter-Kaush, M., Klein, D., Coplerud, E., & Farr, D. (1981). A biobehavioral paradigm for identifying persons at risk for bipolar depressive disorders: A conceptual framework and five validation studies. *Journal of Abnormal Psychology Monograph, 90,* 381–437.

Feighner, J. P., Robins, E., Guze, S. B., Woodruff, R. A., Winokur, G., & Munoz, R. (1972). Diagnostic criteria for use in psychiatric research. *Archives of General Psychiatry, 26,* 57–63.

Fieve, R. R., & Dunner, D. L., (1975). Unipolar and bipolar affective states. In F. Flach & S. Draghi (Eds), *The nature and treatment of depression.* New York: Wiley.

Goodwin, D. W., & Guze, S. B. (1984). *Psychiatric diagnosis* (3rd ed.) New York: Oxford University Press.

Hamilton, M. (1960). A rating scale for depression. *Journal of Neurology, Neurosurgery, and Psychiatry, 23,* 56–62.

Jamison, K. R., & Akiskal, H. S. (1983). Medication compliance in patients with bipolar disorders. *Psychiatric Clinics of North America, 6,* 175–192.

Klerman, G. I. (1983). Psychotherapies and somatic therapies in affective disorders. *Psychiatric Clinics of North American, 6,* 85–103.

Kupfer, D. J., & Thase, M. E. (1983). The use of the sleep laboratory in the diagnosis of affective disorders. *Psychiatric Clinics of North America, 6,* 3–40.

Kupfer, D. J., Pickar, D., Himmelhoch, J. M., & Detre, T. (1975). Are there two types of unipolar depression? *Archives of General Psychiatry, 32,* 866–871.

Leckman, J. R., Weissman, M. W., Merikangas, K. R., Paula, D. L., & Prusoff, B. A. (1983). Panic disorders and major depression: Increased risk of depression, alcoholism, panic and phobic disorders in families of depressed probands with panic disorder. *Archives of General Psychiatry, 40,* 1055–1060.

Liebowitz, M., & Klein, D. (1979). Hysteroid dysphoria. *Psychiatric Clinics of North America, 2,* 555–575.

Robins, E., & Guze, S. B. (1972). Classification of affective disorders: The primary-secondary, the endogenous-reactive and the neurotic-psychotic concepts. In T. A. Williams, M. M. Katz, J. A. Shields (Eds.), *Recent advances in the psychobiology of the depressive illness.* Washington, DC: US Government Printing Office.

Rosenthal, T. L., Akiskal, H. S., Scott-Strauss, A., Rosenthal, R. H., & David, M. (1981). Familial and developmental factors in characterological depressions. *Journal of Affective Disorders, 3,* 183–192.

Sheard, M. H., & Marini, J. L. (1978). Treatment of human aggressive behavior: Four case studies of the effect of lithium. *Comprehensive Psychiatry, 19,* 37–45.

Spitzer, R., Endicott, Jr., & Robins, E. (1979). *Research diagnostic criteria (RDC) for a selected group of functional disorders* (4th ed.). New York: Biometrics Research Division, New York Psychiatric Institute.

Stone, M. H. (1979). Contemporary shift of the borderline concept from a schizophrenic disorder to subaffective disorder. *Psychiatric Clinics of North America, 3,* 517–594.

VanValkenburg, C., Akiskal, H. S., Puzantian, V. R., & Rosenthal, T. L. (1984). Anxious depressions—Clinical, family history, and naturalistic outcome comparisons with panic and major depressive disorders. *Journal of Affective Disorders, 6,* 67–82.

Weissman, M. M., & Myers, J. K. (1978). Affective disorders in a U.S. urban community. *Archives of General Psychiatry, 35,* 1304–1311.

Chapter 5

Schizophrenia

Herman V. Szymanski and Stuart L. Keill

Introduction

Between 0.23% and 0.47% of the total population of the United States (or between 500,000 and 1 million people) is likely to receive psychiatric treatment for a schizophrenic illness during any year. Sixty-two percent of these will be hospitalized for this condition during that year. In addition, about 1% of the persons in the U.S. population will develop schizophrenia during their lifetime (Babigian, 1980).

These figures identify schizophrenia as a major public mental health problem. Given the frequency and seriousness of this disorder, a student preparing for a career as a mental health clinician in any of the mental health professions must be cognizant of the criteria for this diagnosis and of interview techniques for arriving at the diagnosis. The assignment of such a diagnosis to a patient has considerable ramifications for understanding the patient's subjective experience of his or her illness, for treatment, and for prognosis.

General Description of Schizophrenia

There are a number of systems for making a diagnosis of schizophrenia. Not surprisingly, there is partial overlap between the systems,

HERMAN V. SZYMANSKI • VA Medical Center and Western Psychiatric Institute and Clinic, Pittsburgh, Pennsylvania 15206.   STUART L. KEILL • State University of New York, VA Medical Canter, Buffalo, New York 14215.

and each system identifies a small number of patients who are not counted as schizophrenic in any other diagnostic system (Brockington, Kendell & Leff, 1978; Deutsch & Davis, 1983; Gift, Strauss, Ritzler, Kokes, & Harder, 1980; Overall & Hollister, 1979). Thus, in the absence of any definite evidence proving the etiology of schizophrenia, it is not desirable to recommend one diagnostic system above another based on its ability to identify patients with a homogeneous etiology.

Given such considerations, we recommend that the reader learn the criteria published in the American Psychiatric Association's (APA) *Diagnostic and Statistical Manual of Mental Disorders* (DSM-III) (American Psychiatric Association, 1980) because they are the most widely used criteria in clinical settings in the United States. These criteria are presented in Table 1. Note that DSM-III divides the illness into prodromal, active, and residual phases. In order to make a diagnosis, the interviewer must be aware of the marked differences in clinical presentation among these phases. For instance, psychotic symptoms may be present in the residual phase but are not prominent.

Schizophrenia must be distinguished from other functional or organic disorders. Delusions and hallucinations also occur in organic brain syndrome, but the latter manifests disorientation, memory impairment, and impairment in intellectual functions such as information, calculation, abstract thinking, reasoning and judgment not seen in schizophrenia (APA, 1980, pp. 188–190).

Psychotic symptoms often occur in major depression or in a manic episode—the two types of major affective disorders. Distinguishing these disorders from schizophrenia is usually possible if the interviewer is aware of the DSM-III criteria for all three disorders. However, there are a number of patients who manifest symptoms of both schizophrenia and mania or both schizophrenia and major depression. Using these criteria, one would classify these patients as having an affective disorder if the affective symptoms preceded the schizophrenic symptoms and there was no period of time when schizophrenic symptoms occurred without affective symptoms. That is, a patient with schizophrenic symptoms followed by affective symptoms or with schizophrenic symptoms alone at any time would be classified as schizophrenic. In DSM-III, psychotic symptoms occurring along with affective symptoms are not part of schizophrenia if the psychotic symptoms are mood congruent. That is, if the patient is depressed, mood-congruent psychotic features would include delusions or hallucinations consistent with "themes of personal inadequacy, guilt, disease, death, nihilism, or deserved punishment." If the patient is manic, mood-congruent psychotic features would include delusions or hallucinations consistent with "themes of inflated worth, power, knowledge, identity, or special relationship to a deity or famous person," (APA, 1980).

Table 1. DSM-III Criteria for Schizophrenia

A. At least one of the following during a phase of the illness:
1. Bizarre delusions (content is patently absurd and has no possible basis in fact), such as delusions of being controlled, thought broadcasting, thought insertion, or thought withdrawal
2. Somatic, grandiose, religious, nihilistic, or other delusions without persecutory or jealous content
3. Delusions with persecutory or jealous content if accompanied by hallucinations of any type
4. Auditory hallucinations in which either a voice keeps up a running commentary on the individual's behavior or thoughts or two or more voices converse with each other
5. Auditory hallucinations on several occasions with content of more than one or two words having no apparent relation to depression or elation
6. Incoherence, marked loosening of associations, markedly illogical thinking, or marked poverty of content of speech if associated with at least one of the following:
   a. blunted, flat, or inappropriate affect
   b. delusions or hallucinations
   c. catatonic or other grossly disorganized behavior.
B. Deterioration from a previous level of functioning in such areas as work, social relations, and self-care.
C. Duration: Continuous signs of the illness for at least 6 months at sometime during the person's life with some signs of the illness at present. The 6-month period must include an active phase during which there were symptoms from A, with or without a prodromal or residual phase, as defined next.
   • *Prodromal phase*: A clear deterioration in functioning before the active phase of the illness not due to a disturbance in mood or to a Substance Use Disorder and involving at least two of the symptoms noted later.
   • *Residual phase*: Persistence following the active phase of the illness, of at least two of the symptoms noted next not due to a disturbance in mood or to a Substance Use Disorder.
   Prodromal or Residual Symptoms
   1. Social isolation or withdrawal
   2. Marked impairment in role functioning as wage earner, student, or homemaker
   3. Markedly peculiar behavior (e.g., collecting garbage, talking to self in public, hoarding food)
   4. Marked impairment in personal hygiene and grooming
   5. Blunted, flat, or inappropriate affect
   6. Digressive, vague, overelaborate, circumstantial, or metaphorical speech
   7. Odd or bizarre ideation, or magical thinking, e.g., superstitiousness, clairvoyance, telepathy, "sixth sense," "others can feel my feelings," overvalued ideas, ideas of reference
   8. Unusual perceptual experiences, for example, recurrent illusions, sensing the presence of a force or person not actually present.
D. The full depressive or manic syndrome (Criteria A and B of major depressive or manic episode), if present, developed after any psychotic symptoms or was brief in duration relative to the duration of the psychotic symptoms in A.
E. Onset of prodromal or active phase of illness before age 45.
F. Not due to any Organic Mental Disorder or Mental Retardation.

Note: From *Diagnostic and Statistical Manual of Mental Disorders* (3rd ed., pp. 188–190) by American Psychiatric Association, 1980, Washington, DC: American Psychological Association. Copyright 1980 by the American Psychiatric Association. Reprinted by permission.

One of the criteria for determining the validity of a diagnostic system is whether it identifies a group of patients who are relatively homogeneous for etiology and prognosis (Neale & Oltmanns, 1980). Whether DSM-III accomplishes this more than other diagnostic systems is not known. Although this chapter focuses primarily on DSM-III criteria, it is important for the student to be aware of other diagnostic systems, which some professionals still feel are more valid. The relationship between some of the diagnostic systems and DSM-III will be described. In this way, the rationale for some of the DSM-III criteria will become clearer.

History of the Concept of Schizophrenia

The history of the concept *schizophrenia* began with the recognition of a psychosis whose *outstanding* features did not include the memory difficulties seen in the organic brain syndromes or the "affective excess" seen in depression or mania. This distinction was made to a greater or lesser extent by a number of writers during the 19th century such as Pinel, Haslam, Morel, and Kahlbaum (Neale & Oltmanns, 1980).

Kraepelin. The writing's of Emil Kraepelin begin the modern era of psychiatry. In 1883, he published his *Compendium of Psychiatry*, which over the next 40 years was published in a series of ever-enlarging editions. The concept of *dementia praecox* appeared in the fourth edition in 1893 and was expanded in later editions (Kraepelin, 1919/1971). Kraepelin pointed out the difficulty in determining which psychiatric symptoms should be criteria for membership in a particular diagnostic category. He recommended grouping patients according to course of illness. Once this was done, it might be possible to identify symptoms shared in common by the patients with a particular prognosis, and the diagnostic system would at least be valid in terms of identifying a group of patients with a homogeneous prognosis. The same rationale lies behind DSM-III's requirement of at least 6 months duration of illness. That is, DSM-III uses not only symptoms to define schizophrenia but also prognosis. Use of prognosis as a way of validating a diagnostic system is particularly important because the etiology of the illness is not much more apparent now than it was then.

Kraepelin's second major conceptual contribution, also incorporated into DSM-III, is the emphasis on description of observable signs or symptoms of the illness, rather than on inferences about the psychological defect underlying the illness. The first DSM-III criteria (bizarre delusions such as delusions of influence) reflects the Kraepelinian tradition that delusions of influence are infrequent in affective disorder, though modern studies (Carpenter, Strauss, & Muleh, 1973) have found them in up to 25% of manic patients.

Bleuler. In contrast to Kraepelin's emphasis on description, Bleuler in *Dementia Praecox or the Group of Schizophrenias* attempted to specify the underlying psychological "disease processes" involved in schizophrenia (Bleuler, 1911/1950). This was hypothesized to be the "splitting of the psychic functions" or a breaking of associative threads. The hypothetical construct *associative threads* referred to the psychological process of linking together words, thoughts, and actions.

Bleuler (1911/1950, p. 9) proposed four fundamental symptoms (the "four *A*'s") arising from this basic disease process:

1. Associative disturbance—"The process of association often works with mere fragments of ideas and concepts. This results in associations which normal individuals will regard as incorrect, bizarre, and utterly unpredictable. Often thinking stops in the middle of a thought" (or blocking).
2. Autism—A predilection during a major part of waking life toward fantasy "in opposition to reality."
3. Affective disturbance—Flat, silly or incongruous affect.
4. Ambivalence—Although all people experience contradictory impulses or ideas, in schizophrenia these are more intensely and frequently experienced, and there is a rapid changing from one extreme impulse or idea to another.

In Bleuler's system, symptoms such as delusions or hallucinations are secondary to the fundamental symptoms.

Symptoms described by Bleuler such as loose association and blunted affect appear in DSM-III, though not with as much emphasis. The distinction between primary and secondary symptoms is not used in the relatively atheoretical DSM-III.

Schneider. The continuance of the Kraepelinian emphasis on description is illustrated by Kurt Schneider's list of delusions or hallucinations, any one of which, if present, was thought to be pathognomonic for schizophrenia. These include hearing one's thoughts spoken aloud; hearing two voices conversing about oneself; hearing voices commenting on one's behavior; believing external forces can alter one's body functions; believing one's thoughts can be withdrawn, that another's thought can be inserted, or that people can read one's thoughts; ideas of reference; believing that perceptions have personal significance in the absence of reasonable justification for such a belief; and believing that feelings, impulses, or motor actions are controlled from outside the body (Lehmann, 1980). Though any one of these symptoms, when present, indicated schizophrenia, Schneider did not believe that their absence ruled out schizophrenia. The Schneiderian influence on DSM-III is obvious in Criteria A-1 and A-4.

Others. A number of more modern systems of diagnosis use elements of the Kraepelinian, Bleulerian, or Schneiderian approach: The New Haven Schizophrenia Index (Astrachan *et al.*, 1972), the Flexible System (Carpenter, Strauss, & Bartko, 1974), and the Research Diagnostic Criteria (RDC—Spitzer, Endicott, & Robins, 1978). To elicit information concerning the RDC criteria, a structured interview—The Schedule for Affective Disorders and Schizophrenia (Endicott & Spitzer, 1978)—was developed. DSM-III criteria for schizophrenia are based to a large extent on RDC criteria. There is also a British system for diagnosing schizophrenia—the British Glossary of Mental Disorders, (General Register Office, 1968), and a British structured interview—the Present State Exam (Wing, Cooper, & Sartorius, 1974).

Procedures for Gathering Information

Even prior to the interview/examination, there are other valuable sources of information to arrive at a diagnosis of schizophrenia. Family, friends, charts, or other records should, whenever possible, be reviewed first. These may provide essential data that the patient may be unable or unwilling to provide. In instances where informants such as family members or police have been interviewed prior to the patient, Sullivan (1954) recommends telling the patient what information has been given (without including any pejorative attitudes expressed by the informants) and then asking the patient for his or her version of events. This is especially important with patients who tend to identify the interviewer as a critical authority like those who brought him or her in and subtly implies that the interviewer is on the side of the patient.

In most cases, the interviewer will not know the patient has schizophrenia but only that the patient is psychotic. Thus, the "decision tree" on pages 340 and 341 of the DSM-III (APA, 1980) will be useful to keep in mind because it illustrates the differential diagnosis of psychosis.

The general principles of interviewing have been presented in a previous chapter, but some are of particular importance in the interview of a patient having schizophrenia. The interviewer's relationship with the interviewee is ordinarily that of an expert from whom the patient hopes to derive some benefit (Sullivan, 1954). Many schizophrenic patients, however, have, for much of their lives, experienced interpersonal contact as painful or unpleasant and therefore expect a repeat of such experience with each new contact. It is therefore crucial that from the very beginning, the interviewer establish an aura of (a) genuine respect for the interviewee and concern for his or her discomfort; (b) comfort in the role of the professional; (c) a nonjudgmental approach; and (d) a sincere wish to be helpful. A useful device for the interviewer is to imagine his or her reactions if the patient's perception were actually true and then to estimate what the interviewer would feel and do in the patient's place. This kind of introduction is often therapeutic in its initial approach.

Because of the schizophrenic patient's general apprehension about interpersonal relationships and because the psychiatric interview of necessity investigates anxiety-laden topics, it is important for the interviewer to monitor the patient's level of anxiety and level of suspiciousness or hostility toward the interviewer. On occasion it may be necessary to end the interview before completing it and return later.

The paranoid schizophrenic patient has particular difficulty with interpersonal relationships. Beneath the mistrust of a paranoid schizophrenic patient are deep fears of a close relationship. The interviewer must not try to allay these fears by falsely reassuring the patient that he or she is a trustworthy advocate or friend of the patient. This would be similar in the patient's view to establishing a social relationship or suggesting agreement with the delusions. If the patient expresses mistrust for the interviewer, the interviewer should agree with the patient that he or she is unknown to the patient and that he or she can understand the patient's difficulty trusting him or her. Be recognizing the patient's feelings, the interviewer is beginning to establish a professional relationship—with empathy yet appropriate professional distancing—rather than a social one (MacKinnon & Michels, 1971).

Many patients with paranoid schizophrenia will have much less difficulty describing their complaints if the interviewer at first focuses on their somatic complaints. This tends to be better accepted than direct inquiries about the patient's mental health, which often only activate the patient's paranoid defenses. "The royal road to the paranoid is through the body" (Small, personal communication, 1983).

Another element in the relationship between interviewer and patient that is of particular importance in dealing with the schizophrenic individual is countertransference. As with most human beings, the interviewer is subject to emotional reactions, based on his or her earlier life experiences that may be entirely irrelevant to the patient at hand. The sensitive, experienced clinician will often note that certain patients bring out inappropriate feelings in him or her, such as arrogance, protectiveness, erotic fantasies, or fear. Recognizing this he or she will, of course, not act on the feelings but may use them to assist in arriving at a diagnosis.

Assessment of the patient begins with observation of the patient's dress, activity, facial expression, posture, and so forth. The general demeanor toward the interviewee will give clues about whether the patient is suspicious, frightened, angry, confused, and so forth.

The benefit that a patient expects to derive from the interview very seldom consists of arriving at a DSM-III diagnosis describing his or her psychopathology. Thus, the first task of the interview is to determine the patient's version of the interview's purpose. For this reason, it is best to begin the interview by asking the patient a general question about what is presently ailing him or her, for example, "What brings you here?" or "What can I help you with?" For the angry patient who was brought in against his or her will, it might be necessary to begin with "I gather you would prefer not to be forced into coming here."

Patients come to the initial interview with a story to tell. The interviewer should let the patient tell it, saving more specific questions untill later (Strayhorn, 1982). In this way the interviewer conveys his or her interest in hearing the patient's view of his or her situation. This helps to avoid giving the patient the impression that the interviewer is interested only in the technical issues of establishing a psychopathological diagnosis. Another problem with excessive direct questioning at the beginning of the interview is that it establishes a pattern in which the patient does not volunteer information without being directly asked (Strayhorn, 1982).

During the time the patient is telling his or her story, it is crucial for the interviewer to convey empathy to the patient. This can be accomplished by noting the patient's distress about whatever is bothering him or her with statements such as "that must have been difficult for you" or "I can see that you were upset when that happened." This approach is particularly important with patients who have little or no insight and may have been brought to the interview involuntarily. Furthermore, the subjective experience of psychosis often includes feelings of perplexity, isolation, depression, terror, loss of identity, and self-esteem (Strauss & Carpenter, 1981). Empathic understanding is especially important for these patients who will not give diagnostic information to an interviewer who, in their view, may further injure their already fragile self-esteem.

Many patients with schizophrenia, particularly the paranoid subtype, will implicitly or explicitly ask the interviewer to agree with their delusions, and some interviewers mistakenly believe that this is part of the empathic process. The interviewer must not do this and should simply indicate that he or she does not have enough information yet and would like to know more details. There is much written about psychotherapeutic approaches to delusions (Arieti, 1974; Fromm-Reichmann,

1950; Sullivan, 1954), but such treatment is generally beyond the scope of a diagnostic interview.

After the patient has been allowed to tell his or her story, for patients who can give a history, the interviewer should obtain an account of the development of the patient's symptoms and of deterioration of work, social relations, or self-care. Then the interviewer should proceed to a discussion of the patients' earlier life, covering topics such as family, education, socialization (or lack of it), vocational success, and previous physical or emotional illness in the patient and his or her family.

Many patients with schizophrenia will have loose associations or *circumstantiality*. These signs should be noted by the interviewer because, in and of themselves, they are diagnostic criteria. However, they can make it difficult to inquire about other diagnostic criteria. If this occurs, the interviewer must tell the patient in a noncritical way that he or she is "not entirely understanding you" or "I'm not following you." Avoid statements such as "You're not being clear" or "You're not making sense" (MacKinnon & Michels, 1971). If this does not help, the interviewer may have to cut short the first part of the interview (consisting of the patient's story) and interrupt the patient with more specific questions.

Table 2 presents some suggested questions to inquire about DSM-III criteria for the active phase of schizophrenia. Other questions are possible and may be more appropriate given the context. The interviewer must interview according to the principles described previously in Chapter 1. Only inaccurate information can come from presenting the patient with a list of memorized questions.

Most questions used by the interviewer should be open ended, that is, not have simply *yes* or *no* as an answer, in order to encourage the patient to explain himself or herself at length.

Case Examples

Patient in the Active Phase of Schizophrenia

The first case illustrates some of the difficulties interviewing a patient who is in the active phase of the illness.

History, Chief Complaint, Onset of Present Illness

I: What brings you here to the hospital?
P: My mother brought me in her car.

Table 2. Questions Used to Inquire about DSM-III Criteria in Table 1

Criterion	Questions
A-1	Does it sometimes seem as if anyone or anything else can control your thoughts against your will? Can take away thoughts or give them to you through telepathy or mind control? Do you feel that anyone or anything else can control your actions, as if you were a robot? Do you feel that your thoughts are repeated on the television or radio?
A-2	How is your physical health?
Somatic delusions	Do you have any headaches? Do you have any pains or burning feelings or feelings like there's electricity in your body?
Grandiose delusions	Do you have any talents or abilities that are above average?
Religious delusions	What are some of your religious beliefs?
Nihilistic delusions	How do you feel about the future? How badly do you feel things are going now?
A-3, A-4, A-5	Do you sometimes hear voices when there's no one around? What do the voices say? Do they describe what you're doing as soon as you do it? Do the voices talk to each other? How often do the voices occur?
A-6	Do you sometimes have trouble thinking?

Comment. This patient's concrete response to the interviewer's first question does not prove that the patient is *generally* concrete but raises the interviewer's suspicion that he may be so, and the interviewer makes a mental note to watch for other signs of concreteness throughout the interview.

I: I mean, what sort of problems bring you here?
P: There's no problems. My mother [patient now raises his voice] is being vicious toward me. I'm not going to talk to you any more.
I: Why do you suppose your mother's acting this way?
P: Because she's vicious, that's all. That's all there is to it.
I: Vicious?
P: She's a part of the whole scheme of things, including what they said about the food on the TV.
I: What did they say?
P: They warned me about the food and what it could do to a person.

Comment. The patient's initial insistence about not talking anymore could have ended the interview had the interviewer not recognized the patient's feelings about being brought to the hospital. The interviewer then invites the patient to present his viewpoint: "Why do you suppose your mother's acting this way?" Phrasing the question this way amounts to a paraphrase of the patient's story but not an outright agreement with the patient's view. The patient still resists giving information, answering only with short declarative sentences. The interviewer recognizes that the patient is likely to speak at greater length only about the reasons for his anger because then the patient will feel he is being given a chance to vindicate himself.

I: What could the food do to a person?
P: Anyone with any brains at all would know this. [Suspiciously] Why are you asking me these questions?
I: I'm concerned about how your health is. Did something happen to your health?
P: The warnings were right about the F force. It affects only the right side of my head. It starts with causing brain pressure, then electrical forces in the scalp.

Comment. Even when the patient says insulting things ("Anyone with any brains at all would know this"), rather than becoming defensive, the interviewer describes his or her concern about the patient's "health," leaving it open as to whether he or she means mental or physical health. This makes it possible for the patient to describe a somatic delusion, which meets DSM-III Criterion A-1.

I: That must have been an uncomfortable experience. When all this started happening, did you feel sad or blue?
P: I was really depressed [appears angry]. Man, that really got me down.
I: How does it feel to you when you're depressed?
P: They were criticizing me and thought they could make me take the food. They had me down. But then I got up again when I realized that those bastards can never get me down.
I: How did you feel when you felt down?
P: They were trying to control me but couldn't.
I: How did you feel when you felt up?
P: I stopped eating. They can't get me down if I don't eat.

Comment. It is always important to inquire about what a patient means by terms such as *depression, feeling down, up,* or *high.* Here the interviewer discovers that this patient used *depression* to describe his frustration at being under control and *feeling up* when he felt control had been returned to him by not eating. A less inquisitive interviewer might have accepted the patient's use of the term *depression* as accurate, and then regarded the patient's refusal of food as a sign of lack of appetite, as observed in major depression.

I: How long has all this been going on?
P: For a long time.
I: How long is that?
P: For some months, I guess.
I: Well, was it present before last Christmas?
P: No.
I: Before last summer?
P: I guess it started just before last summer [10 months ago].

Comment. When asking about duration of illness, for patients who have difficulty remembering, it is useful to try to date the onset in relationship to well-known holidays.

I: When all this started happening last spring, did you find you didn't feel well enough to do some of the things you used to do?
P: What do you mean?
I: Well, for example, did you work prior to last spring?
P: Yes.
I: Are you working now?
P: No.
I: Did you find that when you weren't feeling well, you didn't feel up to seeing friends?
P: I have lots of close friends.
I: How often do you see them?
P: Very often. Whenever we feel like getting together.
I: When did you last get together?
P: Oh, I guess it was the spring [10 months ago].

Comment. The interviewer tries to determine whether there has been a deterioration from previous level of vocational and social functioning. The first questions about this are general, and only when the patient cannot or will not respond do more specific questions become necessary. In assessing deterioration of functioning in areas such as work, social relations, and self-care, it is important to start off with general questions because the interviewer knows neither the preillness nor current level of functioning. Deterioration can occur in a multitude of different ways, and inquiry about each of these possibilities would be inefficient.

The brevity of the patient's responses and their poverty of content remind the interviewer that the patient is still suspicious of the interviewer, and he or she must be careful not to sound critical. The response of the patient, however, "I have lots of close friends," is very common and should never be taken at face value.

Mental Status

Where possible, of course, there is a considerable amount of time and energy expended on earlier history to note patterns of similar (even if less acute) behavior. When the interviewer feels that enough initial historical data has been accumulated, it is well to move on to the examination of the patient's cognitive and affective state, formally known as the mental status part of the examination. It is essential to arrive at a differential diagnosis.

Many inexperienced interviewers find the questions of the mental status examination elementary and fear they may be perceived as insulting to the patient. If, however, the questions are asked within the context of a professional examination of the circumstances surrounding the patient's discomfort, the patient will almost invariably accept this.

I: Since you've been having these difficulties, has it interfered with your thinking?
P: Yes, it's not like it used to be.
I: Well, I would like to ask you some questions to measure the difficulty that you are having with thinking. Do you know what the name of this place is?
P: It's the City General Hospital [correct].
I: Can you tell me the date?
P: Yes, it is January 15, 1984 [correct].
I: Can you tell me who the president is?
P: Yes, it's President Ronald Reagan [correct].
I: Do you know who the presidents before him were?
P: Yes, Jimmy Carter, Gerald Ford, Richard Nixon.

Comment. Individuals with organic delusional syndromes often demonstrate disorientation with grossly inaccurate dates or locations. The patient with schizophrenia, in answer to the question of "Do you know where you are?" may give a general answer such as "This is the Palace of Murder." This need not be an indication of disorientation but a delusional interpretation of the function of the place. Oftentimes, these patients, when pressed as to the actual name of the facility, will give the correct answer.

If you gave the man in the post office a dollar and asked for three 20-cent stamps, how much change would you get back?
P: Forty cents, but I would have to be careful that some poisonous substance had not been put on the back of the stamp.
I: Would you begin with 100 and subtract 7 and subtract 7 from that until I tell you to stop?
P: 93, 86, 79, 72, etc.

Comment. Organic patients or highly distractable patients have difficulty with this kind of question. Most schizophrenics who do not have an organic deficit and who are not having secondary organic states from oversedation will have little difficulty, providing they agree to be cooperative.

I: If you found an envelope in the street that was sealed and addressed and had a new stamp, what would you do with it?
P: I would put it in the mailbox.

Comment. The schizophrenic ordinarily knows what to do with the envelope. Those with paranoid or sociopathic overtones may give such answers as "I would open it to see if there was any money in it" or "Oftentimes signals are left by those who are trying to harass me." Those with acute organic delusional syndromes will often be perplexed by the question and give bizarre or inappropriate answers. There are a number of other tests of cognitive function that can be used, but this type of question will give an immediate estimate.

It is always worthwhile with schizophrenic patients to note bizarre communications, either persecutory, delusional, or peculiar concepts that the patient utilizes. Bruch (1974) notes that bizarre communications always have a meaning, although it is often not possible to discover what the meaning is: "Schizophrenese represents communication on a different level of abstraction . . . more concrete than ordinary language, often rich in puns, unusual analogies and unlabeled metaphors. With appropriate medications and experience with the patient, less time will be necessary to clarify them."* A recent example that one of the authors encountered was a patient who had been brought to the hospital by his brother. The patient stated, "My brother is trying to kill me; he has brought me here to be poisoned." Investigation of the case revealed that the patient had been a major source of problems to the brother who had been responsible for his welfare for a number of years. The brother, at one point, reluctantly admitted that there were times when he had a fantasy that his life would be much better if the patient would have died early. The second portion of the patient's delusion is explained by the fact that on previous admissions, the medication had resulted in a number of uncomfortable neurological side effects. These had been explained by another patient as the poisonous results of the medication being dispensed. Thus, the bizarre statement is clearer. Although this

---

*Freud (1911, p 387) referred to patients who "possess the peculiarity of betraying [in a distorted form it is true] precisely those things which other neurotics keep hidden as a secret."

example of bizarre communication was somewhat easier to interpret, it is often worthwhile for the interviewer to contemplate possible further explanations relating to history or diagnosis.

Patient in the Residual Phase of Schizophrenia

The degree of insight of patients in this phase, their memory of the active phase, and their willingness to talk about either phase varies greatly. The following dialogue illustrates a patient who has difficulty in all these areas. The patient came to the hospital emergency room at midnight. The only available datum is the nurse's note on the emergency room intake form, "Patient says he's nervous." The patient is 40 years old and has had five previous psychiatric admissions, but the chart is unavailable because the medical records staff cannot find it.

I: What brings you to the hospital?
P: I need to be in the hospital.
I: Why?
P: Nerves. My nerves are very bad.
I: What does it feel like when your nerves are bad?
P: You know. Everybody known what that means. You know, bad nerves, feeling nervous. I'm having a nervous breakdown.
I: What do you mean by nervous breakdown?
P: Things have been too much for me lately.

Comment. The interviewer's goals are to establish a helping relationship with the patient, to understand why the patient has come to the emergency room at this time, to establish a diagnosis, and to begin treatment. One of the patient's goals is to be hospitalized, so the interviewer, once he has learned this, inquires about it. He then attempts to clarify what the patient means by *bad nerves* or *nervous breakdown*. The patient's statement that "things have been too much for me lately" is an important turning point in the interview because it invites the interviewer to next inquire about the patient's environment rather than his mental status or diagnosis. The interviewer knows that inquiry into this area will further all of his goals including making a diagnosis. An inpatient interviewer at this point would have begun asking directly about DSM-III criteria, thus frustrating the patient and almost certainly obtaining less reliable information.

I: What do you think made you feel nervous?
P: I don't know.
I: Has anything stressful or unpleasant happened to you in the past few months?

P: Nothing. I just got nervous.

Comment. Early into the inquiry about the patient's environment, it becomes evident that the patient has little idea what makes him anxious, so the interviewer resorts to more specific questions.

I: Did you have trouble with finances?
P: No.
I: How are you getting along with other people?
P: Very badly. My landlady said I have to leave by the end of the month [in 2 weeks].

Comment. As with the first patient, the interviewer inquires about how things seem from the patient's viewpoint. Too often, inexperienced interviewers ask questions from their own viewpoint as a mental health professional. For example, the interviewer should ask "How are you getting along with other people?" rather than "Has your relationship with anyone else been strained?" The former question inquires about the patient's subjective experiences; the later inquires about a well-established hypothetical construct in mental health literature—interpersonal relationships.

I: When did she say you had to leave?
P: This morning.
I: Why?
P: She says I pray too loud.
I: How much do you pray?
P: I pray all day. I could pray better If I had a house in the country, where no one could interrupt. Sometimes I pray during the meals with the other tenants. Especially sacred is prayer during the breaking of the bread.

Comment. Note the preceding tangential association.

I: Do you pray out loud at meals?
P: Sometimes.

Comment. Inquiry about the reasons for a major recent event in a patient's life such as impending eviction can be quite informative about the patient's symptoms and functioning, as it is here. If the life event consists of an important figure doing something to the patient, it would be helpful for the interviewer to understand the possible reasons. In this case, the interviewer puts himself in the place of the landlady and the other tenants and asks whether the patient's prayer disturbs their meals or sleep. Sometimes beginning interviewers lose track of other possible perspectives.

At this point, the interviewer knows that the patient has bizarre behavior (Criterion C-3) but does not know if there are any delusions or hallucinations underlying this behavior. He then inquires about these symptoms.

I: What effect do you hope your prayer will have?
P: I hope the words rise to heaven. I'm on the third floor. I pray for a more universal bond between men, for a resolution to the struggle between good and evil.
I: I don't quite understand what you mean.
P: I just hope for better communication between all men.
I: It sounds like you feel you're pretty good at prayer.
P: I'm just average at it.
I: Do you have any other spiritual abilities?
P: No.
I: Do you sometimes feel you have a mission from God?
P: No.
I: Do you ever hear God's voice?
P: No.

Comment. The patient's bizarre behavior with regard to prayer makes it likely that delusions or hallucinations, if present, would involve religious themes, and so the interviewer focuses many of his questions around the patient's religious thinking, including some questions about whether he has any grandiose religious delusions. The patient denies any, but much more inquiry and observation would be necessary to rule out current psychosis in this patient.

The interviewer now inquires about social withdrawal.

I: How often do you see the other people in the building?
P: Just about never. Only at meals. She serves the meals.
I: Do you talk to them at meals?
P: No. I don't like talking.
I: What is your day like? What do you do all day?
P: Nothing. I eat and I pray, that's about all.
I: Do you ever go out of the house?
P: No.

Comment. Asking the patient to describe a typical day often reveals much about the patient's environment and relationships with others, and in this case uncovers the patient's social withdrawal.

The interviewer then asks about past psychiatric history.

I: You mentioned that you're having a nervous breakdown now. Have you had nervous breakdowns before?

P: Yes.

I: What were they like?

P: I was very nervous. I was praying a lot. That's all I remember. I went to the hospital.

I: Did you go to the hospital yourself or did someone bring you?

P: The police brought me.

I: Why?

P: I was lying in the street. I was very nervous, and I thought if I stayed in the street, I'd be O.K.

Comment. Questions about active symptoms during previous hospitalizations are so far inconclusive: lying in the street may have been bizarre behavior only, or behavior resulting from a delusion. Hence the interviewer asks for more about the patient's thinking at that time.

I: What made you feel safer in the street?

P: I'd be away from everyone.

I: Whom did you most want to be away from?

P: The people I was living with.

I: What about them makes you say you wanted to be away from them?

P: I thought the people I was living with were sending shock waves through the walls so that I couldn't sleep.

I: How do you feel about that now?

P: It's not possible for someone to do that.

Note that in the preceding interchange, the interviewer avoids questions beginning with "why" (e.g., "Why did you feel safer in the street?" or "Why did you want to be away from everyone?") because they are often viewed by patients as critical. Many "why" questions imply that the patient should have more insight about his or her behavior. A patient could well respond with "Doctor, I thought that was for you, the expert, to figure out."

Contrasting previous active symptoms with the patient's present state ("How do you feel about that now?") can sometimes help to determine if the patient is presently psychotic. At this point, the interviewer could continue to obtain historical data or proceed to the mental status or terminate the interview.

I: I'd like to talk to you again soon (preferably a specific date and time) about the problems you're having with nervousness and try to understand more about you so that we can try to do something about it.

Comment. The termination of the interview illustrates how evaluation is only the first step of a therapeutic process that involves both patient and therapist.

In summary, to establish the diagnosis of schizophrenia in these patients, more interviewing is needed to establish duration, absence of the full depressive and manic syndrome, and deterioration from a previous level of functioning. However, this patient has the "clinical feel" of a patient with residual schizophrenia. Patients with residual schizophrenia often present as did this patient, with bizarre behavior, social withdrawal, thinking that borders on the psychotic, and contact with the mental health system following a life event consequent to their bizarre behavior about which they have little insight.

Summary

The diagnostic interview with the patient with schizophrenia has many features in common with interviews of other patients, but several interviewing skills must be emphasized. These include sensitivity to the experience of psychosis, and the lifelong difficulty most schizophrenic patients have with interpersonal relationships. With patients who have loose associations, it may be necessary for the interviewer to resort to a more structured series of specific questions.

When carried out in the proper fashion, not only can a diagnostic interview with a patient with schizophrenia gather reliable data for making the diagnosis, but it also can take the first step in establishing a therapeutic relationship.

References

American Psychiatric Association (1980). *Diagnostic and statistical manual of mental disorders* (3rd ed.). Washington, DC: Author.

Arieti, S. (1974). *Interpretation of schizophrenia* (2d ed.). New York: Basic Books.

Astrachan, B. M., Harrow, M., Adler, D., Brauer, L., Schwartz, A., Schwartz, C., & Tucker, G. (1972). A checklist for the diagnosis of schizophrenia. *British Journal of Psychiatry, 121,* 529–539.

Babigian, H. M. (1980). Schizophrenia: Epidemiology. In H. I. Kaplan, A. M. Freedman, & B. J. Sadock (Eds.), *Comprehensive textbook of psychiatry III* (pp. 1113–1121). Baltimore: Williams & Wilkins.

Bleuler, E. (1950). *Dementia praecox of the group of schizophrenias* (Joseph Zinkin, Trans.). New York: International Universities Press. (Original work published 1911)

Brockington, I. R., Kendell, R. E., & Leff, J. P. (1978). Definitions of schizophrenia: Concordance and prediction of outcome. *Psychological Medicine, 8,* 387–398.

Bruch, H. (1974). *Learning psychotherapy.* Cambridge: Harvard University Press.

Carpenter, W. T., Strauss, J. S., & Muleh, S. (1973). Are there pathognomonic symptoms in schizophrenia? *Archives of General Psychiatry, 28,* 847–852.

Carpenter, W. T., Strauss, J. S., & Bartko, J. J. (1974). Use of signs and symptoms for the identification of schizophrenic patients. *Schizophrenia Bulletin, 2,* 37–49.

Deutsch, S. I., & Davis, K. L. (1983). Schizophrenia: A review of diagnostic and biological issues. I. Diagnosis and prognosis. *Hospital and Community Psychiatry, 34,* 313–322.

Endicott, J., & Spitzer, R. (1978). A diagnostic interview. Schedule for Affective Disorders and Schizophrenia. *Archives of General Psychiatry, 35,* 837–844.

Freud, S. (1959). *A case of paranoia (dementia paranoides).* New York: Basic Books. (Originally published 1911)

Fromm-Reichmann, F. (1950). *Principles of intensive psychotherapy.* Chicago: University of Chicago Press.

General Register Office. (1968). *British glossary of mental disorders.* London: Author.

Gift, T. E., Strauss, J. S., Ritzler, B. A., Kokes, R. F., & Harder, D. W. (1980). How diagnostic concepts of schizophrenia differ. *Journal of Nervous and Mental Disease, 168,* 3–8.

Kraepelin, E. (1971). *Dementia praecox and paraphrenia* (R. Mary Barclay, Trans.). Huntington, NY: Robert E. Krieger. (Original work published 1919)

Lehmann, H. E. (1980). Schizophrenia: Clinical features. In H. I. Kaplan, A. M. Freedman, & B. J. Sadock (Eds.), *Comprehensive textbook of psychiatry III.* Baltimore: Williams & Wilkins.

MacKinnon, R. A., & Michels, R. (1971). *The psychiatric interview in clinical practice.* Philadelphia: W. B. Saunders.

Neale, J. M., & Oltmanns, T. F. (1980). *Schizophrenia.* New York: Wiley.

Overall, J. E., & Hollister, L. E. (1979). Comparison of research diagnostic criteria for schizophrenia. *Archives of General Psychiatry, 36,* 1198–1205.

Spitzer, R. L., Endicott, J., & Robins, E. (1978). Research diagnostic criteria: Rationale and reliability. *Archives of General Psychiatry, 35,* 773–782.

Strauss, J. S., & Carpenter, W. T. (1981). *Schizophrenia.* New York: Plenum Press.

Strayhorn, J. M. (1982). *Foundations of clinical psychiatry.* Chicago: Year Book Medical Publishers.

Sullivan, H. S. (1954). *The Psychiatric Interview.* New York: W. W. Norton.

Wing, J. K., Cooper, J. E., & Sartorius, N. (1974). *Measurement and classification of psychiatric symptoms.* London: Cambridge University Press.

Chapter **6**

Personality Disorders

Paul H. Soloff

Introduction

Personality is the sum total of an individual's enduring patterns of perception, cognition, and action in the interpersonal world. It is a habitual and predictable style of thinking, feeling, and acting, arising from the integration of constitutional endowment, early life experience, developmental achievement, interpersonal, social, and cultural influences. The word itself has been traced to the Greek *persona*, a mask to portray character in ancient drama. By convention, the term *personality* has come to represent the whole person, the totality of his or her habitual psychological functioning. The term *character* has been reserved for those personal qualities reflecting the person's attitudes and adherence to moral and social values, and *temperament* for the biologic potential of the individual (Millon, 1981). We know our personality only in interaction with others, and our limitations only when circumstances prove our patterned responses inadequate. A *disorder* of personality is defined as a chronically maladaptive pattern of interpersonal functioning, habitual patterns of thought, feeling, and action that repeatedly result in significant social impairment and personal distress. The diagnosis is fundamentally a social commentary on behavior deemed disturbing, eccentric, or excessive by the standards of the social milieu and must be defined relative to a given social and cultural context.

PAUL H. SOLOFF • Department of Psychiatry, Western Psychiatric Institute and Clinic, University of Pittsburgh School of Medicine, Pittsburgh, Pennsylvania 15213.

Traditionally, personality has been conceptualized as a cluster of traits related along opposing dimensions of interpersonal behavior, or, as a series of categories, typologies, or prototypes. The dimensional approach is favored by empiricists and the categorical by clinicians. Empirical psychologists, utilizing advanced statistical analyses, have produced a bewildering array of two dimensional models of interpersonal behavior. Patients are rated for severity on opposing dimensions such as dominance versus submission, control versus affection, active versus passive, intraversion versus extroversion. With increasing complexity and statistical sophistication, a multiple array of two-dimensional factors can be arranged in a circle around orthogonal axes (usually dominance or power vs. affiliation) to yield a circumplex model (Wiggins, 1982). As the complexity of the model increases, related dimensions fuse into crude approximations of clinical typologies.

For the clinician, the categorical model holds the greatest appeal and utility. Efforts to classify behavior according to prototypic patterns date back (at least) to the four humoral personalities of Hippocrates. The modern concept of personality disorder derives from 19th century efforts to classify patterns of eccentric, asocial, and deviant behavior as forms of "moral insanity" and relate them to hypothetical biologic defects. Although the organizational principles around which prototypes are classified vary greatly (from the "psychopathic degeneration" of Cesare Lombroso to Freud's instinct theory), each prototype approximates an easily recognizable clinical entity.

Our most recent classification of personality disorders, included in *The Diagnostic and Statistical Manual of Mental Disorders* (3rd ed.) (DSM-III) (APA, 1980) is an amalgam of dimensional and categorical approaches. Eleven prototypic disorders are defined without reference to any etiologic principles. Instead, in an effort to enhance reliability of diagnosis, specific trait criteria are defined for each category—representing dimensional factors most often associated with the prototype. A quantitative structure is imposed to assure that sufficient dimensional traits are present to warrant a categorical diagnosis. In deference to the obvious overlap of traits among real people (not ideal types), multiple personality diagnoses are allowed. This quasi-empirical classification enhances the *reliability* of diagnoses based upon observable data at the expense of a common sense understanding of the unity of personality. With few exceptions, these quasi-empirical diagnoses have yet to stand the test of research validation. Nonetheless, the DSM-III offers a valuable clinical framework to illustrate the techniques and complexities of diagnostic interviewing of patients with personality disorders.

The essence of personality is its predictability: that is, an habitual pattern of response in affect, thought, and action to the stimuli of the interpersonal world. The diagnostic task begins with a search for this pattern as it is manifested in the patient's developmental, social, and vocational history. The therapist is very much a detective, uncovering his or her patient's modus operandi (i.e., the "track record"). The data for the search are to be found in the *content* of the patient's history, past and present, and in the *process* of the clinical interaction itself. The patient's recall of his or her own historical past is subject to the distortions of his or her adult perspective and his or her needs within the interview. Nonetheless, the interaction with the clinician represents a characteristic interpersonal exchange available for study at a process level. Both process and content of the interview provide "clues" to discovering dimensions or traits of personality that define the patient's predictability. The general task of diagnosis is to identify those key dimensions of personality that are defined by and give structure to the patient's perception, thought, and action. This task begins with a historical reconstruction of early life experiences (albeit through the bias of retrospective distortion) and, more specifically, the history of interpersonal relationships through childhood, adolescence, and adulthood. To add order to the investigation, the clinician may utilize one of many theoretical or developmental schemata to conceptualize milestones or critical phases in interpersonal development. The development models of Erickson, Sullivan, and Freud are particularly useful in that they provide specific anchor points in a life history for evaluation of mastery of that particular psychosocial phase. At each phase, the dominant personality traits may be identified until a pattern emerges through life.

By definition, *personality disorder* is a chronic *maladaptive* pattern of functioning. This is represented in the history by a track record of interpersonal failures. The personality-disordered patient "wears" his or her maladaptive attitudes, defenses, and coping styles like a suit of armor (Reich, 1945). His or her rigid and stereotyped responses to interpersonal relationships are apparent throughout adult life and are manifest in the relationship with the clinician. We recognize the limits of his "character armor" through the patient's inability to respond to a wide variety of interpersonal demands with flexible adaptation. In reviewing the history, the examiner looks for a pattern of maladaptive stereotyped responses to the normal developmental stressors of life: separations and loss, sexuality and intimacy, social and vocational identity, parenting, and the like. Prominent personality traits may be differentiated from personality disorder by the degree to which the traits are clearly and repetitively maladaptive or lead to interpersonal and social impairment. Also important is the degree to which the traits are rigidly related, with a specific presentation of affect, highly selective cognitive mode, defenses, attitudes, and response patterns. The diagnostic process is a careful examination of how the patient experiences his or her inner and outer worlds.

The Personality Disorders

The eleven DSM-III personality prototypes are conceptually grouped into three thematic clusters: a dramatic group, an anxious-fearful group, and an odd or eccentric group (Table 1). Within each group, one may define specific cognitive modes: that is, characteristic styles of experiencing and thinking about the world, related affective styles, and interpersonal response patterns (Shapiro, 1965). Although available through history, these diagnostic indicators are more reliably demonstrated in the interview behavior of the patient and will be illustrated by actual excerpts from clinical interviews.

The Dramatic Group

The Histrionic Personality. The best studied of the "dramatic group" are the histrionic personalities: flamboyant, theatrical individuals who experience the world as a series of intense emotional stimuli. Their perception is highly distractable and easily captivated by emotionally laden stimuli, and their cognition is marked by a defect in sustained intellectual concentration and an impressionistic mode of thinking (Shapiro, 1965). The patient does not examine or analyze the content of perception but reacts emotionally to an initial impression as though it were final reality. The result is a superficial experience of the real world in which details are lost in an overly romanticized, exaggerated affective picture. The patient experiences the sense of self in a similar manner: an exaggerated, untempered impression of a romantic or tragic figure. The impressionistic intake of the world has its parallel in the uncontrolled spontaneity of the patient's emotional output. Feelings are expressed (or reported) with exaggerated intensity but are usually of

Table 1. DSM-III Personality Disorders

Dramatic group	Anxious-fearful group	Odd/eccentric group
Histrionic	Compulsive	Paranoid
Antisocial	Avoidant	Schizoid
Narcissistic	Dependent	Schizotypal
Borderline	Passive aggressive	

short duration and are more superficial than profound. In response to stress, the impressionistic cognitive style leads to increased (defensive) disorganization of thinking, increased intensity of affect, and often a loss of behavioral controls (colloquially referred to as *hysterics*).

In the diagnostic interview, one is struck by the degree to which the patient controls or manipulates the clinician through affect and behavior. The patient creates an illusion of instant rapport and emotional contact, sets a highly emotional tone to each session, and leads the interview by dramatic, angry, sad, or sexualized cues. The histrionic patient presents with a theatrical quality that dominates and controls the flow of the interview, manipulating the attention of the clinician, conveying an impression of great distress with little substantive detail. Because the patient experiences the world impressionistically, the historical narrative is more a collage of affects than facts. The examiner is drawn away from the details of history into a coquettish social banter of "pseudointimacy" as stimulating as it is deceiving. A loud, angry, but poorly focused tirade may serve the same defensive purpose. A lability of mood and explosiveness of affect betray the pressure of underlying issues that the patient avoids through manipulation of the interview. As in theatrical dialogue, the patient may utilize an "aside" or "stage direction" to assure the examiner that things are not quite as bad as they appear, that she or he is fully aware of the performance quality of the presentation. The end result of such an interview is a broad display of affect but little intellectual understanding of the patient's concerns.

Example. This is the sixth interview with Mrs. A., an attractive, socially prominent woman who entered therapy following the termination of an affair. The patient is asked into the office with customary gesture and welcoming smile. By the clock, the session is beginning 5 minutes late, a departure from previous experience. The patient walks quickly into the room, takes her place, and, before the therapist is seated, begins to speak: "You can wipe that smug smile off your face. I know you don't mean it. It's so condescending." She has in her hand a ladies magazine from the waiting room. "I once saw Dr. T. and hated him. I found an article in a magazine in his waiting room and wanted to take it home, but he wouldn't let me do it. I guess it was part of his method, the little shit. I want you to read this unless it's totally against your method, but it's only one or two paragraphs and it says it all." (The article is about sex from the man's point of view. The paragraphs in question discuss the deceptions practiced by men in pursuit of sexual favors.) While the clinician glances at the paragraphs, the patient begins blowing her nose and says, "I know this is disgusting, but it can't be helped." Throughout the session, she continues intermittently blowing or wiping her nose accumulating the bulk of a box of kleenex in her lap. "I don't mean to be so nasty today, but I feel sick." [Doctor] "You notice that you've been angry with me." [Patient] "Why not? You don't care anyhow, that's part of your method so why shouldn't I take it out on you. I can't get angry with anyone else in my life." She goes on to a rambling discussion of all of the injustices she can recall beginning with "being born a blonde in a family of fat farmers from Nebraska." The bulk of the session is taken up by her sarcasm and criticism of her family and their treatment of her. She never intellectually connects her anger with men in general to the breakup of her affair or today's outburst to the lateness of her session. At the last minute, she brings up a topic that requires further discussion and cannot be delayed, namely some concerns about medication. This prolongs the session 10 minutes overtime. As she walks out of the interview her mood changes abruptly. She says brightly, "You know I don't hate you."

The factual history—when finally obtained—will reveal characteristic disturbances in interpersonal relationships reflecting the same style. Histrionic patients typically view their partners as uncaring, unreliable, rejecting, or emotionally unresponsive. They, in turn, are described (by the partner) and experienced (by the clinician) as demanding, manipulative, and dependent. The famed seductiveness of the hysteric proves to be an interpersonal maneuver to evoke interest and secure a dependent tie. Anger or even sadness may serve a similar manipulative function and are far more prevalent than the seductive stereotype.

The challenge in interviewing the histrionic patient comes in resisting the seductiveness of the patient's affective style for the task of obtaining the facts. A stubborn and sustained insistence on the historical details behind the affect supports the diagnostic process and offers a measure of cognitive structure—and limits—to the patient's impulsive affective excess. With the hysteric, the clinician must play detective and get the facts, though this task can be exasperating—as in the next clinical vignette.

Example. (Third diagnostic session—Mrs. A.).
Mrs. A. (P) walks in and begins talking immediately, even before sitting down. She speaks with intensity and angry gestures.

P: I just got on the elevator and a girl got in, 6 foot tall, blonde, and thin. She stood as close to me as she could to show me how pretty she is, the little bitch . . . [Pause] Well? Aren't you going to ask me anything, or should I begin?
T: How are you this week?
P: [Loudly] I've been starving myself, haven't eaten for days—food is absolute poison. Sugar makes me depressed, and preservatives are the worst! You're going to laugh, aren't you? Why doesn't someone write these things down?
T: Why are you so worried about food?
P: Look, I'm 43. It's hard enough when you're 30, but 43! You've got to look as

good undressed as you do outside. Don't you know there are nine women for every man. Don't you ever read anything? And they're all cheats, all of them.

T: Even John [the ex-lover]?

P: He was big and beautiful and male. He was my size. And he's such a liar and cheat and every woman wants him. He's the worst. He has women everywhere and he fell for that big dumb secretary—she's only 24 and thought he was so great—she's big, dumb and tall.

The overall effect is dramatic and stimulating. The therapist is captivated by the patient's anger and theatrical flair. She controls the interview with her loud, rapid speech and angry tone. Without limits, she will wander from topic to topic, venting her affect without discussing the facts of the matter at hand. Her style entertains, intimidates, and manipulates the clinician away from the key dynamic issues—in the case of Mrs. A.—the lost relationship. The clinician may provide limits by focusing on the facts of history or interpreting the process of the interview (e.g., "You're angry that John left you for another woman. Tell me what happened between you?"). At a more process level—"You wander from topic to topic with a lot of angry feelings but don't talk about what brought you here. Why won't you talk about your loss?" The Boston analyst Elvin Semrad taught that hysterics suffer from a "separation of head and heart." The clinician reopens this communication by encouraging the reluctant patient to look at the *facts* of her history and her behavior.

The Antisocial (Sociopathic) Patient. The impulsive dimensions of personality that characterize the dramatic group appear to be transmitted across generations and expressed through a cultural pattern of sex typing into female histrionic and male sociopathic personality styles. Although the relative roles of nature and nurture have yet to be clearly defined in this transmission, the increased prevalence of male sociopathy and female hysteria within the same families suggests a close diagnostic relationship.

The male antisocial patient experiences his perception, thinking, and action as dominated by irresistible internal impulses or commanded by external stimuli. His cognitive style is passive and reactive, easily attracted by opportunity for immediate gratification of prevailing needs, without reflection on consequences. As a result, the patient often complains that he has no control over his action. Impulse is immediately translated into action without delay or reflection on prior experience, values, or morality. The sociopathic patient rarely has any long-term interests and acts to gratify short-term needs according to current mood and opportunities. Because the patient lacks a background of sustained or continuous interests, his behavior lacks a sense of purpose in relation to any long-term goals. The inability to reflect, delay gratification, or inhibit impulse is expressed socially as a lack of conscience, morality, or values. The patient presents himself with a casual insincerity that betrays a lack of critical reflection on his behavior. As with the histrionic patient, the sociopath views the diagnostic interview as an opportunity to impress the clinician with his own point of view. He is often less interested in what he says than in how he says it (Shapiro, 1965).

The "performance" quality of the patient's interview poses a unique challenge to the clinician. Both patient and doctor understand society's condemnation of the antisocial behaviors that characterize the sociopathic patient. How does one obtain factual history from a patient who is more intent on making a favorable impression than talking "straight?" Furthermore, when the history is a catalog of socially offensive behaviors (some of which may still carry legal consequences), the interview itself becomes a threat to the patient.

Fortunately, most sociopathic patients are less defensive about the past than the present. The impulsive pattern of the adult has a long track record extending back into adolescence. Major manifestations of the disorder are clearly evident before the age of 15 and are found in histories of truancy, fighting, running away, and juvenile delinquency. To obtain this history, the interviewer must not only adopt a nonjudgmental attitude but actively encourage a complete rendition by implying that childhood behavior "no longer counts." The patient is encouraged to talk freely about his "wild times," his "pranks," appealing to his sense of bravado, supporting his self-esteem. He is assured that no stigma is attached to his childhood "hell raising"; indeed, that the interviewer understands and is empathic with his account. The interview takes on a casual atmosphere, the doctor "giving permission" for admission of deviant behavior:

> "Lots of kids play hooky from school—did you? Ever play pranks on animals? How about fights? Ever have to put somebody in his place—stand up for yourself in school? How about making it with the girls? Ever get in trouble?"

The purpose is diagnostic—not therapeutic; the method is manipulative. One risk is that the patient may actually embellish his account to please the clinician. Nonetheless, the traditional interviewer's "position of neutrality" will fail with the antisocial patient, who interprets the examiner's "blank screen" as judgmental. All dramatic patients actively manipulate a response from the clinician. Interviewing the sociopathic patient is one of the few clinical situations where these roles may be reversed.

Having confirmed the diagnosis through a nonjudgmental review of childhood, one may then return to adult behavior to identify the interpersonal consequences of sociopathy. The patient lacks an ability to sustain interpersonal relationships, parental responsibilities, or vocational stability. The inability to reflect on a stable system of values or morality is manifest in an absence of empathy for others, a lack of loyalties and disregard of social norms. At the extreme, the sociopath is criminal, in milder form, a chronically irresponsible, inadequate individual. The inadequacy of the patient is most glaring in interpersonal relationships.

Example. A 24-year-old single man was referred for psychiatric evaluation in preparation for a legal defense on felony charges of aggravated assault, involuntary deviate sexual intercourse, and unlawful restraint. The patient was accused of picking up a teenage girl in his car, forcing her to commit sexual acts, then attempting to choke her with a belt while stabbing her superficially in the stomach. This was a first arrest for this man, who prior to arrest, was well thought of in the community and worked as a police dispatcher, a volunteer fireman, and a volunteer rescue paramedic. He was casually dressed, polite, and cooperative for the interview. Although denying the allegations against him, the patient created a distinct impression concerning his relationships with women. This was the only topic of his history presented with strong feeling and language.

T: When did you begin dating?
P: Around 17.
T: Was that early or late for your crowd?
P: It was pretty late, I guess. I was pretty shy.
T: When did you begin your sexual life with women?
P: I knocked up my first piece of ass in high school. She got pregnant right away.
T: You didn't take any precautions?
P: Well, she didn't seem to care, so I didn't either.
T: What happened to the pregnancy?
P: She was opposed to abortion so we got married.
T: How long did that last?
P: Oh, about 9 months. She would always call the cops on me, and her father would come over and beat me up.
T: Why?
P: She didn't like my going out drinking with the boys, wanted me to stay at home all the time . . .

[The patient goes on to describe a second relationship of 2 years' duration that ended for similar reasons. He views himself as being used and overly controlled in a long-term relationship.]

T: Have you seen anyone recently?
P: No, I'm tired of getting fucked, so now I'm out just to get a piece of ass.
T: Did you know Jamie? [the alleged victim]

P: Yeah, she was a young punk dope smoker, hung around with the low life crowd. A hard-looking chick.

T: Were you ever interested in her?

P: We all knew better, she's only 16, jail bait . . .

T: Have you ever been involved sexually with guys?

P: No doc, I'm strictly straight, everything's just average, nothing kinky or unusual.

T: Have you ever been worried about being attacked sexually?

P: Well, me being smaller, the smaller guys are the ones who always get shit on.

T: Has that always been true for you?

P: Yeah.

T: How about now?

P: Well, I'm scared to death of jail, you know, being meat.

In dealing with the sociopathic patient, the clinician must attend not only to what is said—but how it is said. The patient is trying to convey an impression through language, tone, and gesture. An independent perspective, obtained through corollary history from family or friends is imperative to understand the full meaning of the patients' presentation. In this case, family provided a critical perspective.

By history, he was the youngest and least successful of four children born to a middle-class family. As a child, he participated in minor delinquent activities such as fire setting and teasing animals but had avoided any arrest. He was sensitive to the fact that he was physically smaller than average and took great pride in his masculine appearance and activity. In addition to working with the police, fire, and rescue squads of his local community, the patient also participated actively in karate and rifle club activities. The coarseness of his language was in striking contrast to his mild and pleasant social manner, his presentation of himself as a bright, middle-class young man. In light of his history, his presentation suggested an exaggerated defense of his masculinity, a defense motivated both by unconscious factors and by the wish to impress upon the examiner his "straight" masculine orientation as well as his rebuttal of the implication of sexual inadequacy in the charges against him. His sociopathic style of relationship is clearly manifest in a lack of empathy and sexual exploitation of his partners as well as the overt manipulation of the interviewer. Despite the functional veneer, his interpersonal style betrayed a sociopathic orientation.

The Narcissistic Personality Disorder. The narcissistic personality shares with the sociopathic a disregard for the needs and expectations of others. They are specialists in looking to themselves for support and reward. Unlike sociopathic patients, the narcissistic patients' motivations are not dominated by active pursuit of gratification but by a pervasive overvaluation of the self that assures them that they are entitled to have their needs met and need not pursue reinforcement actively (Millon, 1981). It is the hallmark of this egotistical pattern that these patients flatter and reward themselves, that perception, cognition, and action serve the purpose of supporting their inflated self-images. Such patients with a pretentious, pompous disdain for others that borders on arrogance. They selectively interpret others' behavior toward them as supporting their self-importance and discount or deny experience to the contrary. The egotistical pattern is often seen as a defensive posture, reactive to a vulnerable self-esteem and to feelings of worthlessness or inadequacy barely beyond awareness. Confronted with reversals in reality, these patients make even louder demands on others to acknowledge and support their overinflated presentation of self. When all else fails and reality seems unavoidable, the narcissistic patient resorts to fantasy and the restitutional healing of the day dream. With continued intolerable stress, depression and transient psychotic symptoms may appear.

The attitude of the patient in the interview reflects this general style. He is often self-assured and pretentious, unwilling to adopt even the rudimentary cultural deference customary to the patient role. Although referral generally emanates from a failure of the patient's egotistical defense, there is little acknowledgment of fault. Humility and self-searching criticism are not part of the narcissist's psychological makeup. The patient behaves as though he is indifferent to the clinician's perspective. Eventually, the grandiose exaggeration of self, attitude of entitlement, and devaluation of the clinician evokes anger in the interviewer, offering valuable insight into the functioning of the patient in the interpersonal world.

Example. Mr. D. was a 39-year-old schoolteacher who was referred by his psychiatrist for hospital admission for excessive drug and alcohol abuse following separation from his wife. The precipitating event leading to admission was his learning that his wife had "moved in" with another man shortly after their separation, resulting in depression and suicidal ideation. The patient's presenting complaint was couched in a long angry tirade about his wife's infidelity. There was no spontaneous concern about his resort to drug or alcohol abuse or any apparent sincerity in his suicidal statements. We were most impressed, however, by his accent—a distinct South African accent—in a man born and raised in West Virginia! Inquiry revealed that Mr. D. had worked in South Africa for 3 months many years earlier and had adopted the accent that appeared only at times of stress. In his initial interview, the patient (straight faced) asked if we had any medical explanation for the episodic slurred speech, staggering gait, and loss of coordination that alarmed his colleagues at school. He seemed surprised to hear of his drug problem.

When he finally admitted the problem (with little emotion), he berated the clinician for the "primitiveness" of the treatment offered. Each approach was rejected as inadequate to his level. For example, group therapy was rejected because "other patients have nothing to teach me" and "the staff is poorly read"; behavioral approaches to relaxation were "for amateurs," the patient noting that "I studied meditation with a yoga master." Mr. D. left the hospital against advice after 10 days, indignant at the ignorance of the university hospital but no longer concerned about his wife. The South African accent had also disappeared.

The Borderline Patient. The borderline patient is the most extreme and thereby the most impaired of the dramatic group. Defined by pathologic vulnerability in the areas of impulse, affect, and cognition, the borderline disorder represents a conceptual "border" with more severe psychiatric syndromes, including those of psychotic proportion. Given structure and support in the interpersonal sphere, the patient functions at the level of intellectual capacity, with apparent control of cognition, impulse, and affect. Under stress, especially perceived loss or rejection, the inherent instability of the patient is manifested in brief but extreme reactions. The history of the borderline patient is a pattern of "stable instability," with crisis and calm alternating in response to the stress of the patient's interpersonal relationships.

Example. The following transcript is part of a taped interview with a 39-year-old well-educated woman who has been in treatment for borderline disorder for years. She was admitted to hospital following a serious overdose precipitated by a perceived rejection—the discovery of her therapist's 2 month pregnancy (and intent to take a 3 month maternity leave following delivery). The diagnostic interview elicits a history of impulsive-destructive behaviors and affective experience characteristic of borderline patients. The process of the interview is equally revealing. The patient sits slouched in her chair, staring straight ahead. Her remarks are made in a casual, sarcastic, and occasionally flippant manner.

T: How often have you been in the hospital in the past 2 years?
P: Somewhere between four and six.
T: What causes you to be admitted each time?
P: Suicide attempts or trying to avoid suicide attempts.
T: Well, how often in the past couple of years have you attempted to kill yourself?
P: Twice.
T: Okay, and how did you do that?
P: Overdose.
T: So there have been two overdoses in the past 2 years?
P: Yeah.
T: Okay. If we go back further than that, have you overdosed before then?
P: Yeah.
T: Earlier in your life?
P: Yeah, not nearly as serious. I mean life threatening.
T: But there have been attempts?

P: Yeah.

T: Could you tell us how often that's happened in your life, in your earlier years?

P: Well the first one was at age 6 and then there was a sprinkling of them when I was a teenager and probably four or five since I was 30 which would be the last 10 years.

T: Okay, you said that some of your admissions to the hospital were trying to avoid suicide attempts.

P: Yeah.

T: Do you give warning that you're thinking suicidally? That you're thinking about harming yourself? Do you tell people?

P: Sometimes.

T: Do you ever threaten to do it even though you have no intention at that moment of doing it, tell people that if things don't get better you're going to kill yourself if they don't straighten up or if they don't change what they're doing?

P: I don't think so.

T: Not even in a veiled sense?

P: I certainly have when things have been going bad with people. I have said, you know, I am feeling so bad I am thinking of killing myself.

T: Do you think that would be characteristic of you, I mean if we talked to your friends would they say, yeah, when things are going bad she often talks like that. Would your friends recognize it as characteristic or would it sort of surprise them each time?

P: I don't talk about it to people anymore very much.

T: Okay. How about hurting yourself other than suicide.

P: Yeah. What about it. I do it. [Laughs]

T: Okay. Can you describe a little bit about what you do to yourself. How often that happens?

P: Well, let's see. I bang my head a lot. Sometimes bang my fists, but that isn't as good. Umm, I burn myself, I cut myself. Umm, I scratch myself.

T: Do you have any understanding of what this is all about, what that does for you?

P: Umm, yeah, I think so. Part of it is a release of anger, part of it is a release of frustration, part of it is a substitute of a tangible kind of pain for an intangible kind of pain. Part of it is a communication of pain.

T: How often do you do this in one form or another?

P: It varies. I go through periods where it's a lot and then it can be months before something happens again.

T: If you look at the past 2 years, which is our framework, how often would you think you've done things to yourself? Are you talking about many, many times? Or once or twice a year?

P: Certainly not once or twice a year. Umm, in the past two years I've probably added two or three major cuts, maybe 15 burns.

T: Pretty frequent event.

P: Clustered, but this has been a very bad two years.

The patient's tense, single-word replies force the clinician to pursue each answer, to tangibly demonstrate his interest. It is a hostile and demanding manipulation of the clinician's attention.

T: Let's talk about feelings then and focus on the past 2 to 3 months. Have you been depressed in the past 2 to 3 months?

P: Yes.

T: How about being anxious? Have you been more anxious than usual in the past 2 to 3 months or about the same as always for you?

P: About the same.

T: Have you ever been so anxious that you had to just tear out of a place. That you felt if you didn't get out you were going to suffocate or die, heart racing real fast, felt panicky?

P: Umm, I've never had the heart attack panic symptoms, but I've fairly commonly thought that if I don't get out of here right now some huge disaster will strike. Including fantasies that people will do me in, or I will absolutely lose it and make a fool out of myself.

T: Have you had that experience in the past 2 to 3 months?

P: No. I've had the dullest past 2 or 3 months that you could imagine.

T: How would you characterize the way you usually feel, again the past 2 to 3 months. What has it been like to be you? What does it feel like?

P: Like not being a person at all.

T: Can you explain that a little more?

P: Umm, people live, they do things, they think things, they feel things, they interact with other people, they have goals, they have rights, they're real.

T: And you?

P: Pardon?

T: And you?

P: Umm, not really. A nothing.

T: Do you experience a feeling of emptiness inside of you?

P: Yes.

T: What is that like?

P: Are you asking what it feels like or a description of it?

T: Either.

P: Umm, sometimes the emptiness is like there's something gnawing inside. Umm, sometimes it's just a feeling of enhanced depersonalization. Umm, sometimes it's like a, like being pumped full of pressurized air so that the tension is tremendous for explosion, and sometimes it's an emptiness which has a vacuum kind of thing where there would be an implosion. Umm.

T: Do you have it a lot. Or is it there all the time?

P: It's there all the time. Again, I try not to experience it.

T: How about the loneliness? Is it there all the time?

P: Oh, yeah.

T: Do you experience a sense of boredom with life?

P: Yeah.

T: A lot?

P: A lot.

T: Have there been any times say in the past 2 to 3 months that you felt satisfied or fulfilled?
P: Possibly after I took the pills. But I don't remember.
T: After the suicide attempt that brought you in? Why would that make you feel satisfied or fulfilled?
P: It would have ended it.
T: Okay.

The patient tells her story with a self-conscious awareness of the bizarreness of her behavior but not much distress. It has been said that such patients are more disturbing than disturbed. The intent is to manipulate interest.

When first seen, the patient will most likely be in crisis. The affect of the borderline patient is generally angry or depressed, with marked lability. A recent history of dramatic, impulsive behavior is usually evident. These behaviors are self-destructive and include drug overdose, wrist cuts, self-mutilation, or loud suicidal threat. Anger directed against others presents as real or threatened assault, temper tantrums, or destruction of property. More subtle but equivalent impulsive behaviors include binges of alcohol or drug use, sexual promiscuity, or compulsive eating. The behavior appears both self-punitive and manipulative. The impulsive-destructive response invariably follows a perceived loss or rejection, arising out of a chaotic pattern of interpersonal relationships that are marked by intense, unstable attachments. The relationships of the borderline may be overly dependent and masochistic or hostile and sadistic, but all betray the manipulation of the partner in a characteristic manner. The patient uses others to gratify needs with little regard for their individual and separate needs.

In the crisis interview setting, the patient may be angry and demanding or depressed and withdrawn, both presentations coercing care from the clinician. The borderline is the most extreme of the dramatic characters and most prone to loss of control. As with the hysteric, the more dramatic demands must be countered with direct limit setting (e.g., shouting, screaming, throwing objects are unacceptable if the interview is to proceed). Similarly, self-abuse (in front of the clinician) is not tolerated. Once the ground rules for the interview are made verbally explicit, the clinician focuses on details of history, limiting affective demonstrations by structured questioning. The history of the borderline patient will reveal a pattern of repeated chaotic and intense relationships with dramatic separations, impulsive-destructive reactions, and replacement of one love with an equally loved but superficial relationship.

If the patient is unable to discuss the current crisis (presumably a perceived rejection) without loss of affective and behavioral control, the clinician should focus on the past "track record" for details, reserving the most painful exploration for a more controlled time or setting. Common sense should prevail in how far to push for details of the current stressor, taking into account the patients' vulnerability, the setting, and the purpose of the interview (e.g., current history may not be as necessary in making the characterologic diagnosis as in judging whether the patient needs medication or hospital care).

Although the history of episodic impulsive-destructive reactions and chaotic interpersonal relationships are the most discriminating diagnostic criteria, the borderline patient reveals many enduring traits during periods of relative calm. Borderline patients complain of not having a good sense of self, of identity, values, and goals. As with other patients sharing severe dependent needs, a sense of separateness is often sacrificed in the wish to be part of someone else. The exquisite rejection sensitivity of the borderline patient is based on chronically low self-esteem, heightened by the patient's wish for dependent nurturance. The patient complains of an inner sense of emptiness, an internal void experienced primitively as a true physical sensation, prompting often frantic efforts to "fill" the void. (These include excessive alcohol and drug use, binge eating, or sexual promiscuity.) The patients describe a hunger for companionship, an intolerance of being alone. They tend to identify with those less fortunate in life circumstances and go out of their way to involve themselves with the sick and needy. By identifying with the object of their care (projective identification), they meet some of their own needs for nurturance in a socially accepted pattern. Stray dogs and cats may also become the beneficiaries of this dynamic. In relationships with others, the patient tends to present only one aspect of personality, typically keeping separate the hostile or competitive traits from the tender and submissive ones. This defensive process, termed *splitting*, results in the creation of dyadic relationships that are grossly inconsistent but—taken together—represent the totality of the patient's needs. The borderline patient is a very different person to each significant other. In the hospital setting, as in the patient's friendship circle, this splitting process can produce conflict among the dyadic partners, an internal conflict that is acted out outside the patient. In interview, the splitting is problematic because the therapist sees only one perspective of the patient without "outside" help.

Borderline patients use primitive defenses such as splitting and projective identification as part of their characteristic style. Under duress, cognition may become further disrupted, and truly psychotic defenses appear, resulting in distortions of perception (derealization, depersonalization) referential thinking, and paranoid ideation.

The Anxious-Fearful Group

The Compulsive Personality. Although "dramatic" personalities make loud demands upon others and manipulate the environment through affect and behavior, the anxious-fearful group are defined by excessive inhibition and self-control. The best studied of the group are the obsessive-compulsive personalities, whose efforts at self-control produce a rigidity of thought, a formality of affect, and deliberateness to action unequalled by others. The compulsive person views the world with a degree of intellectual effort and deliberateness that controls all spontaneous affect. This style is manifest by a rigid control over perception and attention, an intense preoccupation with details, and an analytic mode of cognition. Impulse and affect are the enemy of the compulsive and are contained by a set of rigid moral directives or "rules" for action that tend to be overbearing and inflexible. The compulsive develops an internal bureaucracy of conscience, with rules and regulations governing thought, affect, and action. Authoritarian dogma in the cognitive realm is matched by a lack of spontaneity in the affective sphere. Without rules, the compulsive becomes paralyzed by choices, an ambivalence that makes free choice intolerable. They avoid novel situations where creative solutions are required. Rigidity of thinking prevents creativity. At the extreme, the compulsive is a caricature of control, a technocrat obsessed with details, unresponsive to the affective value of a situation, unable to appreciate spontaneous impulse or creative choice (Shapiro, 1965).

The interview style of the compulsive patient is marked by an intellectual monotony. The patient recounts his or her history in lengthy detail, somehow missing the point. There is often a glaring incongruity between the content of conversation and the patient's affective tone. Highly emotional issues and conflicts may be presented with characteristic intellectual calm, whereas seemingly trivial events produce an outpouring of righteous indignation. The affect associated with personally hot issues is typically "isolated away," the issue "intellectualized," until the affect can be "displaced" onto another (impersonal) target. The patient defends against experiencing emotion in the interview by focusing on details, by intellectualizing or rationalizing events, or, when all else fails, by obsessing. Under real interpersonal pressure, the patient may fall silent and count books on the clinician's shelf, solve a mind puzzle, contemplate world events—all far removed from the emotional situation at hand. The compulsive shares with the histrionic patient a "separation of head and heart." Where the hysteric is dominated by affect and is blind to reason, the compulsive is dominated by thought.

The more painful the emotion, the more rigid, dogmatic, and intellectual the obsessive defense.

Example. A 40-year-old engineer recently learned that his wife has been unfaithful to him. The therapist tries to elicit some emotional response.

T: What did she tell you?

P: Everything, the whole thing. You know, now I understand why she's been so nervous lately. I thought she was a little crazy or something.

T: How do you feel about it?

P: Well, it sure helped me see a lot that I missed before, you know, put the pieces together. Now they all fit—like a puzzle.

T: What was it like for you?

P: At first I tried to figure out why she did it. If she was unhappy, why didn't she say something. Then I figured she must have met him at the convention. Maybe she was lonely or something. She's not a drinker. Maybe she had too much to drink.

T: She said that to you?

P: No, but there's got to be a reason. She never said anything. It's not like we've been fighting or anything.

T: Must have been a surprise.

P: I try to see things from her point of view. Maybe she just wanted a change, things are too dull.

T: [Insistent] So your wife tells you she has an affair—so how is it for you?

P: That's what I've been saying. I understand more of what's been happening at home. It's like that book up there [refers to a textbook on the shelf], *Hazards of Medication*—hazards is right.

T: What? I don't understand.

P: Well that's what happened to her—all the nerves at home—from the affair— a hazard.

T: [Laughs] I'm trying to get you to talk, and you're reading my books! Look, how would you tell this to a really close friend, I mean, what would you say?

P: What kind of friend. I have all kinds, friends at work, neighbors, at the train club. Talking to a psychiatrist is not exactly easy. Not like talking to a friend, you know.

T: So how would you tell it?

P: Well, I'd find out what went wrong. The way I understand it, I'm responsible for a kind of fault, too, ah, a kind of social infidelity, and she's responsible for a sexual one. I admit it. I've been a lump for a number of years. So I asked myself what was meant by love. I figure there are three parts—understanding, companionship, and passion. So I've decided to unlump myself, exercise regularly, lose some weight, go out more. I told her we would take the week off from work and just spend all the time together. We'll talk it over and figure out what went wrong. We need a second honeymoon. I figure we can go out to dinner every night—like a real honeymoon and straighten this out.

T: Are you angry? Hurt?

P: I suppose. It was quite a surprise, but it really explained everything.
T: You suppose! You don't know?

The session ends without any real expression of feeling, despite the obvious exasperation of the therapist. The following day the patient phoned to ask the therapist to clarify what he meant by "talking to a friend." ("I wanted you to know that I do have friends, but talking to a psychiatrist is different.") This example illustrates the defensive use of intellectualization and rationalization as the patient avoids his painful feelings. Because of deep-seated conflicts concerning powerlessness and dependency, interpretation of the patient's responsibility for his problems will be viewed as critical judgments by a powerful authority. Even the therapist's attempt to be disarming with humor and mild sarcasm (to evoke an affective response) is met by a rigid, stubborn insistence on an alternative intellectual solution. In our example, the patient has a new "understanding" of his wife's nervous behavior—rather than a gut reaction to her infidelity. He works out a plan to deal with the problem rather than responding emotionally. The irrelevance of his rambling rationalization is obvious from his preoccupation with the therapist's meaning in asking about his friends. The compulsive patient will often wander far away from the emotional business at hand in a long-winded litany of endless and meaningless detail. In the extreme case, the patient may actually confront the therapist with a written agenda, notes in hand, in an effort to control the interchange and defend against spontaneous feeling.

To work with an obsessional requires an active intrusive process. The clinician must "follow the affect" and encourage its expression. A quiet reflective position merely complements the patient's defenses. The interview deteriorates into an academic, intellectual exercise in which the patient's motivation is defined and explained but not changed. The role of patient is inherently uncomfortable for the compulsive, whose concerns with dependence and power require keeping the therapist at a distance. The clinician should avoid being drawn into meaningless intellectual arguments, power struggles in which the patient views the therapist as a hostile, critical opponent. On the other hand, the clinician must actively "cut through" rambling discourse to expose the affective issues. A light-handed, uncritical sense of humor, and emotional spontaneity are strong assets for those who would deal with the compulsive patient.

Avoidant, Dependent, Passive-Aggressive Personality Disorders. Although less well established, the remaining three disorders of the anxious-fearful group are defined by conflicts involving a desire for social approval and fears of rejection—the dimension of intimacy versus distance in interpersonal relations. These personality disorders are each organized around a single behavioral dimension, raising the theoretical issue of whether they should more properly be considered trait disturbances. With the understanding that overlapping patterns exist, the authors of DSM-III have represented each separately.

Avoidant individuals suffer from "social" anxieties, fears of rejection, humiliation, and criticism. Although desiring to be accepted, they actively withhold themselves from the social setting, creating sufficient distance to feel "safe." They suffer from a lack of self-confidence, expressed in a passive, unassertive, fearful life-style, avoiding competition and aggression. At the core of the personality is a low self-esteem.

In the interview setting, the patient presents as shy, fearful, and awkward. Rejection sensitivity is apparent from the patient's scanning observational style and painful self-consciousness. Affect and physical movement are overly controlled in a consciously deliberate manner. The patient is hesitant, awkward in speech, and unspontaneous. He or she appears sensitive, mistrustful, and vulnerable.

The dependent person has a similar need for approval and dread of rejection. His or her solution is total submission to the wishes of a benefactor. He or she is the master of the "inferior role" (Millon, 1981). Motivated by a fear of rejection, disapproval, and abandonment, he or she inhibits assertiveness and initiative in the service of maintaining the dependent bond. At the extreme, the dependent individual presents as self-effacing, ingratiating, and helpless. At best, the patient earns his or her position by complementing the partner's needs for dominance, power, or benevolence, masking his or her own degree of dependence by loyal service.

In the interview, the dependent person is deferential to excess, overly cooperative, and eager to please the therapist. Angry feelings or resentful thoughts are suppressed, even when justified (e.g., when the clinician is late, cancels, or changes appointment times on short notice). The absence of initiative is apparent in the context of the interview. The clinician feels pressed to lead the patient, to keep the flow of the interview moving. Without explicit direction, the patient waits. Once the clinician's "interests" are apparent, the dependent patient will elaborate this topic despite absence of relevance in his or her life. The interview may deteriorate into a repetitious account of behavior that the patient feels the clinician wishes to hear. The passivity and submissiveness of the dependent patient must themselves become the focus of work.

A variant of the same theme is presented by the passive-aggressive patient. This individual desires the approval of others but is covertly resentful of the degree of compliance needed to guarantee results. He or she is torn between being passive or assertive to meet dependent or autonomous needs. It is the intensity of these conflicting dynamics that makes the pattern pathologic. As a result, his or her behavior is erratic and vacillates between sullen acquiescence and contradictory, often covert, opposition. Demands by others are met with a negative, resistant attitude as though all are unreasonable. The patient makes a great show of effort to please others or engender guilt at apparent suffering on their account. The martyr role invariably masks a manipulative, often malicious intent. Despite the overt display, the passive-aggressive patient typically manifests resentment through studied inefficiency and intentional ineptness. The patient may be pessimistic, discontented, complaining, or sullen but rarely risks the overt display of anger that threatens dependent ties.

> *Example.* A 28-year-old dental hygienist was admitted to hospital for depression associated with a fight with her roommate of long standing. The roommate was soon to be married, wanted the patient to move out of their apartment in favor of the couple. The patient responded to loss of the interpersonal tie by fighting over the apartment. She describes her method:
>
> P: I'll kill her with kindness. I'll be so sickeningly sweet. She hates that. Anyhow, she can't throw me out when I'm in the hospital.
> T: Why don't you ask her to move in with Don?
> P: She would see that as a rejection, after all, she is supposed to be my best friend.
> T: But she *is* getting married.
> P: She doesn't have to be so nasty about it.

In the interview setting, the passive-aggressive patient complains about the degree to which he or she serves the needs of others, the little received in turn, and how little he or she is appreciated. These attitudes extend to the clinician. The patient complains that he or she is given too little direction, but when suggestions are made, each is found to be unacceptable. He or she is simultaneously demanding, yet rejecting of help.

If the clinician suggests a specific course of action (e.g., psychological or vocational testing), the patient may grudgingly comply but accepts no responsibility for the decision. If the project fails—perhaps due to lack of real effort on the patient's part—he or she accepts no blame. The passive-aggressive patient shrinks from responsibility, preferring the security of a dependent position—reserving the right to complain. A low self-esteem is apparent in the patient's depressive, pessimistic outlook on life but serves the purpose of luring the clinician into further efforts to be directive and helpful. The patient is envious of others—including the clinician—and complains that others are withholding and can give more. As with all dependent individuals, the complaining stops short of actual anger; the aggression is passive and masked. A spilled ashtray or cup of coffee in the doctor's office conveys the message of discontent despite profuse and abject apologies from the patient.

The "Odd/Eccentric" Group. The paranoid, schizoid, and schizotypal personalities comprise the odd or eccentric group. Characterized by social and emotional distance and peculiarities of thought, patients in this group bear a distinct but superficial resemblance to those with psychotic disorders (e.g., paranoid and schizophrenic disorders). All share profound deficits in their ability to relate warmly in personal relationships or form enduring, trusting ties to others. Their oddness and isolation derive primarily from peculiarities of perception and thought rather than social anxiety or shyness.

Among the eccentrics, the paranoid is the most striking and the most functional. His or her perception and interpretation of the interpersonal world is organized around a basic mistrust and a suspicious attitude. Suspiciousness is a style of thinking brought to bear on all interpersonal events and is served by a vigilant, hypersensitive, searching mode of attention. The paranoid scans the world, seeking out potential sources of external threat, discounting the "face value" of events in favor of an interpretation of "hidden motives" allied to the patient's suspicions. He or she approaches novel situations with controlled affect and movement, "ready for action," as though each interaction posed a threat to self-esteem, autonomy, or control. Much of the patient's thought is occupied with a fear of being dominated or controlled by others. Warm, spontaneous emotions are suppressed as indicators of vulnerability (to external control) whereas fearful affects are projected, leading to the perception of threat from others. The patient's inner experience of emotion is restricted, the outward expression of feeling controlled (Shapiro, 1965).

Where the paranoid's mistrust may lead to aggressive defenses and confrontational tactics, the schizoid individual withdraws from emotional interactions, appearing to function with little or no affective spontaneity. Described by Bleuler as "people who are comfortably dull, at the same time sensitive," the schizoid perceives any affective arousal as distressing, avoids interpersonal ties that demand or stimulate emotion (Siever, 1981). The patient may elaborate an inner fantasy world, an autistic environment to which he or she retreats for comfort from the threatening emotional world of interpersonal reality.

The schizotypal individual is one step closer to autistic functioning and experiences true distortions of reality in response to affective arousal. Not only do such individuals experience the world as threatening but defend themselves from it with near-psychotic dissociation (derealization, depersonalization), referential thinking, and mild paranoid ideation. The world is perceived through a cognitive style subject to autistic distortion under stress.

An interview with a paranoid, schizoid, or shizotypal patient is marked by the absence of emotional rapport or even superficial trust that characterizes most doctor–patient exchanges. The clinician feels the suspicion of the paranoid, the emotional distance of the schizoid, and the bizzareness of the schizotypal patient. The scanning hypervigilance of the patient makes the clinician uncomfortably aware that his gestures and words are being examined for hidden meaning or signs of threat.

Success in interviewing the paranoid patient hinges upon one's ability to be open and candid in the face of suspicion and mistrust. While the patient seeks hidden meanings to validate his or her beliefs, the clinician must respond with detailed and explicit discussion of all areas under suspicion, however trivial they may seem. The patient's initial testing of the relationship may begin with the mechanics of arranging the first interview. The operation of the office (or clinic), the hours available, clinician's expectations, and fee may provide an early focus for suspicion. The negotiation of the first visit may represent a first test of power dynamics. With a little forewarning, the clinician anticipates these concerns, explains the format as openly as possible, and gives the patient as much choice as possible—wherever possible (e.g., office hours).

The paranoid patient's need to maintain distance and resist the dependency inherent in the patient role may lead to confrontations, argument, or challenging of the clinician's authority, knowledge—and even credentials. Reasonable inquiry should be answered directly, before asking why the question was asked. (It is wise to delay the investigation of the patient's motivation until it is clear that he or she will remain a patient!) A light-hearted sense of humor, uncritical and benign, helps with the more blatant confrontations. The paranoid patient is fearful of being controlled and humiliated in the relationship with any authority. A mild, soft-spoken manner and physically unassuming presence is reassuring to the patient. It is important for the clinician to be emotionally visible and responsive. The "blank screen" of analytic lore only provokes projection by the paranoid patient. The therapist's silence will be interpreted as hostility. The patient wishes to know "where you are" emotionally and physically. To form a therapeutic alliance, one must "let him know."

To this point, our discussion assumes the patient is cooperative and not severely impaired, that the interview has been scheduled with some opportunity for preparation. In the emergency setting, or in crisis intervention, the patient may be functioning with less control of reality testing. The more impaired the patient, the more explicit the clinician must be about the realities of the interview situation. In the extreme case, where the patient is using psychotic projection and distortion to deal with stress, the clinician must actually help the patient test the reality of his or her fears and set limits on the use of the psychotic defenses. Ideas of reference and persecutory fears can be tested directly, for example, "Who is talking about you? How do they know you? Why you?" and so forth. If the patient is anxious or agitated, offer to change the routine to meet his or her needs (within reason). For example, a patient fearing attack may be interviewed in an open area, a waiting room, or an office with the door open. If the patient is fearful that the room is "bugged," he or she should be encouraged to look until satisfied that there are none. The paradoxical method forces the patient to confront his or her own delusional perception without direct challenge by the clinician. The paranoid patient—even in crisis—should be able to test the reality of his or her distortions given the cognitive structure imposed by the inter- viewer and a nonthreatening, supportive atmosphere. If the patient is unable to test the reality of his or her perceptions, the diagnosis war- rants revision.

Whereas the paranoid patient establishes distance and control in the interview through a suspicious and argumentative style, the schiz- oid shrinks from any affective arousal, appearing insensitive and indif- ferent to interpersonal relationships. The patient does not respond with the casual social graces that are taken for granted by others. Social pleas- antries, greetings, jokes, "small talk" in the office that precede or follow a session fail to bring the customary responses. The clinician is faced with an unresponsive, bland patient whose emotional tone seems re- duced to a bare minimum. An eerie feeling of being out of contact, not on the same "wave length" characterizes this interview.

The schizoid patient's withdrawal and isolation provide a focus for investigation in the interview. If the clinician assumes this to be a moti- vated defensive adaptation, the work of the interview lies in uncovering the painful origins of this life-style. Engaging the patient in this process takes considerable enthusiasm and activity on the part of the clinician. A spontaneous, emotionally active approach is needed to stimulate, ma- nipulate, and even provoke the schizoid patient into recalling painful events. Whenever possible, the clinician labels and encourages the pa- tient's expression of emotion. For example, "You look sad. That must have been painful for you. It's okay to cry," and so forth. The patient may be "given permission" to express feeling. For example, "That would have made anyone angry—how did you feel about it?" When a socially expected response is inhibited, the clinician can get his or her point across with a well-timed exaggeration—"You weren't angry? Not at all? Not even a little bit?")—followed by the more tactful inquiry "If not, why not?" One pokes and prods the schizoid patient, cajoling and coercing until the historical origins of the social withdrawal are clarified and the affect associated with them appropriately acknowledged and felt.

The schizotypal patient differs from the schizoid in the presence of overt manifestations of mild thought disorder. Although research has uncovered no clear empirical evidence for a biologic link between the schizoid personality and schizophrenia, the schizotype appears to be in a genetic spectrum shared by the more severe forms of thought disorder. Schizotypal patients share the paranoid's mistrust and the emotional isolation of the schizoid but demonstrate true cognitive slippage under emotional duress.

The patient appears to suspend reality testing transiently under stress, only to correct the distortions in a conflict-free time or place. In the realm of perception, the schizotype experiences dissociative episodes (derealization/depersonalization), illusions and even non-Schneiderian (e.g., nonschizophrenic) hallucinosis under duress.

Example. A 24-year-old inpatient with mixed borderline and schizotypal personality disorders (by DSM-III criteria) had an argument on the phone with her father that greatly upset her. She spent the day sitting on her windowsill staring down on an adjoining rooftop. She became alarmed when she saw a large snake emerge from a puddle on the roof. The snake opened its mouth and spoke in her father's voice. Although she couldn't make out the words, the message was angry. The experience was transitory (a few seconds) but reappeared once again in a similar fashion a few days later following another confrontation with her father.

A more fanciful distortion occurred as the patient explored her anger toward her father in therapy. She felt her Teddy bear (a constant companion on the ward) had turned against her and was staring at her with hostile intent. The transformation of her transitional object into a "killer bear" (her words) provided an opportunity to demonstrate to the patient her defensive suspension of reality testing and use of psychotic projection.

Writers who view the schizotype as one step removed from schizophrenia point to the patient's cognitive distortions and autistic thinking as a primary process, whereas the more dramatic quasi-delusional symptoms appear in response to stress in interpersonal relationships. The schizotype's difficulties in achieving satisfaction (anhedonia) or resolving conflicting desires (ambivalence) may be indicators of a general distortion of the personality in the direction of schizophrenia. The many earlier terms for this disorder convey the same message: latent, ambulatory, pseudoneurotic, and borderline schizophrenia.

Psychotic Symptoms and Personality Disorder. With the odd, eccentric personality group, the patient's symptoms resemble milder forms of more severe paranoid and schizophrenic phenomena. Although the DSM-III restricts the use of the term *psychotic* to "gross impairment in reality testing" as manifested by the presence of either delusions or hallucinations, it is clear that the psychological function of reality testing appears particularly vulnerable in some pateints with "nonpsychotic" personality disorders, especially the odd, eccentric groups and the dramatic cluster. In particular, paranoid and schizotypal patients appear to have frequent cognitive distortions reflecting a tenuous hold on reality, whereas the borderline, histrionic, and narcissistic types require significant interpersonal stressors to reveal transient loss of reality testing. Psychoanalytic writers make a distinction between the absolute loss of reality testing in the true psychotic and a diminished *sense* of reality (or the "suspension" of reality testing) in the stress-vulnerable personalities. The distinction is important diagnostically and is testable in the clinical interview. With the structure of the interview, the stress-vulnerable personality will reorganize and repudiate irrational "micropsychotic" experience. The truly psychotic individual cannot.

The clinician must look specifically for schizotypal features on both process and content levels of the interview. Such inquiries are not comfortable to most outpatient clinicians. A typical survey of schizotypal symptoms can be phrased as follows:

> [*Perceptual symptoms*] Do your senses ever play tricks on you? Do you sometimes see or hear things that turn out not to be real—like a voice calling your name or an illusion, a shadow that looks like something else? How about walking into a room and feeling like someone else is there—but no one is? Do you ever feel "spaced out," unreal, like you're outside of yourself watching from a distance, or like part of you is changing and isn't real anymore? Ever feel like you're not part of the world around you, like there's a pane of glass or a cloud between you and other people?
>
> [*Cognitive symptoms*] Ever feel people talk about you behind your back—even strangers? Do people make reference to you or give you special signals? Do you ever feel you can make things happen by thinking about them, or have special intuition about the future? Ever lose control of your thoughts, have your mind go blank or drift out? How about day dreams? Ever spend a lot of time with day dreams? Anything really violent or exceptional?
>
> [*Behavioral*] Are you really sensitive to criticism? Prefer to be by yourself?

Do's and Don'ts

Diagnostic interviewing is not therapy. Although the effect may be therapeutic, the intent of the interview is to gather data from the content and process of the interview to make an accurate assessment. Because time is often limited, the methods of diagnostic interviewing may be more active, intrusive, or even manipulative compared to long-term psychotherapy. Unlike the therapist, the diagnostician has a structured format for his or her thinking (predetermined categories used to sort developmental history, symptom presentation, and interview observations). He or she actively includes or "rules out" diagnostic categories as the patient presents his or her problem. An initial impression leads to formulation of a differential diagnosis and a list of related disorders to be considered. Resolution of the differential diagnosis requires active investigation for historical or symptomatic criteria needed to make specific diagnoses.

The clinical approach to the patient must be adapted to the patient's dominant defensive style. Patients from the dramatic group must have a more structured interview to elicit factual history and contain lability of affect and flights of fantasy. Just as the process of therapy with the dramatic patient teaches cognitive control, the diagnostic interview uses the cognitive limits of structured questioning to help the patients organize the thoughts behind their experience in a coherent manner. In contrast, the anxious-fearful patient suffers from cognitive overcontrol and must be pressed for affective responses in painful areas to complete the diagnostic process. The odd/eccentric will need an open, accepting, and uncritical clinician to develop trust enough to relate history. With each interview, the diagnostician reviews his or her "checklist" of criteria until satisfied by the fit between data and diagnosis.

Personality disorder is not episodic. One must examine the life experience of the patient—a longitudinal perspective—to make an accurate diagnosis. The cross-sectional perspective obtained during a hospital admission or crisis interview is rarely sufficient due to distortion by anxieties, depressions, or stress responses superimposed on the personality style. In DSM-III terminology, Axis I disorders often obscure and confound the differentiation of coexisting Axis II personality disorders. One is occasionally embarrassed by the "disappearance" of an Axis II personality disorder along with remission of Axis I depression. On the other hand, one must not "biologize" behavior: that is, force the affective and cognitive reactions of the personality into artificial biologic constructs. Not every depression is a major affective disorder or every cognitive slip an underlying schizophrenia.

Accuracy of diagnosis is proportional to the number of perspectives. The patient does not exist in a vacuum but is defined (in so far as personality is concerned) by his or her interactions with others. Additional perspectives should be sought from family and friends to test the experience of the clinician. The patient presents his or her own history in a self-conscious and self-interested fashion. A biased presentation may be unconscious and unintentional, or consciously manipulative, depending on the patient's motivation. The clinician should not hesitate to test his or her own perceptions against the experience of others.

The general task of the diagnostic interviewer is best likened to that of a detective, whose job is to get the facts. It is useful to view the patient's symptoms and defensive maneuvers as forms of self-deception, and avoidance of a painful inner reality. As the diagnostic process unfolds, the clinician helps the patient acknowledge some of these realities, express and bear the associated feelings, and place them in perspective. Success in this process will lead to an accurate diagnosis, psychodynamic formulation, and assessment of potential for therapeutic change.

Finally, personality disorder is more than a matrix for episodic mental illness. It is a disabling disorder in its own right, more devastating for its subtlety and chronicity and all the more deserving of therapeutic effort. To dismiss the symptoms of disordered personality as "problems of living," unworthy of the most serious attention, is to deny the poet's admonition that "character is destiny."

Summary

The diagnostic interview of patients with personality disorder defines those habitual and predictable aspects of interpersonal functioning that repeatedly result in social and personal distress. The clinician is a detective who utilizes the content of the patient's history and the interpersonal process of the interview to reconstruct the patient's modus operandi, his or her characteristic way of perceiving, thinking, feeling, and acting in the interpersonal world. Dimensions of personality are defined and then organized into recognizable clinical categories according to current nosologic fashion. This chapter discusses the diagnostic process within the framework of the third edition of the DSM, an amalgam of dimensional and categorical approaches producing 11 personality prototypes. Within this nosologic classification, three thematic groups are defined—a dramatic group, an anxious-fearful group, and an odd/ccentric group. An understanding of the perceptual, cognitive, and affective vulnerabilities of each group leads to modifications in interview technique that enhance the cooperation of the patient and reliability of the diagnostic process.

References

American Psychiatric Association. (1980). *Diagnostic and statistical manual of mental disorders* (3rd ed.). Washington, DC: Author.

Lion, J. R. (Ed.). (1981). *Personality disorders: Diagnosis and management.* (2d ed.). Baltimore: Williams & Wilkins.

MacKinnon, R. A., & Michels, R. (1971). *The psychiatric interview in clinical practice.* Philadelphia: W. B. Saunders.

Millon, T. (1981). *Disorders of personality. DSM-III: Axis II.* New York: Wiley.

Reich, W. (1945). *Character analysis* Vincent R. Carfagno, Trans.). New York: Farrar, Strauss & Giroux.

Shapiro, D. (1965). *Neurotic styles.* New York: Basic Books.

Siever, L. J. (1981). Schizoid and schizotypal personality disorders. In J. R. Lion (Ed.), *Personality disorders: Diagnosis and management* (2d ed.) (pp. 32–64). Baltimore: Williams & Wilkins.

Wiggins, J. S. (1982). Circumplex models of interpersonal behavior in clinical psychology. In P. C. Kendall & J. N. Butcher (Eds.), *Handbook of research methods in clinical psychology* (pp. 183–221). New York: Wiley.

Chapter 7

Alcoholism

Glenn R. Caddy

Introduction

Although diagnostic interviewing of individuals experiencing emotional and behavioral pathology inevitably requires sophistication and attention to detail on the part of the interviewer, there are particular problems that the clinician dealing with alcohol abusing patients must face. Various present-day conceptualizations regarding the very nature of alcoholism raise questions about the validity of the conceptual framework used in the evaluative schema. Similarly, the existence of a variety of classification procedures, which are in some respects related to the aforestated conceptualizations, also bear on the validity matter. And then there are the numerous manipulations and strategies exhibited by many alcohol-abusing individuals as they either submit to or resist the collection of credible evaluative data. This chapter provides a perspective on the special problems that must be addressed and overcome if the diagnostic interviewing of alcoholic patients is to result in a valid outcome, thus setting the stage for a reasonable prospect of therapeutic success.

Conceptualizing Alcohol Problems

Throughout history, alcohol-related difficulties have been variously conceptualized and the drinker variously dealt with, largely as a result

---

GLENN R. CADDY • Department of Psychology, Nova University, Fort Lauderdale, Florida 33314.

of the prevailing social understanding of the condition or conditions involved. The way alcohol-related problems are viewed, of course, is crucial to any effort to classify (diagnose) the various levels of problem(s) in an individual case. Equally, the process(es) employed in the diagnostic endeavor always depend on the framework around which a disorder is conceptualized. Irrespective of one's predilection regarding either the concepts of alcohol-related difficulties or the views of the assessment process, however, clinical interviewing inevitably provides the primary means to achieve the goal of comprehensive diagnosis/assessment.

Although over the last 50 years there have been various conceptualizations of alcohol abuse and dependence (Caddy, Goldman, & Huebner, 1976a, 1976b; Siegler, Osmond, & Newell, 1968), in recent years the univariate disease orientation (Jellinek, 1960; Mann, 1968) and the multivariate behaviorally based perspectives (Caddy, 1978; Pattison, Sobell, & Sobell, 1977; Wanberg & Knapp, 1970), though not readily compatible, have come into prominence. Briefly, the disease orientation proposes that alcoholism is a progressive and irreversible condition characterized by an inability to abstain and/or a loss of control over alcohol; that alcoholics are different from nonalcoholics; and that this difference either leads to or includes psychological/sociological and/or biochemical/physiolgical changes in the alcoholic. This traditional view dictates that treatment must emphasize the permanent nature of the alcoholic's difference and, in doing so, stresses that the disease can be arrested only by abstinence that must be lifelong. The disease concept applies only to the diagnosis of alcoholism. Drinking difficulties that are not deemed to involve loss of control, for example, typically are neither conceptualized within the disease framework nor viewed as necessary or probable precursors to alcoholism.

Pattison, Sobell, and Sobell (1977) have summarized the recent evidence supporting a multivariate approach to understanding alcohol dependence and have concluded, in part, that (a) alcohol dependence summarizes a variety of syndromes defined by drinking patterns and the adverse consequences of such drinking; (b) these syndromes exist on a continuum from nonpathological to severely pathological; (c) a variety of factors may contribute to differential susceptibility to alcohol problems. These factors *per se* do not produce alcohol dependence. Any person who uses alcohol can develop a syndrome of alcohol dependence; (d) the development of alcohol problems follows variable patterns over time and does not necessarily proceed inexorably to severe or fatal states; and (e) alcohol problems are typically interrelated with other life problems, especially when alcohol dependence is long established.

Classification of Drinking Difficulties

Various classificatory systems have evolved in response to the differing conceptualizations of alcoholism as well to changes that have occurred more generally in our understanding and classification of mental disorders. Traditionally, the diagnostic methodology employed in classifying drinking individuals has involved examining the specific diagnostic criteria deemed to establish the nature and degree of the drinker's difficulties. Thus, for example, Jellinek (1960) categorized pathological drinking into the following varieties: (a) alpha alcoholism, that drinking employed to relieve physical or emotional distress, but without loss of control; (b) beta alcoholism, characterized by overt physical signs of the consequences of drinking but without physical or psychological dependence; (c) gamma alcoholism, involving increased tissue tolerance and alcohol-withdrawal symptomatology, psychological dependence on alcohol, and loss of control over drinking; and (d) delta alcoholism that is similar to gamma, but whereas gamma alcoholics experience periods of abstinence, delta alcoholics cannot willfully terminate their drinking (see also the similar diagnostic schema developed by the American Psychiatric Association, 1968).

Another diagnostic approach based on specific diagnostic criteria but in this instance focusing more on the presence or absence of multiple symptoms was introduced by the National Council on Alcoholism (NCA, 1972). The NCA system employs major and minor criteria across two tracks (physiological and clinical and behavioral, psychological, and attitudinal) with a total of three diagnostic levels possible. Individuals who fit the Level I criterion must be diagnosed alcoholic; those who satisfy the Level II criterion are under strong suspicion of alcoholism; and those who show Level III symptomatology present signs that are common in alcoholics but do not, by themselves, give strong indication of its existence.

Diagnostic systems such as the preceding tend to imply that attributes such as alcoholism, excessive drinking, and the like exist in the unitary fashion implied by the terms. Moveover, labeling a drinker as functioning within a particular category does very little to add real understanding either of the individual drinker or his or her behavior. It is because of these perceived limitations of the more traditional assessment approach that behavioral assessment approaches have been introduced to the recent alcoholism literature (see the reviews by Briddell & Nathan, 1975; Foy, Rychtarik, & Prue, 1981; Miller, 1977). Caddy (1978), in particular, has extended the general behavioral approach to evaluating alcohol-related problems by proposing that such problems may be understood best in the context of behavioral disorders that are established and maintained by the unique direct and reciprocal interactions of behavioral, discriminative, incentive, and social dimensions, all of which function with varying degrees of cognitive mediation. This multivariate method of conceptualizing alcohol problems also provides a framework for the unique assessment of an individual drinker across each of the dimensions under study.

The final classificatory approach to alcohol-related difficulties being presented herein is the multiaxial schema developed for the DSM-III (*Diagnostic and Statistical Manual of Mental Disorders*, third ed., American Psychiatric Association, 1980). The DSM-III approach provided a multivariate perspective somewhat in keeping with that offered by Caddy (1978), though it does not address the primary clinical syndrome in the same degree of detail. The greatest significance of the DSM-III system is, of course, that over the next decade it will be the most widely used diagnostic schema within the United States. The real advantage of the system, however, is the multiaxial format that facilitates the use of concurrent diagnoses on the primary axis reflecting one or more possible clinical syndromes, on Axis II, which provides for the designation of personality and/or specific developmental disorders, and on Axis III, on which physical disorders and conditions are specified.

Within the DSM-III system, on Axis I, alcohol-related problems are listed under the categories of "Substance-Induced Organic Mental Disorders" and "Substance Use Disorders." The Substance-Induced Organic Mental Disorders category includes the alcohol-related subcategories of alcohol intoxication, idiosyncratic intoxication, withdrawal, withdrawal delirium, hallucinosis, amnesic disorder, and dementia associated with alcoholism. These disorders are all a product of the direct, acute, or chronic effects of alcohol on the central nervous system. The primary clinical syndromes associated with alcohol use are listed under the Substance Use Disorders category as either "alcohol abuse," "alcohol dependence" (alcoholism), or, when the problematic use of alcohol is combined with other drug usage, the subcategory "other, mixed, or unspecified substance abuse" may be employed. Of course, almost invariably, individuals who are diagnosed "substance-abuse"-disordered also experience substance-induced organic mental disorders, such as intoxication or withdrawal.

Alcohol use and abuse are distinguished in DSM-III on the basis of three criteria: pattern of pathological use, impairment in social or occupational functioning (caused by the use of alcohol), and duration of use. The essential determinant of abuse involves pathological use in which social and/or occupational functioning is impaired for at least 1 month. Alcohol dependence is distinguished from alcohol abuse in that the essential features of dependence are either a pattern of pathological alcohol use or impairment in social or occupational functioning due to alcohol *and* either the existence of tolerance or withdrawal symptomatology. Finally, as is noted in the DSM-III schema, there are three major patterns associated with chronic alcohol abuse and/or dependence: (a) the regular daily intake of large quantities of alcohol; (b) regular heavy drinking limited to weekends (both these forms are regarded as continuous and are so specified in the DSM-III approach); and (c) long periods of abstinence interspersed with binges of daily drinking, much of it heavy, and lasting perhaps for weeks, even months. This pattern is labeled as *episodic*.

These then are the major classification systems that, together with the various concepts noted previously, provide the framework for diagnostic interviewing of alcoholic individuals.

Considerations and Procedures for Gathering Information

Interviewing alcohol-involved individuals presents quite substantial problems for the clinican for a number of reasons, each of which must be taken into consideration in every case. First, and perhaps what is most obvious, alcohol-abusing individuals rarely, if ever, seek professional assistance unless they consider themselves to be in serious circumstances. It is quite common for these people to have been drinking rather large quantities of alcohol (and to have been taking other drugs concurrently), and they present for the interview in an intoxicated state. Moreover, they may be suffering from a coexistent physical disorder, for both excessive alcohol use and the life-style of the heavy drinker correlate highly with a whole host of physiologically based difficulties. For example, if the patient has been drinking heavily and not eating, he or she may become hypoglycemic, and this condition may produce symptoms resembling those seen in withdrawal (see Freinkel & Arky, 1966). Certainly the state of intoxication and the physical condition of the drinker must be taken into consideration whenever an interview is being proposed or conducted. Under circumstances of a potential or actual medical emergency, for example, when an individual is seen in a condition of extreme intoxication, if he or she is capable of engaging in an acceptable level of verbal responding, it may be appropriate to elicit some limited information regarding his or her consummatory behavior (both alcohol and drugs) over the past 24 hours as well as his or her physical well-being. With the exception of the gathering of such information, however, and any additional contact deemed necessary to obtain the administrative particulars that may be required prior to treatment being provided, it is typically quite useless, in my view, to attempt any interaction with an intoxicated patient beyond providing a general level of concern and support.*

In order to maximize the prospects of the intoxicated patient actually engaging in the therapeutic process (or in the case of inpatient services, maximizing the value of continuity of care), a second visit should be scheduled with the patient as soon as possible after the initial contact; an appointment card should be provided, and the patient should be advised that he or she cannot be effectively evaluated unless he or she is sober. Typically, during such first visits, the drinker (especially if intoxicated) will be accompanied by a relative or friend. In such cases, it may be desirable to obtain some background data from this significant other and, depending on the nature of his or her relationship with the drinker, to focus much of the session on this other individual and the relationship. In any case, during this first visit, if the primary patient is intoxicated, it may be crucial for the clinician to establish some relationship with the significant other in order to maximize the prospects of the latter influencing the patient to return for the second appointment.

A second problem facing the clinician dealing with alcohol-abusing patients is that with the possible exception of abusers of certain other substances many alcohol abusers and alcoholics engage in quite extreme levels of deception and denial regarding their drinking. Paradoxically, such repertoires appear especially under circumstances in which the patient is in some respects under the influence during the interview (see, for example Sobell, Sobell & VanderSpek, 1979). It is well known that alcoholics may forget segments of a drinking episode or not anticipate accurately the consequences of their actions, but such forgetfulness or misjudgment hardly explains the levels of defensiveness noted in the vast number of alcohol-abusing clients. Alcohol abusers routinely lie about the quantity and frequency of their alcohol consumption. Occasionally, they overstate their patterns of consumption, but mostly they understate their alcohol usage. In either instance their misreporting is essentially the outcome of an attempt to manipulate a more positive image of themselves and their drinking in the eyes of other people. Of course, minimizing the aberrant nature of ones' drinking behavior as far

---

*Of course, it may be necessary or at least desirable to know the approximate degree of intoxication of such a person or to explore further his or her physical condition. If the former is required, breath, urine, or blood analyses provide far more accurate indexes both of the patient's state of intoxication and his or her likely recent drinking behavior. If the latter is required, the medical practitioner who ultimately must determine the patient's physical condition inevitably must await the sobering of the patient before a comprehensive and valid physical history can be obtained.

as others are concerned also may permit the drinker to continue to engage in the self-deception that his or her drinking behavior is not, in fact, pathological.

A third major problem that must be addressed in the diagnostic interviewing of alcoholics involves the extent to which alcohol-involved individuals consider both the label *alcoholic* and their view of the underlying alcoholism construct to be stigmatizing. The vast majority of such individuals may either deny or procrastinate with respect to acknowledging their difficulties with alcohol in the early years of their problems, and in so doing they deny the significance of the consequences of their drinking. In the latter stages of their drinking, still a number of alcoholic individuals will deny their alcoholism. I recall one 60-year-old man, for example, who had been in and out of Veterans Administration alcoholism units for more than 20 years who once said to me: "Doc, I may be a drunk, but I sure ain't no damn alcoholic." Still others will engage in what Caddy (1978) has referred to as the *surrender to the diagnosis*. In this surrender, the alcoholic individual presents in the interview a rather overlearned set of repertoires regarding his or her alcoholism, the inability to control drinking, and the lack of responsibility for his or her present distressed condition. Acceptance of the diagnosis and the attendant disease concept, in fact, provides the drinker with an explanation for his or her drinking, albeit circular, and at the same time permits exoneration from the responsibility for the condition.

A final consideration to be noted herein is that when one is interviewing an alcohol-abusing patient, it must be borne in mind that alcohol-related problems are interrelated with other life problems, especially when the drinking difficulties have been well established. Moreover, these problems are variable within an individual over time and also show great variability from one person to another. Further, to this constellation of what may be considered reactive alcohol-related problems must be added personality disorders, the one most commonly associated with alcoholism being antisocial personality disorder, although the anxiety and affective disorders also are common in such patients. All this makes the functional analysis and therefore the comprehensive interviewing of the alcoholic patient a particularly complex and difficult undertaking.

Given the aforestated considerations, then, what are some of the primary procedures employed in the collection of information via the interview? A matter that stems from several of the preceding considerations and one that, in turn, leads to a number of procedures that are designed to address the tendency of many alcohol abusers to attempt to manipulate or deceive the interviewer is worthy of very special consideration. It is absolutely crucial, of course, that such a situation does not eventuate. If it does, the chances are very much against the interviewer's obtaining the quality of information on the prospective client that is necessary to effectively evaluate the alcoholic patient. Moreover, to the extent that such interviews often set the stage for the development of a therapeutic relationship, it is essential that this relationship not be compromised by errors made by the clinician during the early diagnostic interviewing phase. There are various procedures that I use routinely in an effort to collect the best data and minimize the possibility of the patient's lying or otherwise distorting his or her presentation. These procedures include the following:

1. *Employing breath-testing procedures.* Typically, I require all alcohol-abusing patients seeking my services to undergo routine breath analysis at the beginning of every session. Employing breath analysis as a standard operating procedure with all alcohol-abusing patients maximizes the chances that these individuals will, in fact, present themselves at the office for services in a sober state. Such a procedure also maximizes the accuracy of the data being provided by the patient, and in so doing, facilitates the development of an honest dialogue between the patient and the clinician.

Although I will present an example of the approach I use in obtaining breath samples in a case illustration that is included later in this chapter, it is noteworthy, I think, to report that there are very few, in fact almost no professionals in the alcohol field who routinely use breath-testing procedures. There are many alcoholism professionals who appear to disdain the use of breath testing on the basis of its presumed offensiveness to patients. My experience with the procedure does not support such a view. In fact, I have employed routine breath testing with hundreds of patients and have experienced virtually no resistance from them.

2. *Presuming the probability of some initial ongoing drinking.* It is possible to increase the accuracy of the data obtained from interviewing alcoholic patients by ensuring from the outset that the patient sees the interviewer as operating from the assumption that at least some continued alcohol use by the patient may be expected and that the accurate reporting of alcohol use will be accepted rather than negatively judged if and when drinking does occur. Similarly, historically reported alcohol use and its consequences will be viewed as critical information in the development of a functional analysis of the patient, not as an indictment of past indiscretions. All too often, evaluative interviews are conducted with alcoholic patients without first reflecting seriously to them the need for genuineness and honesty during the interview. By reflecting such concern, by avoiding any hint of judgment, by asking even provocative questions in a matter-of-fact manner, and by advising the patient that

collateral sources of information beyond the patient also will be asked to provide their view of him or her, it is possible to maximize the extent to which the patient provides valid data from the interview.

3. *Involving family members or others.* Social and family relationships have routinely been implicated both in etiological and treatment considerations of alcohol abuse and dependence. All too often, however, the family or other important people in the life of the patient are brought into the picture only after the evaluation of the patient has been completed. Such an approach fails to maximize the possibility of a valid and comprehensive evaluative process. Not only does the patient tend to report more accurately during an interview when he or she knows that collateral sources are being tapped to offer their perspective on the matters at hand, but these various perspectives *per se* offer an increased understanding of the functioning of the primary patient and so facilitate the evaluation process.

For these various reasons and also in order to examine the agendas and functioning of the significant others in the patient's life and to attempt to elicit from the outset their assistance in the therapy whenever possible, I routinely begin the diagnostic process by interviewing the patient and other(s) together, initially, and thereafter, separately.

4. *Using a structured interview.* The use of a structured interview format with precise information being gathered across a large number of areas also facilitates the collection of well-considered, more factual, and more comprehensive data from the patient. Certainly, the structured interview is particularly useful in gathering the data for a multivariate functional analysis approach to the understanding of the individual drinker.

The structured interview format that I employ is based on a research instrument, the Life History and Alcohol Involvement Questionnaire (LHAIQ). The instrument, which has been used in several studies (Caddy, Addington, & Perkins, 1978; Caddy, Addington, & Trenschel, 1984) covers the following areas: statistical/demographic data, family data, medical information, marital/interpersonal history and satisfaction, employment history and satisfaction, legal history, subject's self-perceptions and perceptions of alcohol abuse and alcoholism, subject's motivations and expectations, subject's perceptions of therapy and Alcoholics Anonymous, and subject's drinking and/or drug-taking practices. It takes typically between 2 and $2\frac{1}{2}$ hours to administer an interview employing this questionnaire. A parallel but shortened version of this instrument also has been developed for use with collateral information sources, thus permitting a comparability in the data on a patient derived both from himself or herself and from collateral sources. Because the LHAIQ was developed with consideration given to the multivariate assessment model proposed by Caddy (1978), it permits a particularly clear perspective to be gained regarding the behavioral, social, incentive, discriminative, and cognitive domains within which the individual's drinking difficulties may be understood.

Typically, as well as conducting an LHAIQ-based interview, I also undertake some additional formal psychological testing with the patient. Such testing usually is limited to formal personality assessment procedures but, at least occasionally, impressions gained during the initial diagnostic interview also recommend a thorough intellectual and psychoneurological evaluation. From the vantage point achieved by the gathering of these data, it becomes possible not only to offer a differential diagnosis in terms of the DSM-III criteria but also to complete the more detailed multivariate functional analysis of the patient.

There are, of course, methods of assessment of the alcohol-involved patient that do not follow these guidlines nor employ instruments such as the LHAIQ. There are empirically derived indirect scales such as the MacAndrew Scale (MacAndrew, 1965), face-valid direct scales such as the Alcadd Test (Manson, 1949) and the Michigan Alcoholism Screening Test (Selzer, 1971), and sequenced questionnaire and interview procedures such as those employed in the Mortimer-Filkins Test (Kerlan, Mortimer, Mudge, & Filkins, 1971) (see Jacobson, 1975 for a succinct review of these and other alcoholism-assessment devices). There are also concurrent physiological measures (such as indexes of dependence, tolerance, and the like) and behavioral measures (involving operant analysis, choice situations, and experimental taste-testing procedures) of alcohol involvement that have been developed (see the review by Miller, 1976). Further, there are empirically developed questionnaire-based assessment devices such as the Alcohol Use Questionnaire (Wanberg, Horn, & Foster, 1973) and the structured behaviorally oriented interview known as the Drinking Profile (Marlatt, 1976), both of which were developed from a multivariate understanding of alcoholism and facilitate a functional approach to the assessment of the alcohol-involved individual.

A Case Illustration

David T. was a 39-year-old telephone repairman. He had been married to Betty for 14 years and had two children. At the time of my first contact with David, he and his wife were separated, and Betty and the children were living with her parents in another part of the city. David had been referred to me by a criminal attorney following his second arrest for driving while intoxicated. At the time of my initial interview, I had no information on him beyond that provided by a brief introductory letter from the attorney. Appended to this letter were copies of the police reports on both incidents. Of particular significance in this regard was the police finding of a blood alcohol concentration (BAC) of 0.19% at the time of the first arrest and a refusal to submit to breath analysis on the second occasion.

During the telephone scheduling of the initial visit, David was requested not to drink anything on the day of the interview and also to bring his wife to the session. In fact, his spouse Betty did attend. As a general rule, I attempt to schedule the first session for 90 to 120 minutes in order that a reasonable rapport and a fair understanding of the issues of the case can be determined. In this instance, I saw David and Betty jointly for about 20 minutes, then David alone for about 40 minutes, Betty alone for 30 minutes, and then both of them again jointly to close the session. I also made subsequent appointments with both of them separately in order to continue the process of data collection and to determine how I could provide the most appropriate services to them.

After the introductions but before any initial development of the interview, I initiated a breath-testing sequence as follows:

T: David, I have a standard practice in this office whenever I see a person with any difficulties related to alcohol. I have such patients undergo a standard breath-testing procedure so that we can determine if there is any alcohol in their system. I have found that I get neither particularly valuable information nor a sense of progress from patients if they have been drinking, even small quantities, and so I make it a practice to routinely ensure that my patients have not been drinking when they come to see me. Please come over here, and when I tell you to, I want you to take a deep breath and blow into this mouthpiece.

Although slightly surprised by my procedure, David complied with my request without comment. Then, as the breath sample was being analyzed I added:

T: You see, David, it is very important that I know the precise alcohol-related state of my patients. It is also equally important that they level with me regarding their drinking. So important, in fact, that I attempt to minimize the prospects of patients deceiving me about their drinking by employing routine breath analyses. So, how many drinks of what type have you had today, David?

P: I haven't had any alcohol in the last 2 or 3 days.

T: Alright, now just try and recall as accurately as you can the day on which you last drank, what you drank, and just how much you drank.

These questions are asked in a data-oriented manner and are also asked with the presumption that some alcohol use may have occurred. By using such an approach, it is possible to encourage the acknowledgment of drinking rather than provoking defensiveness. Moreover, by taking a rather neutral stance on the patient's statement about his or her drinking, it is possible to minimize the demand characteristics that the patient may infer from the question about the expectations of the clinician. This, in turn, may facilitate more accurate reporting.

Following the request for specific information about David's recent drinking behavior, the interview proceeded jointly with both Dave and Betty. During the remainder of this joint interview, demographic data were obtained as were some emotionally charged data regarding the present state of the relationship between them. Thereafter, I indicated my preference to see the two of them separately so that I might come to understand the perspective that each of them held regarding their difficulties, and to do so in an efficient manner. In order to show some priority to David, however (on the basis of David's being identified as the primary patient), I escorted Betty from the room. I then proceeded with David by first seeking to motivate him to deal with me honestly in order to protect the integrity of the therapeutic relationship that I wished to establish with him. Thus, the interview continued:

T: David, I want to begin our time together today by assuring you that I will do all I possibly can to help you resolve the difficulties you are facing. I cannot do so, however, nor will I be willing to do so, unless you and I can establish a particularly honest and forthright relationship with one another. For that reason, it is particularly important that you make the commitment to yourself to be as honest and accurate as possibly you can regarding the matters we will deal with in the weeks ahead. Do you consider that that is a commitment which you can make to yourself and keep?

P: Yes, I suppose I can.

T: Good . . . . because while it may be quite possible for you to choose not to be absolutely straightforward with me, ultimately it would be you that would suffer . . . . and clearly I want to do all I can to ensure that that doesn't happen.

Then, as I do routinely with both alcohol-abusing and other patients, I continued the interview by beginning a comprehensive history taking that specifically addressed matters other than the alcohol-based presenting problems. I do this in order to ensure a basic understanding of the dynamics of the patient and to develop an understanding of the context for the problems of him or her. Moreover, especially in the case of alcohol-involved individuals, typically there has been so much focus on alcohol abuse that by avoiding an initial focus on this issue it is possible to minimize the possibility of initial defensiveness on the part of the patient. (Of course, sometimes the patient is particularly keen to present his or her problems with some urgency. Nevertheless, if the clinician reassures the patient of his or her desires to handle the needs of the patient but does so in a manner that ensures an orderly and efficient management of the issues involved in the case, typically the desire of the patient to immediately present his or her problems for attention can be dealt with.) In the history taking, I employ a routine sequence of questions to establish the potentially relevant issues of the patient's childhood, adolescence, and adulthood. Developmental history, family relationships, school achievement, social relationships and functioning, sexual and marital history, and presence/absence of physical or emotional conditions symptomatic of difficulties are all examined in the first several interviews in order to establish the framework of the primary problem. Thereafter, I obtain a history of the presenting problem and develop a functional analysis of this primary concern as a basis for treatment planning.

In the present instance, given the time constraints on the initial consultation with David, it was possible to conduct a general history taking but not to direct any focus to David's drinking history or current alcohol-related practices. Such data would not be gathered until the second session.

Turning now to the initial consultation with Betty, my agenda during that first visit was to begin the establishment of a trusting relationship, to offer my assurance that I would do all I could to be helpful to her husband, and to begin to understand her perspective on the relationship between David and her, so that I could determine the extent of her willingness to be a party to her husband's therapy. During this session, I also presented to Betty the fact that I wished to see her at least occasionally during David's therapy, and that just as was true with her husband, I needed her to be particularly forthright with me. Fortunately, Betty revealed right from the outset that despite her current marital difficulties, it was her sincere wish to reestablish a close relationship with her husband and to "try and help him with his alcoholism."

The session with Betty was then terminated, and I brought both David and Betty together in order to indicate that I would be willing to work with both of them in order, initially, to determine the extent of David's drinking difficulties and then to provide treatment to both of them in order to aid David in overcoming these and perhaps other difficulties also. A second appointment was then scheduled with David and Betty to see each separately. In scheduling these second appointments, it was my intention to have Betty see me first, for before I saw

David I wanted to gather data from her on the parameters of his drinking and her perceptions of its consequences. (Such an approach also often contributes to a greater accuracy of reporting from the alcohol-involved spouse, for he or she knows that the clinician already has tapped an important information source.) Moreover, given my observation that the motivation for therapy of many alcohol-abusing clients is frequently only temporary, I arranged to see Betty the very next day and to see David the following evening. Thus, the evaluative process continued for at least another session with each patient.

During Betty's second appointment, she presented her marital history and, we explored in considerable detail both her attitudes and behavior in relation to David's drinking. I then examined Betty's perceptions of David's drinking history. A section of this interview was conducted as follows:

T: Betty, going back to when you and David were first married, how much did David drink then?

P: Well, David has always been a drinker; it has been a problem on and off since we began dating.

T: Tell me, what did David drink in those early days? What type of alcohol did he drink?

P: Well, he has always been mainly a beer drinker; it has only been in the past 3 or 4 years that he has drunk anything else at all, pretty much.

T: Okay, he used to drink primarily or even exclusively beer. Going back to when you first met David, tell me how often you recall him drinking beer during a week? How many days each week would he drink?

P: Well, he didn't get drunk most of the time.

T: No, I appreciate that. But I am asking if you can recall how many days a week that David used alcohol in the early days of your relationship.

P: Well, I really don't know . . . but looking back it seems that he was always having a few beers with his friends after work . . . and it was usually the case that he would drink when we went out together.

T: Alright, now let me ask you if you can recall the amount of beer that he would drink in those early days. How many, say, glasses of beer or cans of beer would David drink during a typical occasion?

P: Actually, he didn't drink all that much when we went out together because he knew I didn't like him getting drunk. But sometimes he would really overdo it. He probably drank half a dozen beers in the course of an evening even then.

T: Thinking back, how did you feel about David's drinking when he did drink that much?

P: It used to upset me a fair bit. My father used to drink a lot up until I was about 16 or 17, and he only quit because he got sick and my mother told him she would leave him if he didn't stop. David knew it used to upset me.

T: Did you become angry with David, did you just get quiet, or how did you act when you became upset?

P: Well, sometimes I would get angry and tell him to stop drinking, and sometimes I would say nothing.

T: Where you ever really consistent in dealing with David as far as his drinking was concerned?

P: Well, I suppose not, not really anyway. Not until I decided I couldn't go on like this any longer.

T: Tell me, Betty, if you experienced a fair degree of upset as a result of David's drinking even then, why did you go ahead and marry him?

P: Well, I have always loved David. He is a very kind person, and I guess I just felt that when we were married he would be with me and not with his friends.

T: Do you mean his drinking friends?

P: Yes.

Even though this session explored David's drinking practices as they were nearly 15 years before and there was some vagueness on Betty's part notwithstanding, it was possible to gain some important data on her perceptions of David's drinking and some insight regarding Betty and the nature of her relationship with David. Such data were achieved, however, only by the interviewer making constant demands of Betty to communicate her perceptions, especially of David's drinking, in quantifiable terms. This was especially the case when data were being gathered on David's recent drinking practices where the parameters of type of beverage, duration of drinking, quantity of intake, and frequency of consumption were all explored in quite considerable detail. During the remainder of the session I continued to add further to my understanding of Betty's views of her husband's drinking and the dynamics of their present relationship, as I changed the focus from the past to the present. By the end of that session I had developed a substantial understanding of Betty's history, of her relationship with David, and of her perceptions of the dimensions of his drinking difficulties. It had become obvious that David was in his wife's eyes an "alcoholic" or well on the way to becoming alcoholic and that for perhaps the past 5 to 6 years the family life had been increasingly distressed by David's patterns of drunkenness. Moreover, I had had the opportunity to understand Betty's perceptions of her husband's personality and of her uncertainty about their future together. But I also began to develop the sense that Betty had a considerable amount of emotional integrity, that her relationship with David was strained but not yet irrepairably damaged, and that she was willing to enter therapy with her husband if such an action would serve either his or her best interests (even though these interests were yet to be clarified). Finally, from this session with Betty I determined her views on the nature of the relationships that existed between herself, David, and their two children and on the extent to which

David's parental role had been colored by his use of alcohol, especially over the past several years. With all these data in mind, I saw David later that day.

Following the administration of a routine breath-testing procedure (which showed a zero blood alcohol concentration), this second session with David focused primarily on the history and current status of his drinking practices, the outcome of these practices, and David's concepts regarding the various aspects of his alcohol involvement. A segment of this interview went as follows:

T: Having developed the details of your drinking history in 5 year blocks beginning with the time you first began drinking, I now want to go on and have
   you detail your drinking practices over the past 5 years, that is, from about
   1978. Firstly, were you still working for Cell Electric in 1978 or was it about
   then that you went to work for Southern Bell?

(Such data are gathered to help place into context the timetable of the patients' drinking in relationship to objectively recalled timelines.)

P: No, I was with the telephone company from 1977.
T: Alright, then given that you changed jobs and that prior to the change most
   of your drinking was done after work with friends from Cell Electric, how did
   going to the telephone company influence the socializing you did as far as
   drinking was concerned?
P: Well, when I was with Cell I would be with a crew, and we did large jobs all
   over the county. So we would stop in at a bar after work near where we were
   working. When I went to the phone company I didn't keep track of most of
   the people from Cell. My hours changed, too, because with the phone company I began doing shift work.
T: Did these job changes alter your drinking in any way?
P: Well, I began going out once or twice a week with people from the phone
   company who were on my shift. We would go drinking after the shift
   finished . . . sometimes about 3 or so in the afternoon, and on the evening
   shift, not until about 11 o'clock. And except for sometimes on the weekend,
   that is when I did most of my drinking.
T: When you went out with these people, how many hours did you typically
   drink?
P: Well, sometimes that would depend on whether I was supposed to be home
   or what I had to do.
T: Let us say that you didn't feel any need to be home at a particular time, how
   long would you then go drinking?
P: Well, it varied from maybe 2 hours to 5 or 6. It would just depend.
T: Would you drink only beer on those occasions, or would you drink other
   beverages too?
P: Mainly beer, occasionally I would have some bourbon and water.

T: When would you drink bourbon and water, after you had been drinking beer?

P: Yes, sometimes I just didn't want to drink more beer . . . I would get really bloated.

T: So, in a typical drinking session, how many ounces of beer would you drink in the first hour?

P: Well, I am not sure. It would depend on how long I was going to be there.

T: If you were anticipating drinking for 3 to 4 hours, how much would you drink in the first hour?

P: Probably four to five beers, on the average.

T: Would you notice that you had been drinking after four or five beers?

P: No, I mean, I certainly wouldn't feel intoxicated.

T: What about during the second hour?

P: Three to four beers, probably about four beers.

T: Would you feel intoxicated after the second hour of drinking?

P: What do you mean, intoxicated?

T: What do you think it means to be intoxicated?

P: To be so drunk that you can't walk straight, and you stumble around.

T: Okay, would you feel intoxicated after the second hour of drinking, after perhaps eight beers?

P: No, maybe a little unsteady but not intoxicated, not yet.

T: How much alcohol does it take before you feel intoxicated?

P: Perhaps two six-packs in a couple of hours.

T: Alright, now what about your typical drinking in the third hour of a 4-hour session?

P: Well, I guess that I would probably have another three maybe four beers then, too. Over the past year or so I have been having a bourbon and water or two about then.

T: A 1-ounce bourbon or a double?

P: Most often a double.

T: How many beers, then, and how many ounces of bourbon would you typically drink during that third hour?

By the end of the interview I had concluded that, in fact, David's drinking practices were reflective of substantial abuse and indicative of some dependence. He reported a current drinking pattern involving drinking virtually every day, some days resulting in blood alcohol concentrations that I calculated to be about 0.08% and on at least 3 days each week, drinking involving quantities that I calculated to produce BACs of perhaps 0.20%.

As is obvious from the foregoing transcription, it is necessary to probe quite extensively and sometimes specifically motivate the patient in order to obtain the desired levels of detail regarding the parameters of a patient's drinking practices. Having obtained the data reflecting David's drinking practices in 5-year segments, I then used this information as a framework for understanding the development of David's present alcohol use pattern. By obtaining such detail on the parameters of the patient's drinking, it is possible to estimate the patterns and elevations of the BAC curves commonly achieved by the drinker. This information, when combined with data on his or her subjectively perceived state of intoxication and the degree of disequilibrium and disinhibition achieved at various points along the BAC curve, provides the interviewer with an important perspective on the possible development of pharmacological tolerance in the patient. It is clear that such data are crucial in an evaluation of the degree of physiological dependence in the patient.

From the perspective derived from such a data base, I proceeded in this interview to explore the extent of the consequences of David's alcohol involvement. David acknowledged, for example, that Betty had been upset about his drinking for, he believed, perhaps the past 4 or 5 years; and that he had essentially ignored her distress until she became "frigid and then walked out." He reported that she would nag him about his drinking "as if I was an alcoholic" because he went out drinking "a few times a week" and that it was not all that long before she left home that he "really got fed up with her bitching at me." At the same time, however, he acknowledged that Betty was basically a fine person, that he was very angry and hurt by her leaving with the children, and that he did not want the family to break up.

Regarding his relationships with the children, David reported a good relationship with the younger girl, but he was having some problems with his son who "had a real mouth at times . . . and was always being protected by his mother." Regarding his social relationships, it was clear that over the past year or two David had spent very little time in social activities with his wife, children, or the extended family, many of whom lived nearby. Rather, he had developed a pattern of socializing that involved almost exclusively his drinking friends. This socializing involved drinking after work an average of 3 weekdays each week for perhaps 2 hours and on several other days much more time, involving heavier drinking episodes. Although David saw himself to be a rather sociable person and rated his social relations to be "adequate," he acknowledged that he did not have any particularly close friends. As for his work, David reported no real problems on the job but indicated that the amount of freedom that he had during the day aided him in covering himself if he had a bit too much to drink while on the job. David acknowledged that in the past 6 months he had called in sick on perhaps six occasions as a result of being hung over. In terms of the physical health consequences of his drinking, David indicated that he viewed his weight to be a problem and that several years ago he became alarmed because he began experiencing periods of memory loss during several occasions when he had been drinking quite heavily. He did not view his drinking as producing a substantial health problem, although he did acknowledge that he was not in particularly good shape and that he did not take good care of himself. David was particularly concerned about the legal circumstances in which he was involved, for he viewed his job as being in jeopardy if his driving license was revoked. Up to the time that he sought my services, however, David had been able to keep his employer ignorant of the charges pending against him. Finally, regarding his concepts of his degree of alcohol impairment, David did not consider himself to be an "alcoholic," nor did he believe he required alcohol in order to function socially. He denied being dependent on alcohol and reported that he could, if he made the effort, substantially reduce his alcohol consumption. He did, however, agree that his alcohol usage had, at least in part, provoked a number of the difficulties that currently he and his family were experiencing and he acknowledged that he was able to drink quite large amounts of alcohol without feeling particularly intoxicated.

Diagnosis

In accordance with the DSM-III criteria, David ultimately was diagnosed as follows:

- Axis I: 303.91, alcohol dependence, continuous; V61.10, marital problem
- Axis II: V71.09 no diagnosis on Axis II.
- Axis III: Diagnosis deferred on Axis III; referral to medical practitioner required
- Axis IV: Severity of psychological stressors: five (severe)
- Axis V: Highest level of adaptive functioning past year: four (fair).

Given, however, that I routinely offer a diagnosis only after I have confirmed my initial impressions in subsequent sessions with a patient, at the end of this second session the diagnosis offered was proposed only as a diagnostic impression. Nevertheless, by the end of the second session, I had developed an adequate source of information on David, and I had explored elements both of consistency and inconsistency in the perceptions presented by both my primary patient and a collateral information source. I had, in fact, conducted the early evaluative process such that not only had I determined a diagnostic impression by the end of David's second visit, but, what is more important, I had developed enough of a functional analysis both of the dynamics of David's drinking and of his family conflicts that I was in a position to begin structuring an individualized treatment plan for David and his family. Finally, I had developed a definite sense in both David and Betty that I was a competent, concerned, and forthright individual, who was willing to engage either of them, and preferrably both, in a therapeutic process designed to aid them in improving the quality of their lives. Thus, within 2 days of the initial consultation an efficient series of assessment interviews had been conducted, and both David and Betty had committed themselves to the therapeutic process.

Summary

Inevitably, the richness of the clinical process is reduced when placed in print. Nevertheless, in this chapter some of the special problems of evaluating alcohol-involved patients have been discussed, and the richness of the process exemplified by the case of David. This case also illustrates the point that a competent evaluative process is not discontinuous from the process of therapy.

References

American Psychiatric Association. (1968). *Diagnostic and statistical manual of mental disorders* (2d ed.), Washington, DC: Author.

American Psychiatric Association.(1980).*Diagnostic and Statistical Manual of Mental Disorders* (3rd ed.). Washington, DC: Author.

Briddell, D. W., & Nathan, P. E. (1975). Behavior assessment and modification with alcoholics: Current status and further trends. In M. Hersen, R. M. Eisler, & R. M. Miller (Eds.), *Progress in behavior modification*. New York: Academic Press.

Caddy, G. R. (1978). Toward a multivariate analysis of alcohol abuse. In P. E. Nathan, G. A. Marlatt, & T. Loberg (Eds.), *Alcoholism: New directions in behavioral research and treatment*. New York: Plenum Press.

Caddy, G. R., Addington, H. J., & Perkins, D. (1978). Individualized behavior therapy for alcoholics: A third year independent double blind follow-up. *Behaviour Research and Therapy, 16*, 345–362.

Caddy, G. R., Goldman, R. D., & Huebner, R. (1976). Relationships among different domains of attitudes towards alcoholism: Model, cost and treatment. *Addictive Behaviors, 1*, 159–167. (a)

Caddy, G. R., Goldman, R. D., & Huebner, R. (1976). Group differences in attitudes towards alcoholism. *Addictive Behaviors, 1*, 281–286. (b)

Caddy, G. R., Addington, H. J., & Trenschel, W. R. (1984). *A comparative evaluation of aftercare technologies in the management of alcohol dependence*. Unpublished Manuscript.

Foy, D. W., Rychtarik, R. G., & Prue, D. M. (1981). Assessment of appetitive disorders. In

M. Hersen & A. S. Bellack (Eds.), *Behavioral assessment: A practical handbook* (2d ed.). New York: Pergamon Press.

Freinkel, N., & Arky, R. A. (1966). Effects of alcohol on carbohydrate metabolism in man. *Psychosomatic Medicine, 28,* 551–563.

Jacobson, G. R. (1975). *Diagnosis and assessment of alcohol abuse and alcoholism.* A report to the National Institute on Alcohol Abuse and Alcoholism. U.S. Department of Health, Education, and Welfare, Rockville, Maryland (DHEW Publication No. ADM 80-228).

Jellinek, E. M. (1960). *The disease concept of alcoholism.* New Haven, CT: Hillhouse Press.

Kerlan, M. W., Mortimer, R. G., Mudge, B., & Filkins, L. D. (June 1971). *Court procedures for identifying problem drinkers* (Vol. 1: Manual). Ann Arbor, MI: Highway Safety Research Institute, University of Michigan (U.S. Department of Transportation Publication No. DOT-HS-800-632).

MacAndrew, C. (1965). The differentiation of male alcoholic outpatients from non-alcoholic psychiatric outpatients by means of the MMPI. *Quarterly Journal of Studies on Alcohol, 26,* 238–246.

Mann, M. (1968). *New primer on alcoholism.* New York: Holt, Rinehart & Winston.

Manson, M. P. (1949). *The Alcadd Test.* Beverly Hills, CA: Western Psychological Service.

Marlatt, G. A. (1976). The Drinking Profile: A Questionnaire for the Behavioral Assessment of Alcoholism. In E. J. Mash & L. G. Terdal (Eds.), *Behavior therapy assessment: Diagnosis, design and evaluation* (pp. 121–137). New York: Springer.

Miller, P. E. (1977). Assessment of addictive behaviors. In A. R. Ciminero, H. Adams, & K. Calhoun (Eds.), *Handbook of behavioral assessment* (pp. 429–459). New York: Wiley.

Miller, W. R. (1976). Alcoholism scales and objective assessment methods: A review *Psychological Bulletin, 83,* 649–674.

National Council on Alcoholism. (1972). Criteria for the diagnosis of alcoholism. *American Journal of Psychiatry, 2,* 127–135.

Pattison, E. M., Sobell, M. B., & Sobell, L. L. (1977). (Eds.), *Emerging concepts of alcohol dependence.* New York: Springer.

Selzer, M. L. The Michigan Alcoholism Screening Test: The Quest for a New Diagnostic Instrument. (1971). *American Journal of Psychiatry, 127,* 1653–1658.

Siegler, M., Osmond, H., & Newell, S. (1968). Models of alcoholism. *Quarterly Journal of Studies on Alcoholism, 29,* 571–591.

Sobell, L. L., Sobell, M. B., & VanderSpek, R. (1979). Relationship between clinical judgement, self-report and breath analysis measures of intoxication in alcoholics. *Journal of Consulting and Clinical Psychology, 47,* 204–206.

Wanberg, K. W., & Knapp, J. (1970). A multidimensional model for the research and treatment of alcoholism. *The International Journal of the Addictions, 5,* 69–98.

Wanberg, K. W., Horn, J. L., & Foster, F. M. (September 1973). A differential model for the diagnosis of alcoholism: Scales of the Alcohol Use Questionnaire. Selected papers. *Proceedings of the General Session, Twenty Fourth Annual Meeting of the Alcohol and Drug Problems Association of North America, Bloomongton, Indiana.*

Chapter 8

Drug Abuse

Jesse B. Milby and Joseph A. Rice

Introduction

Diagnosing drug abuse and dependence is a task complicated by differences among people and the compounds used. Although acknowledging these multiple interactions, common behavior patterns and similarities in the development of a substance use disorder can be seen. These we refer to as stages in the abuse and dependence process. They need to be thoroughly understood by any clinician who seeks to do diagnostic interviewing.

Common Characteristics of Abuse and Dependence

Initiating Use

Reasons for initiating drug use vary with each person's interests, background, and motivation. There is no common etiological factor for all. Some do it for excitement, some respond to peer pressure, and others satisfy their curiosity or anticipate relief from tension. The World Health Organization (1974) has identified seven widely recognized motives for initiating use, and Dohner (1972) has described several others. The most significant phenomenon in first use is that the individual

JESSE B. MILBY and JOSEPH A. RICE • Veterans Administration Medical Center and Department of Psychiatry, University of Alabama, Birmingham, Alabama, 35294.

can be strongly reinforced for his or her initial involvement by the effects of the drug itself and/or social factors that encourage its repetition.

Increased Dosing and Tolerance

As drug use is repeated, various processes begin. One is *tolerance*, which refers to the decreased drug effects with repeated administration. Decreased drug effects lead to increased doses in order to experience the same effect. Thus, with repeated use, tolerance develops, and the dose increases.

Drug Preoccupation and Development of Drug-Seeking Behavior

With repeated drug use, *drug preoccupation* occurs. More time is spent fantasizing about the favorite drug and its effect. The preoccupation motivates the acquisition of new drug-seeking behaviors, including drug knowledge, skills, and language.

Drug Dependence

The next development is a move from drug abuse to dependence. With dependence there is a compulsive need or desire to obtain the drug in order to experience its effect. Many experts distinguish between two types of dependence: *psychic* and *physical*. Psychic dependence occurs where the effects of the drug are pleasing to the individual and a psychological drive develops that motivates the individual to continue using in order to produce pleasure or avoid discomfort. Physical dependence is an adaptive state of the body. It is manifested by physical disturbances when drug use is stopped, known as *withdrawal* or *abstinence* syndromes. Evidence of tolerance or a withdrawal syndrome is the diagnostic criterion for dependence (American Psychiatric Association, 1980, p. 165). There are no clear-cut signs that psychic dependence has developed, but there are several indications that can be used in making a valid and reliable assessment. One sign of dependence is the development of craving, which is a persistent hunger or need for the drug.

During prolonged dependence dose stabilization is likely. A dose plateau is reached, and dose increases level off. Often, abusers who achieve this "plateau" describe their use pattern as the amount of drug it takes to feel "normal," as they no longer strive for the initial drug effects. Another pattern in dependency involves periods of abstinence, during which the individual stops taking his or her primary drug. He or she may cease drug use altogether or only use drugs that prevent or minimize the withdrawal effects. It is important to note that many who are drug dependent at some time try to break their dependency, and this should be evident in their history. Abstinence may also be caused by other factors such as drug shortages, lack of money, incarceration, and the like. As there are periods of abstinence, there also are relapses. Many drug-dependent individuals demonstrate a repeated cycle of dependency and abstinence.

The unique characteristic of physical dependence is the abstinence syndrome, which occurs soon after the last dose. The syndrome's onset varies with the type of drug being used, but there are many signs and symptoms common to abstinence from various drugs. Typical common symptoms include headache, irritability, restlessness, cramps, nausea, vomiting, sweating, diarrhea, sleep disturbance, and nervousness. Because of this commonality, it is often difficult to determine which class of drug has been abused based solely on the abstinence signs and symptoms.

Characteristics Associated with Drug Acceptance and Drug Type

In addition to the previously mentioned patterns of behavior, there are those that are peculiar to types of drug use. Specifically, if the substance is illegal and must be obtained through "black market" strategies, an assortment of other characteristics develop.

One area of behavioral change is the erosion of nondrug interests. As the individual becomes physically dependent, he or she must devote increasing amounts of time to the procurement of the drug supply. This often leads to neglect or loss of interest in activities that may have once been important or rewarding. As this focus on purely drug-related areas increases, the individual usually senses a change in interest and as a result may experience a reduction in self-worth. This may manifest itself in reduced attention to personal hygiene, having poor diet and poor grooming.

If the individual is dependent on illegal drugs, there is a tendency for him or her to engage in other illegal activities in order to obtain drugs or the necessary funds to secure them. Common criminal activities include shoplifting, burglary, robbery, prostitution, and sale of illegal drugs. As a result of these activities, the addict becomes involved in the criminal subculture, and there is a higher probability that he or she will be arrested and incarcerated during his or her depencence history.

This brief overview of drug abuse patterns is meant to demonstrate the wide range of information that needs to be reviewed when making a diagnosis of substance abuse disorder and developing an intervention plan. It is important to understand the various stages of abuse and dependence and to attend to the variety of information that can determine a diagnosis and provide the basis for treatment planning. When assessing drug abuse, it is important to recognize other disorders that may be primary or secondary to a substance abuse disorder (McLellan, Woody, & O'Brien, 1979; McLellan, Luborsky, Woody, O'Brien, & Druley, 1983). Primary disorders are those from which other problems such as drug dependence presumably develop (Halikas & Rimmer, 1974). A good example is depression, where drug dependence may occur when the individual discovers chemical means to treat dysphoria (Robbins, 1974). Another is agoraphobia, where dependence on hypnotic sedatives may provide escape from intense anxiety and avoid panic attacks. Identifying these disorders has important implications for treatment. Primary disorders need to be addressed before or concurrent with the drug dependence and should be a major focus of intervention (Woody, McLellan, Luborsky, O'Brien, Beck, Blaine, Fox, Herman, & Beck, 1984).

Psychopathology can also be secondary to drug dependence. Family estrangement, antisocial behavior, legal difficulties, poor school or work performance, and low self-esteem often are problems that develop from drug dependence and are therefore secondary. These secondary problems imply a different treatment plan that focuses on the drug dependence and supports reestablishment of old adaptive behavior. Of course, drug dependence can be so entangled with other forms of psychopathology that it plays neither a clear primary nor secondary role. Unfortunately, there are no assessment instruments or procedures by which such inferences can be systematically and reliably derived. They depend on the clinician's judgment after sorting through information available. However, they are more likely to be valid and useful when the diagnostic interview follows the format and conceptual scheme suggested here.

Procedures for Gathering Information

Interview

The interview is the main diagnostic tool for assessing drug abuse and dependence. Interview content and strategy vary depending upon the goals of the interviewer and program. The interviewer may work in a screening clinic where referrals for further assessment and treatment are made. There, a good interview would determine the presence of a substance use disorder, what type, associated problems or hypotheses about problems, and treatment acceptable to the client. If the interviewer works in a treatment program and provides the main data base for treatment planning, this interview format must be extended. Additional phenomena, such as family conflict or support, depression, vocational functioning, legal difficulties, sources of current and likely future motivation for treatment should be discovered. Assessment should include positive client characteristics that intervention could build on. If the interview goal is screening and referral, the interview could terminate before gathering detailed information required to develop a treatment plan. Thus, we are recommending a similar diagnostic interview strategy for most sites that would vary only in its degree of focus and amount of detailed information collected. The strategy is analogous to a progressive screen designed to isolate finer and finer particles. The strategy is illustrated in Figure 1.

We recommend use of a structured interview that is guided by a written outline or series of questions in the form of a decision tree. Research has shown that structured interviews produce higher reliability probably by controlling information variance (Helzer, Clayton, Pambakian, & Woodruff, 1978; Hesselbrock, Stabenau, Hesselbrock, & Mirkin, 1982; Mintz, Christoph, O'Brien, & Snedeker, 1980). The interviewer should use this as a tool in a flexible manner so that digressions are made to follow up leads or get details important for treatment planning. When the assessment interview is broad, detailed enough to make finer discriminations among subtypes of psychopathology and non-drug-related problems, and idiographic, it is most likely to be valid and useful.

There are numerous studies that show low reliability and validity of psychiatric diagnoses, especially those derived from interview methods and based on the DSM-III classification scheme (Spitzer & Wilson, 1975). Though DSM-III shows improvement in reliability of diagnoses, its theoretical flaws, modest reliabilities, and often indeterminant validity have received severe criticism (Eysenck, Wakefield, & Friedman, 1983). However, over the last decade the reliability of psychiatric diagnoses has improved substantially, and there is now evidence of robust and clinically useful high levels of reliability usually obtained using structured interviews (Matarazzo, 1983).

In the assessment of substance use disorders, the more careful investigations show relatively good correspondence between interview findings and verifiable data. Inconsistencies seem to be due more to faulty memory and inaccurate police records than to deliberate deception (Amsel, Mendell, Matthias, Mason, & Hocherman, 1976; Bale, Von Stone, Engelsing, & Zarcone, 1981; Bonito, Nurco, & Shaffer, 1976; Cox & Longwell, 1974). When addicts have nothing to gain by giving false

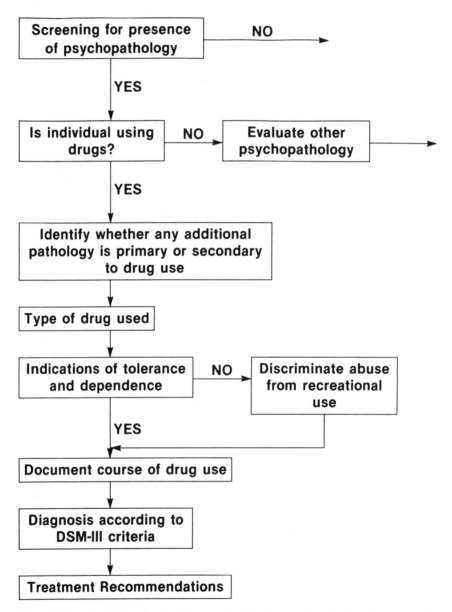

Figure 1. Flow chart of major decisions required in interviewing the drug abuse population.

information, know their records can be checked, and generally if the interviewer gives them no other reason to lie, they have been shown not to distort reports of their drug practices (Stephens, 1972). Though some sensitive material may be suppressed in the first interview, clinically useful and reliable information can even be obtained from court-appointed clients a few days after admission to treatment (Pompi & Schreiner, 1979).

The format for the interview process is presented in Table 1. The outline has been developed in order to assist the interviewer in gaining critical information necessary to make appropriate decisions. This interview strategy should then be integrated with the decision process illustrated in Figure 1, so that the interviewer can meet the goals of his or her respective agency or service.

Table 1. Interview Outline

Presenting complaint
1. Who referred client?
2. Client's view of problem.
3. Other's view of problem.
4. What does client want/expect from assessment and treatment?
General assessment
1. Mental Status Examination
2. Is there evidence for depression, personality or anxiety disorders, thought disorder, hallucinations, etc.?
3. Any indication of organic brain syndrome?
4. Does client report other diseases or disorders? If so, are they related to the drug problem, that is, back injury, chronic pain, and the like? Pursue any positive indications to preceding problems.
Type of drug
1. Identify current drugs used.
2. When was drug use initiated?
3. Amount and frequency of drug used over time.
4. Repeat preceding strategy for all past and present drugs used.
5. Any past periods of abstinence.
6. Past treatment attempts.
Assessing drug abuse
1. Assess client's work history pattern.
2. Assess interpersonal style including quantity and quality of friendships and family interaction.
3. Assess presence of legal difficulties over time.
4. Changes in client's use of free time in a productive and appropriate manner.
5. Assess the "typical" setting in which client uses drugs.
6. Assess indications of dependence—craving, withdrawal, and so forth.
7. Assess overdose history and determine if related to depression or manipulative behavior.
Diagnostic impression (DSM-III)
Treatment or referral recommendations

Presenting Complaint

As presented in Table 1, the first level of evaluation is a review of the presenting complaint. Why is the client presenting for evaluation? Many times clients are responding to some external factor (i.e., legal or family pressure, which may not concur with their own perceptions). Often, drug abusers do not view their drug use pattern as a "problem" yet readily admit to symptoms of anxiety or depression. It is especially important to recognize the existence of other forms of psychopathology that may be concurrent with the substance abuse behaviors. The interviewer must also understand the action of various drugs and their relation to presenting psychopathology. For example, depression may predate the use of drugs or be the result of drug action like amphetamines (McLellan et al., 1979; Robbins, 1974). These factors are critical in terms of assessing the type of drug abused and in the development of appropriate treatment strategies. It is imperative to view drug abuse within the framework of all psychopathologies and to determine which signs and symptoms are the dominant features of the client's adjustment. Whether drug use is primary or secondary to other pathology, the following interview strategy should be a valuable tool in understanding drug abuse behavior and its effects. These data can be collected by use of the mental status examination and questions aimed at detecting depression, anxiety, thought disorders, personality disorders, and organic brain syndromes. The significance of detecting such psychopathology will be to qualify any final diagnosis and to assist in the development of an appropriate treatment plan (McLellan et al., 1983; Woody et al., 1984).

Type of Drug

Once drug use has been identified, it is important to determine which ones have been and are currently used by the client. Clients often progress through use of various drugs, and a thorough drug history is invaluable. During this interview stage it is important to identify drug type, when drug use was initiated, frequency, usual dosage, and so forth. Simply focusing on the current drug of choice may lead to an erroneous assessment of a substance use disorder and inappropriate recommendation and treatment.

A thorough drug history provides information about duration of drug use, changes in dosages, changes in drug types, periods of self-induced abstinence, overdoses, previous treatment attempts, and so forth. In addition to identifying the major drugs of abuse, a drug history provides the first opportunity to document evidence of tolerance, degree of drug preoccupation, and dependence.

Assessing Drug Abuse

A client is considered to be abusing drugs when there is a pattern of pathological use, impairment in social or occupational functioning due to substance use, and the disturbance has lasted for a month or more (American Psychiatric Association, 1980). The goal is for the clinician to assess the degree of impact drug abuse has had on this client's life and level of functioning. Although often denying a "drug problem," many clients can accurately describe their irregular work history, interpersonal conflicts, and legal difficulties. As a result, the clinician should be attentive to reductions in normal social activities. The interview should also explore signs of dependence and an abstinence syndrome. For example, does the client experience "craving"? Does he or she manifest withdrawal signs when drug availability is blocked? Is daily use needed in order to feel "normal"? This focus is needed to determine the extent of dependence and/or dysfunction experienced as a result of drug use patterns.

Use of Assessment Instrument Results in Interviewing

Diagnostic interviewing can be enhanced by additional assessment techniques when results are available for the interview. The following methods are used in drug dependence treatment settings: self-report procedures, reports from significant others, direct observation, saliva, urine, and blood analyses, pharmacological procedures to assess tolerance and dependence, and psychometric procedures.

Self-report includes self-observation, log keeping, questionaires, rating scales, and checklists. A good example of this method is the Addiction Severity Index (McLellan, Luborsky, O'Brien, & Woody, 1980), which is a combined rating scale and structured interview using self-report data. *Reports from significant others* can provide important diagnostic information. They can corroborate self-report, provide new observations and historical detail, and provide important information about the role of relationship factors and the social support available during intervention. However, research has shown that significant others tend to underreport problems and be less aware of dysfunction than clients themselves (Rounsaville, Kleber, Wilber, Rosenberger, & Rosenberger, 1981). *Direct observation* is usually used in research or other special program settings. Observation of the client's appearance and behavior can provide valuable information. For a discussion of diagnostic implications of appearance and behavioral factors, see Milby (1981, pp. 40–61, p. 99) and Sapira (1968). *Saliva, urine, and blood analyses* can provide information on the type of drug dependence and validate self-report. Blood sampling is more invasive and costly and therefore infrequently used. *Pharmacological procedures* are used to assess tolerance and/or dependence on opioids and barbiturates/hypnotic sedatives. Opioid dependence may be indicated by administration of a narcotic antagonist that precipitates withdrawal symptoms. Tolerance may be determined by timed administration of standard drugs like methadone or pentobarbital until signs of intoxication appear. Because this procedure requires careful medical supervision, it is usually employed in a hospital. *Psychometric instruments* much as the Minnesota Multiphasic Personality Inventory (MMPI) are widely used as a screening instrument. They can be helpful in screening for complicating forms of psychopathology (e.g., depression and anxiety-mediated disorders). They also provide the interviewer with hypotheses regarding psychopathology and problems that must be addressed in treatment planning. These instruments can also be used to assess patient response to treatment.

Serial Interviewing

Diagnostic interviewing often involves several interviews over a span of days or weeks. Where interviewing is done in an inpatient detoxification and evaluation unit the clinician(s) often interview over a 1 to 2-week period. In a methadone maintenance program an interview is usually done to diagnose the presence and type of drug dependence so that chemotherapy may begin, that is, detoxification or maintenance. Further interviewing is usually carried out over subsequent days to get more detailed information in order to develop psychosocial aspects of the intervention plan.

We recommend serial diagnostic interviewing by more than one clinician if it is possible and consistent with program goals. Spreading the interview process out allows collection of supplemental data using methods previously described. It also allows clients to remember more relevant material and details and to become more objective in evaluating their strengths and problems. We have also found that serial interviewing, when it includes discovery of client strengths and development of realistic personal goals for treatment, increases self-efficacy and general motivation for treatment. To be useful, multiple interviews, especially by more than one clinician, require good record keeping and communication of findings between interviewers.

Case Illustrations

In this section case studies illustrating common diagnostic problems and our recommended interview strategy are provided. We also include excerpts of diagnostic interviews.

Case of Joan—Multiple Drug Dependence

Joan is a 32-year-old nurse who first presented for treatment after being arrested for forging prescriptions. She also had a long history of stealing Demerol from the hospitals in which she worked. She had been terminated from two positions and lost her license as a result of these activities. The court offered her the opportunity to participate in a supervised treatment program with progress monitored by the court system.

I: How did the hospital find out about the drugs?

P: I wrote a script, which I've done before. But, I wrote a script and I went to a pharmacist I didn't know. He called. I don't know why I did that. I just got to the point where I don't think I much cared one way or the other. Yeah, I didn't really care. I did think that I knew I couldn't ever get away with it for obvious reasons. I knew it was a matter of time.

I: How else were you getting the Demerol other than prescriptions?

P: I had nurses on the team. They brought it to me for menstrual pain and I'd do it every once in a while. And then when I got on a floor where I had tons of it I started walking off with it—couldn't waste it. Then it got to where it wasn't just the waste, it was, you know, if you were going to give 50, instead of taking out 50, you'd sign up for a 100 and waste 50 and take—you'd give the patient 50 and take the other 50. Then it got to where I was signing out when nobody wanted it. It just got worse and worse and worse. And then your tolerance gets such that it takes more. And my tolerance was high to start with, which didn't help. But I was only doing it at home.

I: You were only taking it at home?

P: I never did it at work. Never did. I don't think I could have functioned on it. For one thing, I don't—some people like to take Demerol and then run up and down the hall and work. I don't. I like to keep laid back. Can't do that at work.

I: How much were you using?

P: I was taking home 800, 900 miligrams at a time which really isn't that—that's a lot I guess for some people. It's not for somebody that's doing it all the time. I did it most every day. When I was off work I didn't do it. Had a couple days off, I didn't do it. Which was almost enough to make me want to go back to work, just to get it. I was doing like 2 or 300 milligrams I.V. when I got home, and then I'd do another 2 or 3 a little later in the evening. I was doing it like that. I was doing a lot at once. Tolerance got so that I was—most of the time I didn't want to do it unless I had at least 350 miligrams. Because I didn't want to just be mellowed out a little. I wanted to be really out of it.

Based on this information, it is clear that Joan was opioid dependent although denying having experienced withdrawal. During the interview Joan casually mentioned use of alcohol and other drugs that needed to be pursued.

I: You mentioned drinking a lot before you began nursing school. How much were you drinking back then?
P: Well, it got to the point, before I started nursing school, where I was drinking all night, 3 or 4 nights a week. I don't know how much alcohol. I spent a lot of money. It was nothing for me to drink a fifth or two, you know. But it wasn't affecting me as much. Then I got to the point where I wasn't remembering what I did. That's when I'd start getting in trouble.
I: When was that?
P: Oh, about '76, '77, and then I almost totally quit. People started telling me about the weird things I was doing and I couldn't remember doing it.
I: Like what?
P: Mainly hostility. People trying to get me to quit drinking and go home and I'd get nasty, which was a little bit out of character at that time. I didn't believe them. At first I didn't believe them but so many people said something to me about it, I said they can't all be wrong. So I just quit. And part of it, I hated my job, you know—but I loved drinking, I really loved it.
I: What were you drinking?
P: Everything. I switched around a lot. I'd mix it up.
I: Mostly liquor or wine?
P: Liquor. Always liquor. But it got to the point where it scared me a little bit, so I just quit, and decided to go back to school. I'd still drink like if I went out to eat or I'd meet somebody for happy hour and have a couple drinks, go eat dinner, and I'd have a couple more. But it wasn't anything like that—I didn't get drunk. I've been drinking since I was 17. More of a binge drinker though now. It's like, it's an occasional thing, if I do it, I do it all night or I don't do it at all. There's no such thing as one or two anymore. So I just don't do it because the hangovers are so bad. I don't know if it's age or if it's my body is just tired of it. The drinking's not worth the hangover. They were that bad.

In the following excerpt the interviewer is assessing Joan's mood and the possibility that depression and low self-esteem are contributing to the drug dependence. One question provides a cascade of important information.

I: During your drug abuse history how would you describe your mood usually?
P: It varies. I go through periods of depression. It's related to—probably just to things that I've done to myself. It all started, I think, at a young age. I got out of high school, I was very straight, religious, all the way through high school.

Typical Baptist background. No sex, no drugs, no nothing, very strict background. When I got out of high school, everybody went haywire, all my friends went nuts. I waited about a year after they did to do the same thing and got married. Then, I think it was a combination of being divorced, sleeping with my boyfriend, and drinking and doing all these things I was taught not to do and not feeling particularly good about it. And when my self-esteem went down, I went into a depression and stayed there. And didn't know what to do about it. And didn't do anything about it. Instead of changing my life-style, I kept doing the same old things that just reinforced the low self-esteem. It just got worse, and when I first did all of the drugs that summer, LSD and all that, it was right in the middle of the worse period of depression that I had gone through ever, and I didn't particularly care whether I lived or died. So, naturally, I'd do anything. It was a relief, you know. The MDA [Methylendioxyamphetamine] was a relief because on MDA you really can't give a hang about anything. It's impossible to care. As a matter of fact, I felt really good on it. It scared me. I felt so good on it, I didn't ever want to be straight again. That's when I wanted to stay off on MDA all the time, which I knew was not possible. We would have ended up in jail sooner or later because in order to do that amount of drugs, you've gotta deal, and sooner or later you end up in jail, and I didn't want him in jail. So we quit the drugs, got married, went back to work and did alright except for drinking. The main problem with the drinking was on weekends. It was your typical, you know, married couple living in an apartment, working 5 days a week, getting drunk on Friday and Saturday.

Joan actually was admitted to a hospital and treated with ECT for depression over a 3-week period when she was 22.

This is a good case history because it is typical of the kind of substance use disorders currently extant. Joan abused a variety of substances, hallucinogens, alcohol, and opioids. She was probably dependent upon all of them at different times in her life. She also experienced several different problems that contributed to her substance use disorder, two of which were probably primary: personality disorder and depression. Additionally, family and marital conflict, low self-esteem, job-related stress, and sex-role confusion all contributed to her difficulties, added to her stress level and depression, and increased her motivation for Demerol use that provided escape.

Diagnostic Impression. Two diagnostic impressions are offered for this case. One uses the DSM-III format, which is more useful for epidemiological and general treatment planning purposes. The second is more descriptive of the problems noted, not useful for epidemiological purposes, but more useful for specific treatment planning. The second diagnostic description is included at the beginning of "Referral Recommendations" noted after "Diagnostic Impression." The DSM-III diagnoses are:

- Axis I: 1. 304.01, Opioid dependence, continuous
             2. 303.91, Alcohol dependence, continuous
             3. 305.32, Methylenedioxyomphetamine (MDA) abuse, episodic
- Axis II: 301.83, Borderline personality disorder
- Axis III: None
- Axis IV: 5, Severity of psychosocial stressors, severe
- Axis V: 5, Highest level of adoptive functioning postyear, poor

Referral Recommendations. In addition to the aforementioned diagnoses, it should be noted that Joan has fundamental problems regarding her identity. Her sense of self-worth is extremely low and probably needs further assessment. It is likely that she has insufficient intrinsic criteria for her self-worth; that is, extrinsic criteria predominate and thus could become a major focus in her treatment plan. Additionally, she may have poor gender identity. She has felt attracted to, emotionally bonded to, and supported by a relationship with another woman. Her relationships with men, though sexually satisfying, were not gratifying emotionally or supportive of her sense of self-worth. This is a second major domain for a treatment plan and development of personal goals. Another major problem, related to the two previously mentioned, is periodic depression. During these periods she is most vulnerable to exploitation in quickly developed, intense but shallow relationships, and these are the periods when she is also at risk for substance abuse and dependence. Thus, the treatment plan should include understanding, prevention, or more effective coping with such moods.

Knowing resources and limitations imposed by the court referral, the following specific treatment recommendations were made:

1. Referral to the outpatient drug dependence treatment programs.
2. Monthly, detailed reports to probation officer including results of random urinalyses conducted weekly.
3. Individual therapy with the most experienced and trained therapist available to develop a therapeutic alliance and work toward ameliorating the problems noted previously via establishment of stepwise personal goals.
4. Group therapy to explore personal self-worth, difficulty in relationships with men, and gender identity issues. The general strategy here would be to gain self-understanding and self-acceptance. Secondarily, this group could meet some of her needs for emotional closeness so that she could take risks in developing healthier intimate relationships outside the group with both men and women.

Case of Peter—Cocaine Abuse

Peter is a 22-year-old male presenting himself to a mental health clinic that does not specialize in drug problems. His initial concern is due to long-standing interpersonal difficulties. In addition to much subjective distress in social situations, Peter also admits to regular recreational use of cocaine. In this excerpt, the interviewer is trying to establish the role drug use serves in Peter's life.

I: Could you explain when you usually use cocaine?

P: Well, I use it only once in awhile. You know it's real expensive. I guess I get it every couple of weeks.

I: When do you usually use it?

P: Well, usually I do it alone. I really don't want anybody to know about it, especially my girlfriend. But when I'm feeling real down or bothered I'll start thinking about doing some coke, and I'll try to get some. It makes me feel so good. I guess it just gets me away from all the crap.

I: You mentioned that you use cocaine about once every 2 weeks. What made you choose that rate:

P: Money! I guess I've spent maybe $3,000 on it over the past year or so. Usually, what happens is I get some lump of money, you know, like a student loan check, or I'll work for a couple weeks during vacations, and then I'll start buying some.

I: What happens during those times when you have no money coming in?

P: Well, then I just go without for awhile. If I really feel bad, then I can usually get some money from my folks or somebody, and then I'll get a little.

I: Have you ever had times when you were out of money and you had a strong desire to do some cocaine?

P: Well, just lately. I've been trying to stop using it, and I'm trying to make my relationship with Linda work out. Well, as you know, things have not been so good between us, and I sometimes really feel I need a break. I've been thinking about getting some coke a lot lately. I've been feeling real down. I'm scared that Linda is not going to need me anymore. I really want to get away from all this mess.

I: You mentioned that you have felt this way before. What did you do before you started using cocaine?

P: Well, when I was in high school I was a real loner. I mean I didn't have any friends, and, you know, Linda is the first girl I've ever really gone out with. So, anyway, I got into camping and stuff. I took some survival training and learned how to live in the woods for weeks without any supplies, people, or anything. It's funny, when I came back out of the woods I felt different. I could talk to people, and I felt good. I mean it was something I could do all by myself and I liked it. That would last a little while; then I would feel depressed and lonely, so I would go back into the woods. I haven't been out in a year and now I am afraid I've lost all my skill. I don't think I could make it anymore.

In this interview, it is becoming clear that Peter's periodic use of cocaine is serving as relief for his feelings of depression and insecurity. Further interviewing revealed he is not experiencing severe forms of pathological use, but cocaine is clearly being used to cope with depression and distress. During the past 2 years this drug use has replaced a somewhat more adaptive mechanism, that is, survival camping. His recreational use of cocaine has moved to more compulsive use that is beginning to interfere with the relationship with his girlfriend and to cause him financial difficulties. He is also making increased efforts to exert control but has not effectively controlled his use. Thus, this case illustrates the use of an interview to discriminate recreational use from a diagnosed drug abuse, DSM-III 305.62 Cocaine abuse. The case also illustrates how drug abuse can be diagnosed via interview in a treatment facility that does not specialize in screening, referral, and treatment for drug abuse and dependence.

Case of Carl—Amphetamine Dependence

Carl is a 34-year-old white male who has a high school education and is employed as a diesel mechanic for a large trucking firm. He has recently divorced, and his two children are living with his ex-wife. He is living with his mother. He obtained this job 3 years ago, and it represented an opportunity to significantly raise his income because of higher wages and many opportunities for overtime. Since that time he has raised his income substantially, but his long work hours away from the family, his irritability, and aggressive behavior associated with job stresses have contributed to his marital conflict and subsequent divorce. Since his divorce he has worked even longer hours, felt more lonely, withdrawn, and depressed.

He has had stomach symptoms, insomnia, reduced appetite, and weight loss of 15 lb without intent over the past 3 months. These symptoms reported in the first interview caused him to be admitted to a VA psychiatric hospital with the admission diagnosis of nonpsychotic depression. The excerpt is from a second interview conducted by another staff member and thus illustrates the technique and results of serial interviewing. The interviewer had read the admission note describing the preceding and had briefly discussed the case with the staff person who admitted him. The interviewer's objective was to explore reasons for marital conflict, causes of depression, and to check out the possibility of alcoholism and drug use.

I: You sure have been through a lot lately, Carl. What do you think contributed to your divorce?

P: Work mostly. Long hours, you know, and not spending time with my wife and family. Sarah was getting frustrated with me cause I was never home to help with anything.

I: When you were home, how did you get along?

P: Not so good. She would need help with chores and things, or would ask me to do something with the kids, and I would get irritated with her. She would make me real mad and I'd holler and swear. I also would beat the kids too hard because they'd be so loud and stuff. I slapped her a few times, too, didn't mean to, but I'd just get so mad. I was real irritable because I wasn't sleeping well and I was working a lot of overtime.

I: How did you keep going without much sleep and having to work overtime?

P: Well, one of the mechanics would get some Benzedrine from one of the drivers, and we'd both take them to stay awake and get the jobs done.

I: When did you start to use Benzedrine, Carl?

P: About 3 years ago. Billy and I started working together about 6 months after I began working there, and he started offering them to me. After a while, I started getting "Bennies" for myself, and we started using more and more. We could stay awake and work like a son of a bitch. After a while we got a reputation for really cranking out the work, and our boss would ask us to do more and more special jobs on o.t. We could flat do some work. But we got to the point where we had to take the Bennies to keep up the pace, you know.

I: How many did you have to take to keep going?

P: Well, at first one was enough for me, but Billy would keep taking a couple more during the shift, and I started taking more too. Maybe four to five during the whole 14-hour shift. But just before my divorce I was eating them like candy. They was messing me up too.

I: How did they mess you up?

P: Well, they started messing up my mind. I'd get real irritated and suspicious of everything. I'd start thinking Billy was messing with my tools, and I got into it with him a few times. Then I got to thinking Sarah was stepping out on me when I was working. A couple of times I started hearing voices talking to me, and it scared the shit out of me. I thought I was going crazy. Then I started to really worry about that and I got down. I'd get so bad I'd want to be left alone all weekend and stay in the bedroom. I'd sleep all weekend. I'd even eat in there. Get Sarah to fix me a tray. I was sorry, I'll tell ya.

Further interviewing established that at the end of his first year on his new job, amphetamine use was routine, and in the following year use increased to the point where his wife complained about his abuse and the effects the drug had—his sleep disturbance, irritability, and aggressiveness. In spite of his wife's complaints, his realization that Benzedrine use was causing him difficulty, and his efforts to cut back his use, his abuse continued. The year before his admission for treatment, he showed extensive abuse, and had repeated conflict with his wife who left him for brief periods several times, two of which involved episodes of psychotic paranoid behavior. Prior to his admission he reported eating Benzedrine tablets like candy during the week and then "crashing" and sleeping the whole weekend and starting the pattern again the next week whether or not he had to work overtime.

Admission to treatment was motivated by a warning from his employer to get help or be fired and by repeated urging of his ex-wife to get help and his hope that he might get back together with her. He also stated that he did not tell the staff member who did screening about his drug use because he was afraid he would be rejected for treatment or referred elsewhere.

This case is interesting for several reasons. Carl presented for screening to a general psychiatric facility. During screening he was anxious, dysphoric, tearful, and emphasized his recent divorce and sense of loss of his family with consequent loneliness. He reported he was trying to cope with his loss by working and volunteering for overtime so he could lose himself in his work. He also complained of sleep disturbance, weight loss over the past 6 months, and decreased appetite. The screening diagnostic impression was depression based on the classic symptoms he reported. However, during his first week of admission, serial interviewing revealed the primary role of amphetamine abuse in causing his marital conflict and classic depressive symptoms. More importantly, serial interviewing uncovered the central role of work for his sense of self-esteem and the basic feelings of inadequacy in most other areas of life. Demands of family responsibility for intimacy and increased socialization from his wife made him feel more inadequate. These challenges to his self-esteem were met by doing more of what he could do best (i.e., work and earn more money). Serial diagnostic interviewing thus yielded a more complete assessment of this man. It sorted out multiple problems and discovered the primary personality disorder and the role of amphetamine abuse in his depressive symptoms and divorce. Thus, serial diagnostic interviewing yielded the most complete and accurate assessment from which a strategic treatment plan was derived.

Critical Information Required to Make Diagnosis and Recommendations

Although we think all of the information recommended here is important for a thorough assessment, certain information is critical for making an accurate diagnosis and useful referral. This information falls into three categories: (a) concurrent psychiatric symptoms and disorders; (b) detailed chronological drug abuse history; and (c) what recommendations for treatment the client is willing to accept and implement.

The most common error made in diagnostic interviewing of drug abusers is the failure to assess concurrent psychiatric and physical disorders. If the substance use disorder is accurately diagnosed but concurrent anxiety or depressive disorders remain unrecognized, the diagnostic interview has failed. Thus, we consider making an accurate diagnosis to include concurrent psychiatric disorders and associated physical disorders. Drug abusers often have common physical disorders, which, if they remain undetected and untreated, can be a hazard to the patient and severely interfere with drug abuse treatment (Sapira,

1968). If the interviewer does not have the required expertise to assess physical disorders associated with drug abuse disorders, appropriate referral should be part of the routine for initial interviewing for substance use disorders.

The second critical domain, sometimes neglected in assessing drug abusers, is the detailed chronology of drug abuse development. This information helps discriminate the polydrug-dependent person currently abusing opioids, from the opiate addict who rarely uses other substances. The careful chronological history can detect the opioid addict who is also addicted to alcohol and even the addict who maintains a dual addiction to opioids and barbiturates/hypnotic sedatives. This history can also identify the client at risk for overdose death.

The third kind of critical information seems obvious, but perhaps for that reason it is sometimes ignored or assumed without direct assessment. What treatment is the client willing to accept? What treatment referral is the client most likely to implement (i.e., appear for the initial appointment and become engaged in the treatment offered?). In order to obtain useful information in this area, the client's motivation for treatment must be addressed. Also, where appropriate, treatment choices must be explained and the client involved in the referral process. For example, though the client may meet criteria for referral to a therapeutic community, he or she may wish to maintain his or her job. Referral to a therapeutic community would probably be futile.

Some Practical Do's and Don'ts for Interviewing Drug Abusers

Some practical recommendations for increasing the accuracy and usefulness of the interview are listed next.

Do assess the client's motivation for treatment, especially the court-referred client. If this is not assessed, or if wrong conclusions are derived, the usefulness of other interview data may be wasted. Important here is to determine the source and intensity of motivation. Is motivation intrinsic or extrinsic? Is it based on inner factors of dissatisfaction or wanting to improve current status, or is it based on pressure from the court to engage in treatment or suffer immediate incarceration. Timing of presentation for admission often indicates initial motivation. Did the client recently lose his or her job? Is the client under pressure from family or spouse?

Usually, whatever motivation is present can be enhanced by the interviewer emphasizing choices, options, and responsibility for treatment decisions. This tends to build motivation for active participation in the interview process and subsequent treatment. Client motivation can also be enhanced by including an assessment of strengths. This can help devise more realistic treatment plans, but it can also build client self-respect and intrinsic motivation.

Do use a structured interview format. The research clearly shows structured interviews produce the highest reliability and most accurate data (Matarazzo, 1983; Mintz et al., 1980).

Do assess the efficacy and usefulness of the interviewing process. Monitor the accuracy of diagnoses by doing occasional dual interviews or comparing information gathered via serial interviewing by different staff. Request feedback from programs receiving your referrals. It is useful to obtain data on referral show rates, accuracy of referral diagnoses, and viability of recommendations.

Do not assume that drug abuse or dependence is the main or only problem of a client presenting for substance use disorder treatment. Depression, anxiety, and personality disorders are prevalent in this group. Clients for whom these and other critical problems are not addressed are prime candidates for treatment failure (McLellan, Moody, Luborsky, O'Brien, & Druley, 1982). However, when these concurrent problems are identified and treatment plans implemented to address them, results are much better (McLellan et al., 1983).

Do not assume that laboratory data are correct when there is a disparity between self-report and laboratory data (Bernadt, Mumford, Taylor, Smith, & Murray, 1982). Self-report data usually are fairly accurate except for historical details or where there is an obvious reason for distorting certain information (i.e., illegal activities of a client who is court referred). Unless these circumstances prevail, the assumption that laboratory data are correct can interfere with rapport between the client and the interviewer or other staff and negatively effect the assessment and referral process.

Establishing a differential diagnosis is not easy. Building rapport, motivation for treatment, and developing a realistic and effective treatment plan is not easy. If reliable and valid differential diagnoses are the only products of the interview process when a treatment plan is needed, the interview is not working. The main point here is that the diagnostic interview is a critical phase in referral and intervention. If it is done poorly, the client may never return. It is important enough to command the attention of the most experienced and competent clinicians. It is also important enough to carefully evaluate and use feedback to improve the process.

Summary

This chapter has given a brief overview of common characteristics of abuse and dependence that need to be understood in order to do good diagnostic interviewing. These characteristics include initiating use, increased dosing, tolerance, drug preoccupation, development of drug-seeking behavior, and patterns of behavior dependent upon societal acceptance of the drug and its type.

In addition to careful attention to a structured interview, its strategies, and format, we have also reviewed other procedures for gathering information that can supplement the diagnostic interview: self-report data sources, reports from significant others, direct observation, saliva, urine, and blood analyses, pharmacological procedures, and psychometrics. We strongly recommend use of serial interviewing. Several cases were discussed to illustrate recommended strategies and procedures. Critical information required to make a diagnosis and recommendations were reviewed. Practical *do's* and *don'ts* for interviewing drug abusers were recommended. Last, the importance of the diagnostic interview was underlined, and evaluation of its utility was recommended.

References

American Psychiatric Association. (1980). *Diagnostic and statistical manual of mental disorders*, (3rd ed., pp. 163–165). Washington, DC: Author.

Amsel, Z., Mendell, W., Matthias, L., Mason, C., & Hocherman, I. (1976). Reliability and validity of self-reported illegal activities and drug use collected from narcotic addicts. *International Journal of the Addictions, 11,*(2), 325–336.

Bale, R. N., Von Stone, W. W., Engelsing, T. M. J., Zarcone, V. P. Jr. & Kuldan, J. M. (1981). The validity of self-reported heroin use. *International Journal of the Addictions, 16,*(8), 1307–1398.

Bernadt, M. W., Mumford, J., Taylor, C., Smith, B., & Murray, R. M. (1982, February 6). Comparison of questionaire and laboratory tests in the detection of excessive drinking and alcoholism. *The Lancet,* pp. 325–328.

Bonito, A. J., Nurco, D. N., & Shaffer, J. W. (1976). The verdicality of addicts' self-reports in social research. *International Journal of the Addictions, 11*(5), 719–724.

Cox, T. J., & Longwell, B. (1974). Reliability of interview data concerning current heroine use from heroin addicts on methadone. *International Journal of the Addictions, 9*(1), 161–165.

Dohner, V. A. (1972). Motives for drug use: Adult and adolescent. *Psychosomatics, 13,* 317–324.

Eysenck, H. J., Wakefield, J. A., & Friedman, A. F. (1983). Diagnosis and clinical assessment: The DSM-III. In M. R. Rosenzweig & L. W. Porter (Eds.), *Annual review of psychology* (pp. 167–193). Palo Alto, CA: Annual Reviews.

Halikas, J. A., & Rimmer, J. D. (1974). Predictors of multiple drug abuse. *Archives of General Psychiatry, 81,* 414–418.

Hesselbrock, V., Stabenau, J., Hesselbrock, M., & Mirkin, M. (1982). A comparison of two interview schedules. *Archives of General Psychiatry, 39,* 674–677.

Helzer, J. E., Clayton, P. J., Pambakian, R., & Woodruff, R. A. (1978). concurrent diagnostic validity of a structured psychiatric interview. *Archives of General Psychiatry, 35,* 849–853.

Matarazzo, J. D. (1983). The reliability of psychiatric and psychological diagnosis. *Clinical Psychology Review, 3*, 103–145.

McLellan, A. T., Woody, G. E., & O'Brien, C. P. (1979). Development of psychiatric illness in drug abusers: Possible role of drug preference. *New England Journal of Medicine, 301*, 1310–1314.

McLellan, A. T., Luborsky, L., O'Brien, C. P., & Woody, G. E. (1980). An improved diagnostic instrument for substance abuse patients: The Addiction Severity Index. *Journal of Nervous and Mental Disease, 168*, 26–33.

McLellan, A. T., Woody, G. E., Luborsky, L., O'Brien, C. P., & Druley, K. A. (1982). Is treatment for substance abuse effective? *Journal of the American Medical Association, 247*, 1423–1427.

McLellan, A. T., Luborsky, L., Woody, G. E., O'Brien, C. P., & Druley, K. A. (1983). Predicting response to alcohol and drug abuse treatments: Role of psychiatric severity. *Archives of General Psychiatry, 40*, 620–625.

Milby, J. B. (1981). *Addictive behavior and its treatment.* New York: Springer.

Mintz, J., Christoph, P., O'Brien, C. P. & Snedeker, M. (1980). The impact of the interview method on reported symptoms of narcotic addicts. *International Journal of the Addictions, 15*(4), 597–604.

Pompi, K. F., & Shreiner, S. C. (1979). The reliability of biographical information obtained from court-stipulated clients newly admitted to treatment. *American Journal of Drug and Alcohol Abuse, 6*(1), 79–95.

Robins, P. R. (1974). Depression and drug addiction. *Psychiatric Quarterly, 48*(3), 374–386.

Rounsaville, B. J., Kleber, H. D., Wilber, C., Rosenberger, D., & Rosenberger, P. (1981). Comparison of opiate addict's reports of psychiatric history with reports of significant other informants. *American Journal of Alcohol Abuse, 8*, 51–69.

Sapira, J. D. (1968). The narcotic addict as a medical patient. *American Journal of Medicine, 45*, 555–587.

Spitzer, R. L., & Wilson, P. T. (1975). Classification in psychiatry. In A. M. Freedman, H. I. Kaplan, & B. J. Saddock (Eds.), *Comprehensive textbook of psychiatry,* (Vol. 1, 2d ed., pp. 826–850). Baltimore: Williams & Wilkins.

Stephens, R. (1972). The truthfulness of addict respondents in research projects. *International Journal of the Addictions, 7*, 549–558.

Woody, G. E., McLellan, A. T., Luborsky, L., O'Brien, C. P., Blaine, J., Fox, S., Herman, I., & Beck, A. T. (1984). Severity of psychiatric symptoms as a predictor of benefits from psychotherapy: The Veterans Administration–Penn study. *American Journal of Psychiatry, 141*, 1172–1177.

World Health Organization Expert Committee on Drug Dependence. (1974). *Twentieth report.* Geneva: Author.

Chapter 9

Sexual Dysfunctions and Deviations

Linda J. Skinner and Judith V. Becker

Introduction

Although interest in sexuality is as old as the human race, several significant changes have occurred during the last 35 years that have greatly impacted on mental health professionals' perception of and approach to sexuality.

During this time, research on human sexual functioning has become "respectable" and has increased geometrically, with the result that our knowledge and understanding of sexuality has undergone rapid growth. Second, sexuality has been taken out of the closet. Not only is discussion of sexuality open today, but also satisfactory sexual functioning has become a goal actively sought by both males and females. Finally, as a result of the two previous changes, sex therapy has become an independent therapeutic specialty.

Today more than ever before, mental health professionals are seeing patients seeking treatment in response to dissatisfaction with their sexual functioning. Such dissatisfaction most commonly stems from a sexual dysfunction, but may also be the result of a sexual deviation or the sexual variation of ego dystonic homosexuality. The purpose of this chapter is to offer guidelines for conducting a diagnostic interview with patients whose presenting complaints focus on sexual functioning.

LINDA J. SKINNER • Department of Psychology, University of Hartford, West Hartford, Connecticut 06117.   JUDITH V. BECKER • New York State Psychiatric Institute, New York, New York 10032.

Sexual Dysfunctions

A major category of psychosexual disorders is that of *sexual dysfunctions*. These disorders may interfere with the appetitive phase or the psychophysiological changes characterizing the excitement, orgasm, or resolution phases of the sexual response cycle. However, inhibition in the resolution phase generally is not clinically significant.

Usually a sexual dysfunction is characterized by disturbance in both the subjective sense of pleasure and objective performance. Although most of the dysfunctions first appear in early adult life, patients do not typically seek clinical intervention until in their late 20s or early 30s. The two exceptions to these general observations are premature ejaculation, which frequently begins with initial sexual experience, and inhibited sexual excitement in the male, which commonly has an onset later in adult life.

All sexual dysfunctions can be described in relation to three dimensions. A dysfunction may be lifelong (primary) or acquired (secondary). The lifelong dysfunction appears when an individual first engages in sexual activity, whereas the onset of an acquired dysfunction is after an individual experiences a period of normal sexual functioning. Second, a dysfunction may also be generalized or present in all sexual situations, or it may be situational or specific to particular situations or partners. For example, a woman may be orgasmic with penile-vaginal intercourse but not as a result of oral sex. Finally, a dysfunction may be classified as total or partial. That is, functioning may be completely absent, or it may be reduced in terms of degree or frequency of disturbance.

Although sexual dysfunctions most frequently are manifested in sexual interactions with another person, they may also be present during masturbation. The course of a sexual dysfunction is highly variable. However, these disorders typically do not result in impairment in overall social functioning.

Prior to a discussion of the procedures for conducting a sexual problem history, the seven sexual dysfunctions included in the *Diagnostic and Statistical Manual of Mental Disorders* (American Psychiatric Association [APA], 1980) will be reviewed.

The Nature of Sexual Dysfunctions

Inhibited Sexual Desire. An individual who complains of having no interest in initiating or participating in sexual activity may be given the new DSM-III diagnosis of inhibited sexual desire. It must be stressed, however, that a lack of sexual desire is not clinically significant unless the individual reports being distressed by the condition. Similarly, the fact that an individual engages in sexual activity does not rule out this diagnosis as some individuals with inhibited sexual desire are sexual on occasion and may, in fact, experience sexual arousal.

This diagnosis is warranted if the inhibition of desire is persistent and pervasive and is not caused exclusively by psychiatric or organic disorders. Frequently an individual experiences inhibited sexual desire in conjunction with or as a consequence of one or more of the other sexual dysfunctions. Both males and females may experience this dysfunction.

Inhibited Sexual Excitement. Previously known as *impotence* in males and *frigidity* in females, inhibited sexual excitement is a dysfunction that is characterized by a recurrent and persistent lack of sexual excitement during sexual activity. Erectile difficulties or difficulties with vaginal lubrication and swelling are the diagnostic symptoms for this dysfunction. Before this diagnosis is given, the clinician must determine that the patient engages in sexual activity that is adequate to induce excitement in an individual and that the lack of excitement is not the result exclusively of psychiatric or organic factors.

Inhibited Female Orgasm. The dysfunction *inhibited female orgasm* is characterized by a persistent and recurrent pattern in which a woman does not experience an orgasm subsequent to adequate sexual stimulation and excitement or experiences a delayed orgasm following such stimulation and excitement. This diagnosis is sometimes given in conjuction with inhibited sexual excitement but should not be given if the condition is caused exclusively by psychiatric and organic factors.

Inhibited Male Orgasm. The dysfunction *inhibited male orgasm* is characterized by a delay or absence of orgasm once an erection occurs. It is sometimes found in connection with inhibited sexual excitement. If the condition is exclusively caused by an organic or psychiatric problem, this diagnosis is not appropriate.

Premature Ejaculation. Previously called *impotence,* premature ejaculation is a dysfunction that consists of a persistent and recurrent absence of adequate voluntary control of the ejaculatory response. Typically, the man who is troubled by premature ejaculation is capable of participating in a wide variety of sexual activities but loses ejaculatory control shortly after intercourse begins. This dysfunction is one of the most frequent problems seen in sex therapy clinics (Kaplan, 1974).

Despite the considerable discussion focusing on this issue, no concensus has been reached concerning the definition of prematurity (Kaplan, 1974; LoPiccolo, 1977; Masters & Johnson, 1970). However, a general rule of thumb used by many clinicians is that premature ejaculation exists when the rapidity of ejaculation is reported by the couple to be problematic to their sexual relationship. If the couple feels that the rapidity of ejaculation is not diminishing the quality of their sexual activities, then this diagnosis is not warranted. Additionally, psychiatric and organic factors as the exclusive causes of the condition must first be eliminated before the use of this diagnosis is appropriate.

Functional Dyspareunia. Sometimes called *painful intercourse,* functional dyspareunia refers to recurrent and persistent genital pain during coitus. The onset of the pain can occur anytime from at the start of intercourse until after completion. Although both males and females may experience dyspareunia, it is unusual in males. This diagnosis is not warranted if the condition results exclusively from organic or psychiatric factors. Similarly, if the pain is symptomatic of a lack of lubrication or vaginismus, this diagnosis should not be given.

Functional Vaginismus. A comparatively uncommon problem, functional vaginismus is diagnosed when a woman experiences involuntary contractions of the muscles, primarily the bulbocavernosus and leviator ani muscles, surrounding the outer one-third of the vaginal barrel (Silny, 1980). Interfering with sexual activity, these spasms of the vaginal musculature make penetration by the penis, or even a finger, painful or impossible. This dysfunction is not necessarily related to inhibited desire, excitement, or orgasm, as evidence by the observation that many women with vaginismus enjoy sex and are desirous of intercourse (Kolodny, Masters, & Johnson, 1979). Although a history of having problems using a tampon or a diaphragm may be suggestive of vaginismus, this diagnosis cannot be made with certainty without a pelvic examination and until organic and psychiatric factors have been ruled out as the exclusive causes. There is no sexual dysfunction analogous to vaginismus in males.

General Interviewing Procedures in the Assessment of Sexual Dysfunctions

Rather than using one of the numerous paper-and-pencil instruments that have been developed for assessing sexual function (Schiavi, Derogatis, Kuriansky, O'Connor, & Sharpe, 1979), we prefer conducting a problem-oriented sexual history when working with patients referred as a result of apparent sexual problems. Whereas a general sexual history entails obtaining a complete history of an individual's sexual development and activities, the focus of a problem-oriented sexual history is limited to the problems an individual is experiencing when seen. A problem-oriented sexual history format that is relatively easy for a clinician to use has been developed by Annon (1976) and covers five major topics: identification of the problem, onset and course of the problem, the patient's perception of causes and maintenance factors, previous treatment for the problem and treatment outcome, and the patient's current therapeutic goals and expectations.

Identification of the Problem. In order to be able to arrive at an accurate diagnosis, a clinician must obtain a clear and complete description of the presenting problem. Such a goal is not necessarily easy because most people in our society experience discomfort, embarrassment, and anxiety when having to discuss their intimate sexual behavior. Additionally, many individuals insist upon labeling their sexual problems with terms lacking diagnostic precision, such as the term *frigidity*.

Confusion and imprecision can usually be circumvented if the clinician has the patient describe her or his behavior rather than discuss the problem. Specifically, the patient should be asked to describe in detail exactly what occurs whenever she or he attempts to be sexual. Should the patient begin to stray from the task at hand and use labels rather than behavioral descriptions, the clinician should redirect the patient's attention.

Although it is the clinician's responsibility to assign diagnostic labels to identify sexual problems, it is the responsibility of the patient to determine what is a problem. Although a clinician may consider the absence of orgasms a problem, a patient may be very satisfied engaging in sex without experiencing orgasms, in which case the absence of orgasms would not constitute a sexual dysfunction.

Onset and Course of the Problem. Obtaining a history of the presenting problem is an integral part of taking a problem-oriented sexual history. Relevant information that should be discussed includes (a) the age of the patient when the problem was first experienced; (b) whether the problem onset was gradual or slow; (c) data about any significant events that occurred at the time of problem onset; (d) how long the problem has been experienced; (e) changes in the intensity of the problem; and (f) the circumstances under which the problem occurs. Such information will assist the clinician in determining if the sexual dysfunction is lifelong versus acquired, generalized versus situational, and total versus partial.

Causes and Maintenance Factors. It will behoove a clinician taking a problem-oriented sexual history to ask a patient to comment on the etiology and maintenance of a sexual problem, as very often patients are able to identify with precision the cause of their problems. Knowing the patient's concept of the cause and maintenance factors of a sexual problem may assist a clinician in designing a treatment plan and, in some cases, shed light on a patient's negative response to treatment.

Previous Treatment History. As in the case of any type of presenting problem, when a patient is being assessed for a possible sexual problem, it is important that the clinician obtain a treatment history. Very often patients will have sought treatment previously for their sexual problems or will have used some of the self-help books available on the market. Knowledge about previous treatment and treatment outcome is helpful, again, in the planning of therapy. For example, if the new treatment plan mirrors previously unsuccessful efforts, a patient may resist offered help. On the other hand, a clinician may wish to incorporate previously successful therapeutic components into the present treatment plan.

The previous treatment history should also cover the patient's medical history. Specifically, it is important to determine if the patient has had a medical evaluation since the onset of the sexual problem and, if so, how recently it was performed, the results of the evaluation, who performed it, and any form of treatment prescribed as a result of the evaluation. The thrust of this component of the history is to identify or rule out organic factors that may be impacting on the patient's sexual behavior.

Current Goals and Expectations. Just as it is the patient's responsibility to define what is a sexual problem, she or he is also responsible for identifying treatment goals. However, the clinician has the duty of insuring that the patient-identified goals and expectations are realistic as well as concrete and specific. We have found it particularly useful to have patients define their goals behaviorally rather than emotionally. For example, it is much easier to work toward the goal of experiencing an orgasm as a result of intercourse than toward the nebulous goal of enjoying sex more. With behaviorally defined treatment goals, it is much easier to devise a treatment plan, as well as evaluate therapeutic progress.

Case Illustrations

Depends upon the Situation. Referred by his physician for an evaluation, 40-year-old Joe's presenting problem was that he was having difficulty obtaining a full erection and controlling ejaculation. He and his second wife, 30-year-old Jan, had one child, aged 6.

Session 1. Despite the usual request that he bring his sexual partner to the interview, Joe appeared alone at the first session. He began the interview by indicating that he was very interested in receiving treatment as he loved his wife and wanted to stay married to her. In addition, he did not want to leave his son. Although his wife informed him that she could live a life without sex, Joe was interested in sex.

Joe reported that he and Jan were sexual about once a month, and he was the person who initiated sex. Usually he would undress her and then they would get into bed. In bed she would hold him but would not caress his genitals. He would stimulate her genitals, but usually Jan would be rigidly on her back while Joe penetrated her. A few second after attempting penetration, he would ejaculate.

According to Joe, he first noticed the problem a couple of months after he and Jan were married. The onset was sudden and also occurred when he infrequently masturbated. When asked if there were any situations in which he did not experience this problem, Joe embarrassingly admitted that he had been seeing another woman for about 2 years and that when he was sexual with her, he was able to obtain a full erection and penetrate her about 80% of the time. In contrast, Joe reported that he would obtain only about 50% of full erection when he had intercourse with his wife. When Joe was questioned about his ejaculatory control, he said that he had always ejaculated very quickly and that he considered his rapid ejaculation a problem.

Joe indicated that he did not have any sexual difficulties during his first marriage. He had been able to obtain an erection sufficient for penetration and had maintained sexual interest in his first wife throughout the marriage. He indicated that the marriage ended because his wife was rather reckless in terms of finances.

Joe felt that the problem was caused and maintained by Jan's coldness and her lack of affection. In addition, he felt that her lack of sexual experience and know-how interfered with his excitement. On the other hand, he reported that his girlfriend was quite experienced sexually and knew how to arouse him. Although Joe had not sought any psychotherapeutic intervention for his problem, he had read extensively about sexual problems and had been examined by a neurologist, who was unable to find any organic etiology for the problem. Joe was not taking any medication and had no known illnesses. He reported that he was experiencing morning erections, sometimes having a full erection. Joe's therapeutic goal was to be able to have a full erection when he was being sexual with his wife and to gain control over his ejaculation.

After receiving assurances that information about his extramarital relationship would not be revealed, he made an appointment for his wife to be interviewed.

Session 2. The information given by Jan was consistent with that obtained from Joe. Although she agreed that her lack of sexual experience was contributing to the problem they were having, Jan reported that it was very difficult for them to communicate about sex and that their frequency of sexual activity had been decreasing over time. Jan indicated that she was uncomfortable initiating sex and was concerned that if she did initiate sex and Joe failed to obtain a full erection, the problem would be exacerbated. The wife also reported that she was suspicious that Joe might be involved with another woman. When asked about her husband's ejaculatory control, Jan indicated that usually he was able to effect penetration, with ejaculation occurring within seconds after penetration. Sometimes, according to Jan, Joe would ejaculate before penetration.

Based on the information obtained from this problem-oriented sexual history, Joe's problems were diagnosed as situational inhibited sexu-

al excitement and premature ejaculation. Frequently, these two diagnoses are associated with each other.

In cases of erectile problems, it is imperative that the clinician differentiate organic from psychogenically caused problems. In the preceding
case, it was relatively clear cut that the patient was not experiencing an
organic problem as he was able to obtain full erections upon awakening in
the morning and when sexual with his extramarital partner. Furthermore, the results of a medical examination revealed no history or problem
consistent with a diagnosis of an organically based erectile or ejaculatory
problem. On the other hand, the history provided by Joe included several
factors that are common psychogenic causes of erectile problems including (a) insufficient sexual stimulation by a partner; (b) the "performance
anxiety" Joe felt when he was sexual with his wife; (c) guilt and discomfort Joe was experiencing because of his extramarital affair; and (d) Joe's
worry about his rapid ejaculation. Therapy focusing on both their marital
problems and Joe's sexual problem was recommended.

Just Not Interested. Referred by her gynecologist, Susan, a 26-year-old
single female, stated that she felt as if her sexuality had gone on vacation. When
asked to explain in more detail what occurred when she was sexual with her
partner of 2 years, she reported that she had no desire to be sexual, but when
she did engage in sexual activity, she found penile-vaginal intercourse to be
extremely painful.

According to Susan, she first began experiencing the problem at the age of
24, about the time she had been dating a man who had pressured her into
having sex with him. When asked if she had been pressured into being sexual on
any other occasion, Susan recalled that she had been raped at age 18. A college
student at the time, she accepted a ride home from a male at a party. He drove
her to a deserted area, where the rape occurred.

Susan reported that her consensual sexual experiences prior to the rape
were pleasurable and enjoyable. Subsequent to the rape, she did not engage in
sexual activity for several months. Later, she began to see a gentle and sexually
considerate man with whom she enjoyed sex, experiencing no pain or discomfort. Since she dated the man who pressured her sexually, she had lost her
desire to be sexual and experienced pain during sexual relations. Susan stated
that she was somewhat mistrusting of her current sexual partner as he was very
flirtatious with other women and did not seem to be "in tune" to her sexually.

Susan believed that pain during sex was partially related to the fact when
pressured at the age 24, she was not lubricated and, consequently, the intercourse was very painful. She was uncertain as to why she had lost her desire to
be sexual.

The results of Susan's medical evaluation revealed no organic basis for her
problem, and she was not on any medication and had no illnesses that would
interfere with sexual functioning. She had not received any prior treatment for
her problem.

Susan was experiencing two problems—functional dyspareunia and inhibited sexual desire. The etiology of the dyspareunia was related to the physical pain experienced when she was pressured into being sexual. Additionally, Susan most probably experienced psychological pain during this episode as a result of a sense of reliving her earlier rape. Over time, the painful intercourse caused Susan to lose her desire for sexual relations.

Critical Diagnostic Information

Whenever evaluating a patient for a possible sexual dysfunction, a clinician should make every effort to determine if the problem is organic or psychogenic because the treatment plans may differ considerably for these two classes of problems. Discussions of many of the various illnesses, medical conditions, and medications that affect sexual behavior and performance are available in the literature (Becker & Skinner, 1983; Bray, DeFrank, & Wolfe, 1981; Brouillette, Pryor, & Fox, 1981; Fitz-Gerald & FitzGerald, 1980; Higgens, 1979; Jensen, 1981a, 1981b; Kaplan, 1974; Kolodny, 1971; Kolodny, Kahn, & Goldstein, 1974, Lamberti, 1979; Lilius, Valtonen, & Wikström, 1976; Lundeberg, 1977, 1978; Maruta, Osborne, Swanson, & Halling, 1981; Masters & Johnson, 1970; Podolsky, 1980; Wabek & Burchell, 1980).

Certainly, referral to either a gynecologist or urologist for an examination is essential. In addition, some psychophysiological procedures have been developed that show promise in aiding a clinician making a differential diagnosis.

In males, measure of nocturnal penile tumescence or penile erection during REM sleep periods can help a clinician assess objectively a patient's biological erectile capability (Karacan, 1970; Karacan, Williams, Thornby, & Salis, 1975). Because this assessment sometimes produces equivocal results, current research is investigating the use of adjunctive measures such as penile blood pressure, perineal muscle activity, and penile rigidity. In females, measurement is vascular changes in vaginal responses during REM sleep using a vaginal photoplethysmograph shows promise in making a differential diagnosis (Abel, Murphy, Becker, & Bitar, 1979).

Diagnostic Interviewing Do's and Don'ts

The Do's

1. Have the patient describe her or his sexual problem in behavioral terms.

2. Question the patient as to prior illnesses or sexual traumas that might be interfering with sexual behavior.
3. Be sure to ask the patient what medications or street drugs she or he may be using.
4. Determine if the patient in an ongoing relationship is involved with other sexual partners. Very often guilt about a second relationship interfers with sexual functioning with a primary partner.

The Don'ts

1. Don't assume that the patient will volunteer all the information necessary for diagnosis. Sexuality is a very difficult topic for a patient to discuss.
2. Don't rely on the patient's report if other sources are available. If the patient is involved in a relationship, ask him or her to bring in his or her partner to assist in the history giving. We have found that very often patients misperceive or distort what has been occurring sexually.

Sexual Deviations

A second major category of psychosexual disorders is that of sexual deviations. Although only a very few sexual behaviors may be considered deviant in all cultures, each culture designates some sexual behavior as aberrant, abnormal, atypical, or deviant. In our society, sexual behavior whose goal is something other than consensual intercourse with an adult is considered deviant. Such behaviors include paraphilias, incest, and rape.

The various sexual deviations can be placed in one of three subcategories: (a) deviation in the selection of the sexual partner or object; (b) deviation in the method of sexual functioning; and (c) deviation in both the selection of the sexual partner or object and in the method of sexual functioning.

Deviations in the Selection of the Sexual Partner or Object

Fetishism. Fetishism is a paraphilia that is characterized by some degree of sexual preference for nonliving objects and dependence at least in part on the objects for sexual arousal. Gebhard (1977) has distinguished four degrees of such sexual preference, ranging from a slight preference for the object to the actual substitution of a person as a sexual partner by an object. When the preference is slight or strong, it is likely to be integrated in consensual intercourse with a human partner. However, when the object is a necessity, sexual partners are not likely to be a participant in the fetish, and when actual substitution occurs, the object becomes the target of the sexual activity, making a partner unimportant (Gosselin & Wilson, 1980; Money, 1977).

Two major types of fetishes have been identified: a media fetish and a form fetish (Gebhard, 1977). In a *media fetish*, the focus is on the material, such as the leather or rubber, of which the object is composed. The shape and function of the object is more important in a *form fetish*. Common fetish objects include female undergarments, boots, and shoes.

Partialism. In this variation of a fetish, partialism, sexual arousal is dependent, at least in part, on some particular part of another person's anatomy (Caprio, 1961; Gagnon, 1977). In mild forms, partialism is experienced by most adults in our society and, in fact, is socially acceptable. Consider, for example, the "leg man" and the "breast man." Partialism is generally considered clinically significant when the body part is not one of the accepted sexually arousing body parts.

Apotemnophia or Amputism. Apotemnophia or amputism is a relatively rare variation of partialism in which a person is aroused by amputation. Two forms of apotemnophia have been identified: partner and self. In the partner form, an individual wishes to be sexual with an amputated partner, whereas in self-amputism the individual increases sexual arousal by fantasizing about being amputated. Apotemnophia generally is restricted to fantasy rather than actual activity. However, cases in which individuals have attempted to obtain medically unnecessary amputations to increase sexual satisfaction have been reported (Money, Jobaris, & Furth, 1977).

Transvestism. Although transvestism may involve a deviation in the method of sexual functioning (dressing in the clothing of the opposite sex to derive sexual arousal), it is a paraphilia that is frequently perceived as behaviorally similar to fetishism and, consequently, it is considered a deviation in the selection of sexual partner or object. Much confusion surrounds transvestism stemming from a definition problem. In an attempt to rectify this problem and mirror the different types of transvestite activity, Benjamin (1966) delineated three types of transvestism. The man* with pseudotransvestism cross-dresses for exploratory purposes rather than in response to sexual desires. In fetishistic trans-

---

*Males are considerably more likely than females to manifest the various sexual deviations, with the exception of sexual masochism (Money & Wiedeking, 1980). For this reason, male pronouns will be used throughout this chapter when referring to an individual with a sexual deviation.

vestism, increased sexual arousal results from cross-dressing. The individual with true transvestism cross-dresses as a result of discomfort with his gender and is seeking relaxation rather than sexual arousal. True transvestism should not be confused with transsexualism.

Although females may engage in transvestism, this paraphilia is identified almost exclusively in males. The majority of men so diagnosed are heterosexual, married, or have a regular sexual partner, and report a level of sexual satisfaction with their partners comparable to that of heterosexual males who do not cross-dress (Benjamin, 1967; Gosselin & Wilson, 1980; Prince & Bentler, 1972; Wise & Meyer, 1980). Variations in the pattern of cross-dressing have been reported (Prince & Bentler, 1972). Lingerie are generally the most commonly worn articles of clothing. However, the majority of men with this diagnosis prefer to cross-dress completely rather than wear only one or two pieces of clothing. Additionally, cross-dressing is most commonly done in private.

Bestiality and Zoophilia. Bestiality and zoophilia are two paraphilias that share the characteristic of animals serving as the target of sexual arousal. However, the two deviations do differ in underlying motivation. *Bestiality* involves sexual activity with an animal, usually as a result of curiosity, a desire for novelty, or the unavailability of a human partner (Tollison & Adams, 1979). However, *zoophilia*, sexual activity, real or imagined, with animals is the preferred or exclusive means of producing sexual excitement.

Although these deviations are usually considered rare (APA, 1980), their prevalence may be greater than imagined. Kinsey and his associates (1948, 1953) reported that 8% of the adult males and 3.6% of the adult females they studied had engaged in sexual activity with animals. In fact, of the males interviewed, 17% of those who had lived on farms during their adolescence reported reaching orgasm as a result of sexual contact with animals. Some differences between males and females engaging in these behaviors have been noted. For males, the sexual activity involved farm animals and generally included vaginal intercourse. In contrast, females usually reported contact with household pets, with the contact likely to be restricted to cunnilingus or masturbation of a male animal.

Pedophilia. The defining characteristic of pedophilia is repeated sexual activity with prepubertal children. Although a 10-year age difference between an adult assailant and the victim is sometimes required before a diagnosis of pedophilia can be applied (APA, 1980), this criterion is arbitrary, and clinical judgment should always enter into the making of such a diagnosis. However, the term *pedophilia* is most appropriately used only in cases in which the victim is under 13 years of age.

Virtually any sexual activity that may take place between two people can be found in pedophilia. However, exhibitionism and genital fondling are the most common behaviors. Some form of pressure, coercion, or verbal and/or physical aggression is frequently present in these offenses. In the majority of cases of pedophilia, the assailant is an acquaintance, family friend, or relative of the victim (Christie, Marshall, & Lanthier, 1978; De Francis, 1969; Katchadourian & Lunde, 1975).

Although cases of women engaging in sexual activity with children have been reported (Fritz, Stoll, & Wagner, 1981; Kolodny et al., 1979; Tollison & Adams, 1979), the overwhelming majority of individuals with this diagnosis are males. With regard to the sex of the victims, female children are twice as likely to be victims (APA, 1980).

Heterosexually and homosexually oriented pedophiles have been found to differ from each other (APA, 1980; Finkelhor, 1979; McCaghy, 1980; Mohr, Turner, & Jerry, 1964). Those who are heterosexually oriented prefer 7-to 10-year-old female targets, rarely attempt intercourse, and have a better prognosis. In contrast, those who are homosexually oriented are less likely to be married, prefer slightly older male victims, may engage in mutual masturbation, fellatio, and anal intercourse, and are more likely to identify their pedophilic behavior as affectionate. Those with an undifferentiated sexual orientation prefer younger victims than the previous two groups. Victim age preference is also related to the age of the assailant, with older males assaulting young children and younger offenders seeking out older victims.

Various typologies of pedophilic men have been proposed (Cohen, Leghorn, & Calmas, 1969; McCaghy, 1971). Although gross psychopathology is not common among men with this deviation, personality disturbances are often noted (Gebhard, Gagnon, Pomeroy, & Christenson, 1965). The recidivism rate for this diagnostic category is high, with pedophilia representing a large proportion of known criminal sexual acts (APA, 1980).

Hebephilia. The term applied when the victim of sexual molestation is an adolescent but not an adult is *hebephilia*. The characteristics of this paraphilia are similar to those of pedophilia.

Necrophilia. Little is known about necrophilia, a rare paraphilia that is characterized by an erotic interest in corpses. However, it is frequently associated with severe psychological disturbance (Templar & Eberhardt, 1980).

Mysophilia. In mysophilia, a rare paraphilia, sexual arousal is dependent at least in part on filth. Sexual excitement is increased when sexual activity occurs among filth, real or imagined. On occasion the filth is incorporated into the sexual activity.

Klismaphilia. Individuals with the paraphilia *klismaphilia* receive sexual pleasure by administering and receiving enemas. Such activities are frequently called "water sports."

Urophilia. Also known as *urolagnia*, urophilia is centered around urine or urination. The range of activities includes observing others urinate, being urinated upon (known as "golden showers"), or drinking urine. This erotic interest is sometimes involved in sadomasochistic activity.

Coprophilia. The focusing of erotic interest on feces is coprophilia. This rare paraphilia may range from watching a person defecate to spreading feces on one's body, which is sometimes called saliromania.

Incest. Although incest is not included as a formal diagnostic category in DSM-III, this activity is a deviation in the selection of a sexual partner. Legally, incest is sexual interaction between close blood relatives. However, a clinical definition may be extended to include as incest offenders regular sexual partners of single parents and guardians (legal or otherwise) because these individuals frequently function in the parental role.

The incidence of incest is unknown but now believed to be considerably higher than previously thought. It has been estimated that as many as 50,000 children are sexually victimized by parents or guardians alone each year (Burgess, Groth, Holmstrom, & Sgroi, 1978; Finkelhor, 1979; Summit & Kryso, 1978) and that from 10 to 20 million people in the United States have been incestuously assaulted (Forward & Buck, 1978).

The most common form of incest occurs between brothers and sisters and may range from exhibiting the genitals to intercourse. Fondling of the genitals is the prevalent sexual activity. Sex between siblings generally is not an isolated incident but rather occurs on an ongoing basis and may involve coercion or force. Cousins also are common sexual partners, ranking as the most likely blood-related partner for males and the second most likely partner for females (Finkelhor, 1979).

Although not the most common form, father–daughter incest has received the most attention from researchers as well as clinicians and legal authorities. Three basic patterns of this incest have been identified (Blair & Justice, 1979; Meiselman, 1978). In pedophilic incest, the father is sexually immature and inadequate and engages in sexual activity with his own children as well as other young children. A psychopathic father who is promiscuous with related and nonrelated adults and children is associated with the second pattern—psychopathic incest. Finally, in family-generated incest, disintegration within the family results in the daughter's assuming the mother role, including serving as a sexual partner for the father.

The type of sexual contact in father–daughter incest differs in relation to the age of the daughter (Gebhard *et al.*, 1965). Specifically, genital manipulation and oral-genital activities are the most common forms of sexual contact when the daughter is under the age of 12, whereas intercourse is most prevalent with older daughters.

In contrast to incest involving the father, mother–son incest is rare and usually involves a psychologically disturbed party (Meiselman, 1978). In this form of incest, genital fondling without coitus is the most common activity when the child is under the age of 10. However, intercourse is typically involved with males over the age of 10. Within the nuclear family, mother–daughter incest is the rarest form reported. In the extended family, grandfather–granddaughter incest may account for 10% of intrafamilial contacts (Courtois & Hinckley, 1981).

Deviations in the Method of Sexual Functioning

Exhibitionism. The paraphilia *exhibitionism*, also known as *indecent exposure* and *flashing*, involves repeated genital exposure to unsuspecting strangers for the purpose of deriving sexual arousal. Although almost exclusively a male paraphilia (Smukler & Schiebel, 1975; Stoller, 1971), a few cases of female exhibitionism have been reported (Evans, 1970; Hollender, Brown, & Roback, 1977). This paraphilia accounts for more arrests for sexual offenses than any other single behavior (Allen, 1969; Hughes, 1977) and has the highest recidivism rate for sexual offenders (APA, 1980).

The typical male who exposes himself is under the age of 40, married, above average in intelligence, satisfactorily employed, and sexually inhibited and does not manifest serious emotional problems (Blair & Lanyon, 1981; Kolarsky, Madlafousek, & Novotna, 1978; Langevin, Paitich, Freeman, Mann, & Handy, 1978; McCreary, 1975; Smukler & Schiebel, 1975). Females, particularly adults, are the preferred victims (Langevin, Paitich, Ramsay, Anderson, Kamrad, Pope, Geller, Pearl, & Newman, 1979; MacDonald, 1973). The act itself typically involves exposing at close range of the penis, often erect and frequently while masturbating.

Numerous motivations for exhibitionism have been forwarded (Hendrix & Meyer, 1976; Smith & Meyer, 1980). Yet, the most common motivating factors are a desire to shock the victim, a hope that the victim will enjoy the episode and be impressed by the size of the penis, and a desire to have sexual relations with the woman (Langevin et al., 1979). It is generally assumed that men who engage in exhibitionism are not particularly dangerous in that they do not seek physical contact with their victims (Tollison & Adams, 1979). However, not all such men may be nonviolent as 1 in 10 has thoughts about or has attempted rape (Gebhard et al., 1965; MacNamara & Sagarin, 1977).

Voyeurism. It may be theorized that the popularity of topless bars and the Dallas Cowboys cheerleaders reflect societal acceptance of at least some degree of voyeurism. In fact, Gagnon (1977) suggested that, given the opportunity, most people are voyeurs, and Feigelman (1977) found that such behavior is accepted and expected in some occupations, such as high-rise construction workers. However, when an individual repeatedly obtains sexual pleasure from watching others' bodies, sexual anatomy, or sexual behavior, and the victim is unaware of being observed, a diagnosis of *voyeurism* may be warranted. Masturbation to orgasm during the voyeuristic activity is common. Sometimes the term *scopophilia* is used to describe the act of observing sexual acts and genitalia, whereas *voyeurism* is applied to the act of observing nudes.

By definition, this is a male-only paraphilia (APA, 1980). Men who engage in voyeurism are similar to those who expose themselves in that both groups are typically young and have poorly developed sociosexual skills (Gebhard et al., 1965; Smith, 1976). Strangers are the preferred victims, and the risk of discovery enhances the experience (Tollison & Adams, 1979). Although individuals who engage in this paraphilia have generally been considered to pose no threat to the victim, some such males have criminal histories including rape, burglary, and arson (Gebhard et al., 1965; MacNamara & Sagarin, 1977; Yalom, 1960). The more dangerous males are those who as part of their deviant sexual behavior enter homes or buildings or tap at windows to obtain the victim's attention.

Sexual Masochism. Experiencing sexual pleasure as the result of pain inflicted during sexual activity is not uncommon (Barbach & Levine, 1980; Gebhard & Johnson, 1979; Hunt, 1974; Kinsey, Pomeroy, Martin, & Gebhard, 1953). However, when the preferred or exclusive method of achieving sexual arousal involves being beaten, bound, or humiliated, a clinical diagnosis of *sexual masochism* is appropriate. In addition, participation in even a single sexual episode in which the individual was physically harmed or the person's life was threatened for the purpose of sexual excitement is grounds for this diagnosis.

Sexual masochism covers a wide spectrum of behaviors, from mild forms to extremes. The more common mild activities include humiliation, bondage, biting, spanking, slapping, and pinching. Some of the extreme forms of sexual masochism are whippings, semistrangulation, being trampled, and self-mutilation. Devices and paraphernalia such as leather or rubber clothing, spike-heeled shoes, handcuffs, chains, collars, hoods, ropes, and whips may be used in the sexual activities. Most frequently a relatively low, tolerable level of pain is preferred (Gosselin & Wilson, 1980; Spengler, 1977). This is the only paraphilia that occurs more frequently in females than in males.

Sexual Sadism. The paraphilia *sexual sadism* involves (a) the intentional infliction of psychological or physical pain on a nonconsenting partner in order to derive sexual arousal; (b) humiliating or mildly hurting physically a consenting partner as the preferred or exclusive method of obtaining sexual excitement; or (c) inflicting extensive, permanent, or mortal bodily injury on a consenting partner in pursuit of sexual arousal. The complement of sexual masochism, sexual sadism is less prevalent in general, and males with diagnoses outnumber females (Gosselin & Wilson, 1980). Occasionally, both sexual patterns coexist in the same individual.

Sexual interaction between an individual preferring sadism and one preferring masochism is called *sadomasochism* (S & M). Such activity is frequently associated with bondage and discipline (B & D). A complete industry, including stores, mail-order companies, and advertising outlets, supporting sadomasochism has developed.

Coprolalia. The paraphilia *coprolalia* involves using or hearing certain "dirty" or obscene words in order to obtain sexual arousal. Frequently, crude and vulgar language is used to describe excrement. Although such behavior is sometimes considered acceptable in our society, it becomes clinically significant when such verbal stimulation is necessary for arousal or when it occurs with an inappropriate person in an inappropriate situation.

Telephone Scatologia. Obscene telephoning, a male paraphilia that is called *telephone scatologia*, is a form of coprolalia and entails calling a victim and making sexual and prohibited comments. Frequently, the caller masturbates while engaging in this behavior. Three types of obscene telephone calls have been delineated (Masters, Johnson, & Kolodny, 1982). The most common type of call involves the caller's boasting about himself and his genitalia and explicitly describing his concomitant masturbatory behavior. In the second type of call, the caller makes sexual and aggressive threats against the victim. However, the caller rarely carries out these threats. The aim of the third type of call is to get the victim to reveal intimate information. For example, the caller may ask questions about menstruation, contraception, or sexual activity under the guise of conducting a research survey. A caller may repeatedly telephone the same victim if she responds to his comments and questions. However, the more typical pattern is to call a variety of victims.

Men who make obscene telephone calls are similar to men who expose themselves in that they generally feel inadequate and insecure and have poorly developed sociosexual skills (Nadler, 1968). However, as compared to men who engage in exhibitionism, individuals who are inclined toward telephone scatologia are more anxious and hostile when interacting with females.

Frottage. In this paraphilia, sexual arousal is achieved by rubbing one's genitals against a nonconsenting victim or by rubbing the genitals of such a victim. Usually committed at a high frequency by males, this sexual deviation occurs most frequently in crowded situations, such as elevators, buses, and subways, and with a fully dressed victim.

Rape. Because rape is not generally considered to be the result of a mental disorder, the American Psychiatric Association failed to include it as a diagnostic category in the DSM-III (APA, 1980). However, mental health professionals who work with individuals who rape recognize the necessity of such a diagnosis.

A useful clinical definition of rape would include any form of sexual behavior involving physical contact between the assailant and the non-consenting adult victim and that does not fall within any other diagnostic category. This broad definition covers completed or attempted forced oral, vaginal, or anal intercourse and marital and date rape.

There is much controversy as to whether rape is a sexual or an aggressive act. Several classification schemes focusing predominantly on the aggressive component of rape have been proposed (Cohen *et al.*, 1969; Gebhard *et al.*, 1965; Groth, Burgess, & Holmstrom, 1977; Groth & Birnbaum, 1979). However, ample research data demonstrate the role of both aggression and rape in such assaults and support the consideration of rape as a sexual deviation (Abel, Barlow, Blanchard, & Guild, 1977; Barbaree, Marshall, & Lanthier, 1979; Hinton, O'Neill, & Webster, 1980; Kercher & Walker, 1973; Quinsey & Marshall, 1983).

In a few reported instances, women have aided men attacking another woman and in a few isolated reports, men have been coerced into sexual activity by women. However, rape is overwhelmingly a male behavior.

As a group, men who rape tend to be young (Amir, 1971; McCary, 1978), of lower intelligence but not mentally retarded (Perdue & Lester, 1972; Ruff, Templer, & Ayers, 1976; Verba, Barnard, & Holzer, 1979; Wolfe & Baker, 1980, have previous criminal histories (Smithyman, 1979; Wolfe & Baker, 1980), have difficulty expressing anger and aggression (Rada, 1977), and tend to be involved in an ongoing relationship (Groth & Birnbaum, 1979; MacDonald, 1971). The rape assaults tend to be premeditated (Chappell & James, 1976), include physical force (National Institute of Law Enforcement and Criminal Justice, 1978), and be perpetrated against an unknown victim similar in age, social class, and ethnic background to the offender (McDermott, 1979).

Deviations in Both the Selection of the Sexual Partner or Object and in the Method of Sexual Functioning

Deviations in this third subcategory are characterized by the direction of inappropriate sexual behaviors at inappropriate targets. For example, some men restrict their genital exposure to prepubetal females, whereas other men carry out sexual sadism on animals. Some clinicians have suggested that the man who rapes children is different from the man who engages in pedophilia (Groth & Birnbaum, 1979). Most of the behaviors listed in the second subcategory of sexual deviations can be directed at children, adolescents, and/or animals.

General Interviewing Procedures in the Assessment of Sexual Deviations

Mental health professionals who work with individuals who engage in sexual deviations must realize that this population presents some problems not regularly associated with other patient populations seeking therapeutic intervention. Most of these problems stem from the facts that such a patient must talk openly about sexual behavior, a topic that engenders much anxiety and discomfort in our society, and that the patient will be admitting to behaviors that not only are not socially acceptable but are, in fact, illegal. Failure to appreciate the seriousness of these problems and to take precautionary steps greatly handicaps the work of the professional.

Informed Consent and the Issue of Confidentiality. The success of any diagnostic interview is dependent upon the quantity and quality of information obtained. Whether self-referred or referred by others, individuals who commit sexual deviations have a great incentive to restrict or censor the information they provide. Hence, it is important that the interview situation be structured so as to foster and support self-revelation.

In our work with this patient population, we have found that obtaining informed consent has been useful in setting the desired atmosphere. We routinely use detailed consent forms that delineate the purpose of the assessment, the type of information to be obtained, the procedures to be followed, and the rights of the patient.

The consent forms also include explicit information about the procedures that have been established to protect the confidentiality of the patient and his records. Certainly this patient population is very concerned about the disclosure of self-incriminating information both to the mental health professional as well as to outside parties. Thus, it is imperative that the professional take strong precautionary steps aimed at protecting confidentiality. For example, we use numbers to identify patients and do not include any identifying information in their files. As a result, any person who obtained access to our files through the courts would have to attempt to match known information about a particular patient to the available information in any one of several hundred files, a difficult task at best. This and the other procedures instituted to protect the patient are detailed in the consent form.

Although written informed consent is a necessity with this and any other patient population, the form will be useless unless it is understandable to the patients. Thus, the form should be written in plain English and without professional or legal jargon. As further insurance, we read the consent form to each patient and, on occasion, may "quiz" a patient as to the meaning of a sentence or paragraph if we sense that he has not comprehended it.

Details of Sexual Acts. When interviewing other patient populations, it is generally routine to ask for details surrounding the presenting problem. However, when the reason for referral is a sexual deviation, it is not necessarily in the interest of the clinican or the patient to seek detailed information because the clinician may, at some time in the future, be called to testify in legal action against the patient.

We have adopted the procedure of having our patients provide only general information about their deviant sexual activities rather than the specifics, such as dates, names, and locations. Such a procedure protects both the clinican and the patient because the clinician cannot be expected to retrieve information she or he does not have.

State Laws. A clinician working with this patient population should be familiar with state laws concerning sexual deviation, particularly in relation to the disclosure of information about child abuse. Additionally, as part of the informed consent procedure, the clinician should make sure the patient is aware of and understands the legal responsibilities and obligations of the clinician.

Sexual Language. Regardless of the sophistication or lack thereof of the words used by the patient to refer to sexual organs or behavior, the clinician should not appear shocked by the language. When possible, it is helpful if the clinician uses the same or similar words, provided he or she is not uncomfortable with such words. Additionally, the clinician must insure that the language she or he uses is understood by the patient. Many people are too embarrassed to admit that they do not understand sexual terms and, instead, may answer according to what they think the clinician is asking. Whenever there is reason to question the patient's comprehension, the patient should be requested to describe rather than label the act, event, or body part.

The Posing of Questions. How and in what manner a question is posed influences the answer given. Following the lead of Kinsey, the clinician should ask direct questions, placing the burden of denial on the patient. Additionally, all questions should be asked and responses accepted in a nonjudgmental manner. The patient is usually aware of the seriousness of his behavior and many times is particularly sensitive to the reaction of a professional purporting to provide help.

Multiple Interviews. Whenever possible, it is recommended that a patient be interviewed independently by two clinicians. Many patients are inhibited initially in discussing their socially unacceptable behavior and offer only minimal information while testing the therapeutic atmosphere. Other patients limit their self-revelation as they test the confidentiality procedures. For some patients, the initial interview serves as a catalyst, causing the patient to ruminate about and review his sexual behavior. The usual result of this activity is the provision of additional relevant information during a second interview. Finally, on occasion a patient may feel uncomfortable with the initial interviewer and, subsequently, withhold information. For example, we have found that some patients find discussing their sexual problems with a male interviewer inhibiting, and a female conducting a follow-up interview is able to collect considerably more clinically relevant material. If it is not possible to have interviews done by two clinicians, then, at the very least, the diagnostic interview should require a minimum of two sessions, with time intervening between them.

Additional Sources of Data. Regardless of the skill of the clinician, an individual with a sexual deviation may unintentionally or intentionally provide erroneous information about his behavior. Thus, whenever feasible, other sources of data should be utilized. An excellent assessment technique that has been used with this patient population is the measurement of erection responses to sexual stimuli (Freund, 1967a, 1967b; Freund, Chan, & Coulthard, 1979; Kersher & Walker, 1973; Laws & Holman, 1978; Quinsey, Bergersen, & Steinman, 1976; Quinsey & Carrigan, 1978; Quinsey, Chaplin, & Varney, 1981; Quinsey & Marshall, 1983; Quinsey, Steinman, Bergersen, & Holmes, 1975; Rosen & Kopel, 1977). Such a technique provides precise, objective information on the patient's sexual arousal patterns. An excellent procedural manual for building and operating a sexual behavioral laboratory has been prepared by Laws and Osborn (1983).

Case Illustrations

Just the General Facts. Stressing the importance of not revealing the details of the deviant sexual behavior engaged in by a patient is an important component of the initial interview. Sometimes periodic warnings are necessary, and whenever the clinician thinks that the patient is about to reveal unwanted details, a brief reminder should be given.

Trevor, 34 years of age, had an extensive history of molesting young girls. During his initial interview, the topic of assault details was discussed.

CLINICIAN: Don't tell anyone connected with your assessment the specifics of any illegal act. If you have sexually assaulted someone, don't tell us any of the particulars about it.

TREVOR: So you don't want to hear about my problem? Is that what you are saying?

CLINICIAN: Not at all. In order to determine the nature of your problem, we will have to talk about any assaults you have committed. But we'll talk about them in generalities. I don't want you to tell me any of the particulars about them.

TREVOR: So how do I talk about something without talking about it?

CLINICIAN: For example, don't tell me when an assault occurred, what time of day, where, who the victim was or what she looked like.

TREVOR: So, I can tell you I molested some girl but nothing else. Right?

CLINICIAN: More information than that is needed. For example, I need to know things such as the approximate age of your victim, your behavior during the assault, and the general pattern of them. But instead of saying "I molested by manipulating her genitals a 10-year-old blond female named Suzanne in her house at 122 Hanford last Sunday night at 8:00 P.M.," you indicate that you molested a prepubertal female and the assault involved mutual masturbation or whatever.

During a subsequent meeting, Trevor appeared upset but, at first, refused to talk. Then, without warning he began talking.

TREVOR: I did it again. Last week I stopped to grab a bit to eat at . . .

CLINICIAN: [Interrupting] Wait a minute, Trevor. Remember, I don't want any of the specifics of an assault.

What Did You Say? As with any professional, a clinician becomes accustomed to using jargon and technical terms unknown or confusing to the layperson. When talking to a patient with a sexual problem, a clinician may easily remember that the average person is unfamiliar with words such as frenum, introitus, or pubococcygeus muscle. However, it is also easy to forget that many people do not understand some of the more common everyday sexual words and, consequently, be unaware of the "failure to communicate."

Referred to treatment because of a rape he committed, 16-year-old Neal was very uncomfortable discussing his sexual behavior, making the interview slow and arduous. At times it was difficult to determine if the slowness of the interview was due to his discomfort, his difficulty putting his thoughts into words, or his failure to understand the questions.

CLINICIAN: During the assault, did you ejaculate?
NEAL: Well, of course.
CLINICIAN: At what point?
NEAL: What do you mean? I said I did it.
CLINICIAN: What happens when you ejaculate?
NEAL: Well, I put it in the woman—have sex.
CLINICIAN: Put it in?
NEAL: My penis.
CLINICIAN: What happens when you put your penis in a woman?
NEAL: Nothing.
CLINICIAN: When you put your penis in a woman, does anything come out of your penis?
NEAL: You mean like when I "do" myself?
CLINICIAN: Yes, like then.
NEAL: I don't know.

It was apparent to the clinician that Neal, while understanding the event of ejaculation, was not familiar with the word and equated ejaculation with intercourse. In fact, not only had Neal not ejaculated during the rape, but he had been unable to maintain his erection immediately after intromission.

I Beg Your Pardon. When interviewing a patient about his sexual behavior, close-ended questions provide him with an excellent and easy opportunity to deny his behavior. Self-revelation is usually greater when the patient cannot rely on "yes" or "no" responses.

Steve, a 34-year-old musician, referred himself for treatment after he had attempted to rape a woman. He had been relatively forthright during the interview until the focus changed to his deviant sexual behavior. At that point, he became visibly upset, reporting that he was very embarrassed to have to admit to doing such things. The clinician assured Steve that nothing that was said would upset or alarm the clinician, who was there to help the patient. The clinician then proceeded with the interview.

CLINICIAN: How many times per week do you masturbate?
STEVE: Whoa. I never said I did.
CLINICIAN: I realize that. But since masturbation is a normal activity for most people, I assumed you did.
STEVE: Well, sometimes but not that much.
CLINICIAN: Okay. How many times each week?
STEVE: I don't know. Maybe two or three times a week.
CLINICIAN: When you do masturbate, about what do you think?
STEVE: Oh, making it with my lady or making it on the beach.
CLINICIAN: What percent of your masturbatory fantasies are about rape?
STEVE: Wow! You expect me to answer that?
CLINICIAN: It would help. Most men who have raped also think about rape

sometimes when they masturbate. Some of their masturbatory fantasies are about rape. What percent of yours are about rape?

STEVE: All of them?

CLINICIAN: So everytime you masturbate, you think about rape? But a few minutes ago you mentioned thinking about having sex with your lady on the beach.

STEVE: Well, I think about that, too.

CLINICIAN: Okay, of the last 10 times you masturbated, how many times did you fantasize about having sex with your lady?

STEVE: Oh, four times.

CLINICIAN: And how many times did you think about having sex on the beach?

STEVE: One time.

CLINICIAN: Was it with force or consenting?

STEVE: No force—consenting.

CLINICIAN: And how many times did you think about rape?

STEVE: Five times.

CLINICIAN: Okay. So 50% of your masturbatory fantasies are of rape.

The Second Time Around. For a variety of reasons, patients may reveal, during a second interview by an independent party, relevant information needed in order to make an appropriate diagnosis.

Perry, a 43-year-old writer, had been seen by one interviewer, who had identified that the patient's sexual deviation was rape because Perry reported that he had, on numerous occasions, forced anal intercourse on women. As part of the clinic routine, Perry was interviewed by a second clinician who had no knowledge about the outcome of the initial interview.

CLINICIAN: So your predominant sexual interest is forcing females to engage in sex?

PERRY: Anal sex only.

CLINICIAN: Okay, forcing women to participate in anal sex?

PERRY: Women?

CLINICIAN: What are the approximate ages of the women?

PERRY: Young and old. Anywhere from 10 on.

By the end of the second interview, it became evident that the preliminary diagnosis was not adequate. Rather, Perry's deviation consisted of forced anal intercourse. The age of his victims was irrelevant. In fact, although he had never assaulted a male, he thought the sex of the victim irrelevant as well.

I Didn't Say That. Diagnoses based on a patient's verbal report may be inappropriate or incomplete as a result of a lack of veracity. When assessing individuals with sexual deviations, psychophysiological measures should be obtained whenever possible. Such results are sometimes very enlightening.

A 30-year-old clerk, Ross, was referred for treatment as a result of his ongoing incestuous assaults on his youngest daughter. When interviewed, Ross readily admitted that he had assaulted his daughter but denied committing any other forms of deviant sexual behavior.

As part of his assessment, Ross had his erection responses monitored while listening to a variety of descriptions of deviant and consensual sexual activities. He manifested significant erection responses to three categories of sexual behavior: mutually consenting intercourse with an adult female, sexual behavior with his youngest daughter, and sexual behavior with nonrelated prepubital females.

CLINICIAN: If I understood you, you are not aroused by thoughts of having sex with younger females other than your daughter.

ROSS: That's right—just my daughter.

CLINICIAN: Well, that leaves me a little confused. Remember when you were in the lab and listened to many descriptions of sexual interaction with adults and children while we monitored your penile responses? I looked at the polygraph printout afterwards, and you manifested arousal to only a few types of interactions. I brought the printout with me so let's review it.

Carefully, the clinician examined the printout with Ross, pointing out that definite erection responses were manifested when the patient heard descriptions of sexual interactions with children other than his daughter.

ROSS: I don't believe it.

CLINICIAN: Do you mean that these descriptions were not arousing to you?

ROSS: No, that's not what I mean. I get very turned on thinking about having sex with young girls—any young girls. I've been turned on by little girls since I was a teenager. Now I think about the kids in the neighborhood. But I've never touched them; I've never molested any kids but my own daughter. I've wanted to but never had. I just can't believe you found out. I've never told anyone before, not my wife, my therapist, no one. But it is true.

Critical Diagnostic Information

For most of the paraphilias listed in DSM-III as well as for rape and incest a diagnosis may be warranted if the individual engages in the behavior or if he has fantasies about such behavior. Thus, the type of information necessary for diagnosing the various sexual deviations falls into two categories: the nature of overt sexual behavior and the nature of sexual fantasies.

The Nature of Overt Sexual Behavior. When investigating the nature of overt sexual behavior, it is essential to determine both the method of sexual functioning and the target of the functioning. That is, the method of functioning anything other than consensual intercourse, and, if so, specifically how is it different? In addition, any sexual target other than an adult makes the sexual behavior deviant, with the identity of the target determining in part the specific deviation.

As part of determining the nature of the sexual behavior, there are several additional issues the interviewer should cover. Some measure as to the frequency of the behavior—such as times per week—should be noted. In addition, the patient should be asked how long he has experienced the problem. It is also important to get some sense about the usual situation leading up to and surrounding the deviant behavior. Not only may this information impact on the diagnosis process because some paraphilias, including pedophilia, are not to be diagnosed if the behavior is due to another mental disorder, such as alcohol intoxication, but this information may assist when designing the treatment plan. Similarly, some measure of the degree of physical and/or verbal coercion or aggression is warranted both for making a diagnosis and planning treatment. Finally, ascertaining the patient's current degree of control over his deviant behavior is important. We routinely ask each patient to rate his control on a 0 to 100 scale. This information from the initial interview is particularly useful when later evaluating the effectiveness of any treatment intervention.

The Nature of Sexual Fantasies. Sexual fantasies play an integral part in human sexuality (Byrne, 1977; Carlson & Coleman, 1977; Crépault & Couture, 1980; Hariton & Singer, 1974; McCauley & Swann, 1976, 1980; Mednick, 1977; Moreault & Fallingstad, 1978; Sue, 1979; Wish, 1975). One of the major functions of such fantasies is to enhance sexual arousal or excitement. Briefly, an orgasm, whether the result of self-stimulation or sexual activity with a person or object, is pleasurable and reinforcing. Behavior, odors, thoughts, fantasies, and other stimuli that occur or are present simultaneously with an orgasm can be classically conditioned to take on arousing properties themselves. Each additional pairing may strengthen the conditioned arousing properties. Subsequently, an individual may use sexual fantasies or sexual situations that are not arousing to enhance the sexual experience or to spice up an already arousing situation.

Taken by itself, a fantasy may not be considered indicative of a sexual deviation (APA, 1980). Instead, fantasies have been characterized as a safe means of experiencing illegal or culturally improper urges and discharging inner needs or tensions. Generally, the use of sexual fantasies with paraphilic themes becomes clinically significant when the individual relies heavily or completely on such fantasies as a means of becoming sexually aroused. However, patients who report having sexual fantasies with themes of rape, pedophilia, and/or incest should be considered potentially dangerous regardless of the frequencies of such fantasies.

Just as the method of sexual functioning and the target of the functioning must be determined with regard to overt sexual behavior, these two aspects of sexual fantasies must also be ascertained. This can generally be accomplished by asking the patient to identify the basic themes of his masturbatory and his coital fantasies and then to indicate their prevalence with percentages. Obtaining some indication of the frequency of masturbation, such as times per week, is also important.

Diagnostic Issues

Multiple Diagnoses. In our work with men with sexual deviations, we have found that a large percentage of our patients engage regularly in multiple paraphilias, warranting the assignment of multiple diagnoses. For example, a man who exposes his genitals to both adult women and young girls would be given both diagnoses of *pedophilia* and *exhibitionism*. Recognizing the existence of multiple deviations is important when designing a treatment plan.

Frequency of Behavior. For most of the paraphilias, an isolated incidence of the behavior generally does not warrant the diagnosing of a deviation. Instead, the behavior must be repetitive. When interviewing men with histories of sexual deviations, we regularly use the term *urges* when referring to the desire to engage in a particular deviation. For example, we may ask a patient how strong his control is over his urges to rape. This term conveys the idea of repetition and is immediately understood by the patients.

There are two exceptions to this general rule about repeated behaviors being a diagnostic necessity. The diagnosis of sexual masochism is warranted on the basis of one episode if the individual was physically harmed or had her or his life threatened. On the other hand, a diagnosis of zoophilia is not warranted despite repeated sexual activity with animals if this behavior occurs because a suitable human partner is not available and if sexual fantasies with a theme of zoophilia are absent.

Deviant versus Nondeviant Arousal. It is important to realize that deviant sexual arousal and nondeviant sexual arousal can coexist within a person and that, in fact, these types of arousal may be conceived of as being independent. Thus, a person may have a very satisfactory, mutually consenting sexual relationship with his wife but still rape other women. For this reason, we believe that the diagnostic criteria outlined in DSM-III for some of the various paraphilias requiring that the paraphilic behavior be the preferred activity may be too stringent. For example, a man who reports that sexual sadism accounts for 40% of his sexual behavior and fantasies would not meet the criteria outlined for this diagnosis. In many cases, clinical judgment may be more important than strict adherence to the criteria.

In a related manner, it is misleading to use labels such as *rapist*, *pedophile*, or *exhibitionist* as these labels suggest that the sexual deviation is the patient's only sexual outlet, which we have not found to be true for the majority of patients we have seen. Rather than labeling a patient, it is more appropriate to label his behavior.

Fantasies and Sexual Masochism and Sadism. These two paraphilias serve as exceptions to the procedure of diagnosing sexual deviations on the basis of fantasies alone because sadistic and masochistic fantasies are not uncommon. Acting out such fantasies is necessary before these diagnoses may be applied appropriately.

Additional Diagnostic Information

In order to determine if a patient has a sexual deviation, only information about his sexual behavior and fantasies is essential. However, if the assessment is restricted to these two areas, the clinican will not be able to draw a complete picture of the patient and will be greatly handicapped when designing a treatment plan. In addition to addressing the patient's deviant sexual arousal, the following three other areas should be discussed: (a) nondeviant arousal; (b) any cognitions surrounding his deviant behavior; and (c) his sociosexual skills.

Nondeviant Arousal. As part of a thorough diagnostic assessment, the interviewer should collect information on the level of nondeviant (or mutually consenting intercourse with an adult) arousal experienced by the patient. If a patient reports having no such arousal or a low level of such arousal, he needs to be offered treatment to develop it. In addition to finding out what percentage of a patient's masturbatory and coital fantasies are nondeviant, the clinician should obtain a brief nondeviant arousal history covering the following points: (a) sexual orientation; (b) age at and circumstances surrounding first consensual sexual experience; (c) frequency of nondeviant sexual interactions; (d) satisfaction with nondeviant sexual interactions; and (e) the existence of any sexual dysfunctions.

Deviant Cognitions. The unspoken beliefs and thoughts of a patient may reinforce or support his deviant sexual behavior. For example, it is common for a man who exposes his genitals to believe that his victims are actually aroused by his behavior and to interpret any behavior of the victim as indicative of her arousal. These cognitions are maintained as the patient generally has had no opportunity to test the validity of them. The man has had no reason to modify or eliminate such cognitions. However, when a patient does harbor such thoughts, ample opportunity to test the reality of them should be included as part of the treatment. We have found that irrational cognitions are particularly common among cases of exhibitionism, incest, and pedophilia.

Sociosexual Skills. A complete assessment of a man with a sexual deviation must include an evaluation of his sociosexual skills because these skills are necessary to establish and maintain a mutually consenting sexual relationship with an adult. This assessment can be as simple as having the patient rate his skills as compared to his peers as well as having the clinician rate the skills upon completion of the interview. However, a behavioral assessment such as that described by Becker, Abel, Blanchard, Murphy, and Coleman (1978) would provide more specific data and aid in the designing of a treatment plan.

Ego-Dystonic Homosexuality

The perception of homosexuality in general by mental health professionals has undergone considerable modification. In the original *Diagnostic and Statistical Manual of Mental Disorders* (American Psychiatric Association, 1958), homosexuality was considered pathological sexuality, a subclassification under psychopathic personality, and in the DSM-II (American Psychiatric Association, 1968), homosexuality was listed as a sociopathic personality disturbance. However, in the DSM-III (APA, 1980) homosexuality itself is not considered a mental disorder. Increasingly, homosexuality is being considered a normal sexual variation. This movement away from the classification of homosexuality as a pathological orientation has received considerable research support. In general, findings have indicated that psychologically, individuals with homosexual orientations cannot be differentiated from individuals with heterosexual orientations and that the few differences that have been found are minor and inconsistent rather than indicative of personality maladjustment in individuals with homosexual orientations (Adelman, 1977, Bell, 1974; Freedman, 1971; Gonsiorek, 1982; Green, 1972; Hoffman, 1977; Hooberman, 1979; Hooker, 1957; Marmor, 1980; Masters & Johnson, 1979; Morin, 1977; Reiss, 1980; Sagher & Robins, 1973; Siegelman, 1981; Strassberg, Roback, Cunningham, McKee & Larson, 1979; Thompson, McCandless & Strickland, 1971; Weinberg & Williams, 1974). However, in recognition of the continuing debate among clinicians on this issue, the diagnosis of ego-dystonic homosexuality was

created in DSM-III and included under a third major category of psychosexual disorders, that of *other psychosexual disorders.*

A diagnosis of ego-dystonic homosexuality is considered warranted
if the patient is distressed about his or her homosexual arousal pattern
and wants to have heterosexual arousal. Thus, the person feels that his
or her sexual orientation is incongruent with how he or she wants to be.

Generally, the patient will have little or no heterosexual arousal,
with the result that he or she has a history of being unsuccessful in
establishing or maintaining desired heterosexual relationships. However, some patients will have no history of heterosexual relationships as
their expectation of inadequate sexual responsiveness to an opposite-sex
partner prevents them from making any attempts to establish such relationships. Frequently, a desire for children and a family life is reported
by adults given this diagnosis. A history of unsatisfactory homosexual
relationships is generally present. However, some patients restrict their
homosexual arousal to fantasies as a result of strong negative feelings
regarding homosexuality.

Critical Diagnostic Information

Two diagnostic criteria have been specified for ego-dystonic homosexuality. First, the patient must complain of having weak or no heterosexual arousal and, consequently, significant difficulty initiating or
maintaining heterosexual relationships. Secondly, the individual must
not want his or her homosexual arousal and must experience distress as
a result of this arousal pattern. Homosexual arousal, even if limited to
fantasy, must be present before this diagnosis is appropriate. In brief,
the patient is desirous of eliminating homosexual-arousal activity patterns and replacing them with heterosexual patterns.

It is imperative that the clinician determine that the reported distress is a result of internalized conflict and not a response to situational
factors. For example, distress experienced as a result of being fearful
about losing one's job because of sexual orientation is not sufficient for
this diagnosis. The reported distress considered indicative of ego dystonic homosexuality is sometimes characterized as the result of the inter-
nalization of negative societal attitudes toward homosexuality. In addition, the distress and the subsequent desire to change sexual orientation
must be persistent. Individuals with this disorder are also described as
lonely, and to show guilt, anxiety, and depression in some cases (APA,
1980, p. 281).

The clinician must insure that psychological problems are not the
cause of the reported distress about sexual orientation. For example, a
patient with a major depressive disorder may experience self-hatred and

dissatisfaction that is subsequently directed at his or her sexual orientation. In such a case in which the desire to change sexual orientation is a symptom of the depressive disorder, a diagnosis of ego-dystonic homosexuality is inappropriate.

Homosexuality that is not congruent with these diagnostic criteria is not classified as a mental disorder.

A Continuing Ethical Issue

Much controversy continues to surround the inclusion of ego-dystonic homosexuality in DSM-III. Many clinicians take the position that choice of a consenting adult sexual partner is irrelevant to the diagnosis of a mental disorder and that, therefore, the inclusion of this diagnosis is inappropriate. In contrast, other mental health professionals assert that homosexuality *per se* is an emotional illness and must always be considered pathological.

This controversy is particularly apparent in the various stances taken in relation to the provision of treatment to individuals with a diagnosis of ego-dystonic homosexuality. Some psychoanalytically oriented clinicians assert that, because homosexuality is pathological, all individuals with a homosexual orientation should be treated (Bieber, 1976; Socarides, 1970). Such treatment is considered necessary whether the patient desires to become heterosexual, as in the case of ego-dystonic homosexuality, or the patient is satisfied with his or her sexual orientation. In the opposite camp, mental health professionals assert that treatments to modify sexual orientation should not be available to any homosexually oriented individuals, as the availability of such treatment reflects the belief that homosexuality itself is wrong or abnormal (Davison, 1976, 1978). Other clinicians take a middle-of-the-road position and recommend making treatment available to voluntary patients who want to change their sexual orientation (Masters & Johnson, 1979; Sturgis & Adams, 1978). Still other clinicians assert that a homosexually oriented individual may seek treatment in the belief that his or her sexual orientation is the cause of experienced dissatisfaction when, in actuality, other problems in functioning underlie the distress. Thus, the treatment offered should be directed at improving general functioning and coping skills rather than changing sexual orientation (Coleman, 1982; Hoffman, 1977; Phillips, Fischer, Groves, & Singh, 1976; Sandus, 1980). In fact, Halleck (1976) suggests that this may be the rule more than the exception and that it is imperative that a clinician address this issue in each case of possible ego-dystonic homosexuality.

Clearly, these various positions in relation to the treatment of ego-dystonic homosexuality reflect different ethical perspectives on homosexuality. A mental health professional should consider the various perspectives and their ethical implications and assess his or her own position prior to evaluating patients with homosexual orientations.

Summary

Diagnosing sexual dysfunctions and deviations as well as ego-dystonic homosexuality can be difficult at best because there is frequently no line dividing pathological from nonpathological behavior. This chapter discusses the procedures for conducting interviews with patients who have sexual problems, who engage in sexually deviant behavior, or who have an ego-dystonic homosexual orientation. Whenever possible, psychophysiological assessment should be included to augment the diagnostic process.

ACKNOWLEDGMENTS

The authors wish to thank Claire Silverstein and Suzanne Gattuso for their assistance with this chapter.

References

Abel, G. G., Barlow, D. H., Blanchard, E. B., & Guild, D. (1977). The components of rapists' sexual arousal. *Archives of General Psychiatry, 34,* 895–903.

Abel, G. G., Murphy, W. D., Becker, J. V., & Bitar, A. (1979). Women's vaginal responses during REM sleep. *Journal of Sex and Marital Therapy, 5,* 5–11.

Adelman, M. R. (1977). A comparison of professionally employed lesbians and heterosexual women on the MMPI. *Archives of Sexual Behavior, 6,* 193–202.

Allen, C. (1969). *A textbook of psychosexual disorders* (2d ed.). London: Oxford University Press.

American Psychiatric Association. (1958). *Diagnostic and statistical manual of mental disorders.* Washington, DC: Author.

American Psychiatric Association. (1968). *Diagnostic and statistical manual of mental disorders* (2d ed.). Washington, DC: Author.

American Psychiatric Association. (1980). *Diagnostic and statistical manual of mental disorders* (3rd ed.). Washington, DC: Author.

Amir, M. (1971). *Patterns in forcible rape.* Chicago: University of Chicago Press.

Annon, J. S. (1976). *Behavioral treatment of sexual problems: Brief therapy.* New York: Harper & Row.

Barbach, L. G., & Levine, L. (1980). *Shared intimacies.* Garden City, NY: Anchor Press/Doubleday.

Barbaree, H. E., Marshall, W. L., & Lanthier, R. D. (1979). Deviant sexual arousal in rapists. *Behaviour Research and Therapy, 17,* 215–222.

Becker, J. V., & Skinner, L. J. (1983). Sexual dysfunction. In M. Hersen (Ed.), *Outpatient behavior therapy: A clinical guide* (pp. 203–228). New York: Grune & Stratton.

Becker, J. V., Abel, G. G., Blanchard, E. B., Murphy, W. D., & Coleman, E. (1978). Evaluating social skills of sexual aggressives. *Criminal Justice and Behavior, 5,* 357–368.

Benjamin, H. (1966). *The transsexual phenomenon*. New York: Julian Press.

Bell, A. O. (1974). Homosexualities: Their range and character. In J. K. Cole & R. Dienstbier (Eds.), *Nebraska Symposium on Motivation, 1973* (pp. 1–26). Lincoln: University of Nebraska Press

Benjamin, H. (1967). Transvestism and transsexualism in the male and female. *Journal of Sex Research, 3*, 107–127.

Bieber, I. (1976). A discussion of "Homosexuality: The ethical challenge." *Journal of Consulting and Clinical Psychology, 44*, 163–166.

Blair, C. D., & Lanyon, R. (1981). Exhibitionism: A critical review of etiology and treatment. *Psychological Bulletin, 89*, 439–463.

Blair, J., & Justice, R. (1979). *The broken taboo*. New York: Human Sciences Press.

Bray, C. P., DeFrank, R. S., & Wolfe, I. L. (1981). Sexual functioning in stroke survivors. *Archives of Physical Medicine and Rehabilitation, 62*, 286–288.

Brouillette, J. N., Pryor, E., & Fox, T. A. (1981). Evaluation of sexual dysfunction following rectal resection and intestinal stoma. *Diseases of the Rectum and Colon, 24*, 96–102.

Burgess, A. W., Groth, A. N., Holmstrom, L. L., & Sgroi, S. (1978). *Sexual assault of children and adolescents*. Lexington, MA: D. C. Heath.

Byrne, D. (1977). The imagery of sex. In J. Money & H. Musaph (Eds.), *Handbook of sexology* (pp. 327–350). New York: Elsevier/North-Holland.

Caprio, F. (1961). Fetishism. In A. Ellis & A. Abarbanel (Eds.), *Encyclopedia of sexual behavior* (Vol. 1). New York: Hawthorn Books.

Carlson, E. R., & Coleman, C. E. K. (1977). Experimental and motivational determinants of an induced sexual fantasy. *Journal of Personality, 45*, 528–542.

Chappell, D., & James, J. (1976). *Victim selection and apprehensions from the rapist's perspective: A preliminary investigation*. Paper presented at the Second International Symposium on Victimology, Boston.

Christie, M., Marshall, W., & Lanthier, R. (1978). *A descriptive study of incarcerated rapists and pedophiles*. Unpublished manuscript.

Cohen, M. L., Leghorn, T., & Calmas, W. (1969). Sociometric study of the sex offender. *Journal of Abnormal Psychology, 74*, 249–255.

Coleman, E. (1982). Changing approaches to the treatment of homosexuality: A review. In W. Paul, J. D. Weinrich, J. C. Gonsiorek, & M. E. Hotvedt (Eds.), *Homosexuality: Social, psychological and biological issues*. Beverly Hills, CA: Sage.

Courtois, R. A., & Hinkley, J. A. (1981). Grandfather–granddaughter incest. *Journal of Sex Education and Therapy, 7*, 37–42.

Crépault, C., & Couture, M. (1980). Men's erotic fantasies. *Archives of Sexual Behavior, 9*, 565–581.

Davison, G. C. (1976). Homosexuality: The ethical challenge. *Journal of Consulting and Clinical Psychology, 44*, 157–162.

Davison, G. C. (1978). Not can but ought: The treatment of homosexuality. *Journal of Consulting and Clinical Psychology, 46*, 170–172.

De Francis, V. (1969). *Protecting the child victim of sex crimes committed by adults*. Denver: American Humane Association.

Evans, D. R. (1970). Exhibitionism. In C. G. Costello (Ed.), *Symptoms of psychopathology*. New York: Wiley.

Feigelman, W. (1977). Peeping: The pattern of voyeurism among construction workers. In R. D. Bryant (Ed.), *Sexual deviancy in social context*. New York: New Viewpoints.

Finkelhor, D. (1979). *Sexually victimized children*. New York: Free Press.

FitzGerald, M., & FitzGerald, D. (1980). The potential effects of deafness upon sexuality. *Sexuality and Disability, 3*, 177–181.

Forward, S., & Buck, C. (1978). *Betrayal of innocence: Incest and its devastation.* New York: J. P. Tarcher.

Freedman, M. (1971). *Homosexuality and psychological functioning.* Belmont, CA: Wadsworth.

Freund, K. (1967). Diagnosing homo- or heterosexuality and erotic age-preference by means of a psychophysiological test. *Behaviour Research and Therapy, 5,* 209–228. (a)

Freund, K. (1967). Erotic preference in pedophilia. *Behaviour Research and Therapy, 5,* 339–348. (b)

Freund, K., Chan, S., & Coulthard, R. (1979). Phallometric diagnosis with "nonadmitters." *Behaviour Research and Therapy, 17,* 451–457.

Fritz, G. S., Stoll, K., & Wagner, N. N. (1981). A comparison of males and females who were sexually molested as children. *Journal of Sex and Marital Therapy, 7,* 54–59.

Gagnon, J. H. (1977). *Human sexualities.* Glenview, IL: Scott, Foresman.

Gebhard, P. H. (1977). Fetishism and sadomasochism. In D. Byrne & L. A. Byrne (Eds.), *Exploring human sexuality.* New York: Crowell.

Gebhard, P. H., & Johnson, A. B. (1979), *The Kinsey data: Marginal tabulations of the 1938–1963 interviews conducted by the Institute for Sex Research.* Philadelphia: W. B. Saunders.

Gebhard, P. H., Gagnon, J. H., Pomeroy, W. B., & Christenson, C. V. (1965), *Sex offenders: An analysis of types.* New York: Harper & Row.

Gonsiorek, J. (1982). Results of psychological testing on homosexual populations. In W. Paul, J. D. Weinrich, J. C. Gonsiorek, & M. E. Hotvedt (Eds.), *Homosexuality: Social, psychological and biological issues.* Beverly Hills, CA: Sage Publications.

Gosselin, C., & Wilson, G. (1980). *Sexual variations: Fetishism, sadomasochism, and transvestism.* New York: Simon & Schuster.

Green, R. (1971). Homosexuality as a mental illness. *International Journal of Psychiatry, 10,* 77–98.

Groth, A. N., & Birnbaum, H. J. (1979). *Men who rape: The psychology of the offender.* New York: Plenum Press.

Groth, A. N., Burgess, A. W., & Holmstrom, L. (1977). Rape: Power, anger and sexuality. *American Journal of Psychiatry, 134,* 1239–1243.

Halleck, S. L. (1976). Another response to "Homosexuality: The ethical challenge." *Journal of Consulting and Clinical Psychology, 44,* 167–170.

Hariton, E. B., & Singer, J. L. (1974). Women's fantasies during sexual intercourse: Normative and theoretical explanations. *Journal of Consulting and Clinical Psychology, 42,* 313–322.

Hendrix, E., & Meyer, R. (1976). Toward a more comprehensive and durable client change: A case report. *Psychotherapy: Theory, Research, and Practice, 13,* 263–266.

Higgens, G. E. (1979). Sexual response in spinal cord injured adults: A review of the literature. *Archives of Sexual Behavior, 8,* 173–196.

Hinton, J. W., O'Neill, M. T., & Webster, S. (1980). Psychophysiological assessment of sex offenders in a security hospital. *Archives of Sexual Behavior, 9,* 205–216.

Hoffman, M. (1977). Homosexuality. In F. Beach (Ed.), *Human sexuality in four perspectives* (pp. 167–189). Baltimore: John Hopkins University Press.

Hollender, M. H., Brown, C. W., & Roback, H. B. (1977). Genital exhibitionism in women. *American Journal of Psychiatry, 134,* 436–438.

Hooberman, R. E. (1979). Psychological androgyny, feminine gender identity and self-esteem in homosexual and heterosexual males. *Journal of Sex Research, 15,* 306–315.

Hooker, E. (1957). The adjustment of the male overt homosexual. *Journal of Projective Techniques, 21,* 18–31.

Hughes, R. C. (1977). Covert sensitization treatment of exhibitionism. *Journal of Behavior Therapy and Experimental Psychiatry, 8,* 177–179.

Hunt, M. (1974). *Sexual behavior in the 1970's*. Chicago: Playboy Press.

Jensen, S. B. (1981). Diabetic sexual dysfunction: A comparative study of 160 insulin treated diabetic men and women and an age-matched control group. *Archives of Sexual Behavior, 10*, 493–504. (a)

Jensen, S. B. (1981). Sexual function in 20 younger insulin-treated diabetic out-patients: A two year follow-up study. *Sexuality and Disability, 3*, 61–67. (b)

Kaplan, H. S. (1974). *The new sex therapy*. New York: Brunner/Mazel.

Karacan, I. (1970). Clinical value of nocturnal erections in the prognosis and diagnosis of impotence. *Medical Aspects of Human Sexuality, 4*, 27–34.

Karacan, I., Williams, R. L., Thornby, J. I., & Salis, P. J. (1975). Sleep-related tumescence as a function of age. *American Journal of Psychiatry, 132*, 932–937.

Katchadourian, H. A., & Lunde, D. T. (1975). *Fundamentals of human sexuality*. New York: Holt, Rinehart & Winston.

Kercher, G. A., & Walker, C. E. (1973). Reactions of convicted rapists to sexually explicit stimuli. *Journal of Abnormal Psychology, 81*, 46–50.

Kinsey, A. C., Pomeroy, W. B., & Martin, C. E. (1948). *Sexual behavior in the human male*. Philadelphia: W. B. Saunders.

Kinsey, A. C., Pomeroy, W. B., Martin, C. E., & Gebhard, P. H. (1953). *Sexual behavior in the human female*. Philadelphia: W. B. Saunders.

Kolarsky, A., Madlafousek, J., & Novotna, V. (1978). Stimuli eliciting sexual arousal in males who offend adult women: An experimental study. *Archives of Sexual Behavior, 7*, 79–87.

Kolodny, R. C. (1971). Sexual dysfunction in diabetic females. *Diabetes, 20*, 557–559.

Kolodny, R. C., Kahn, C. B., & Goldstein, H. H. (1974). Sexual dysfunction in diabetic men. *Diabetes, 23*, 306–309.

Kolodny, R. C., Masters, W. H., & Johnson, V. E. (1979). *Textbook of sexual medicine*. Boston: Little, Brown.

Lamberti, J. (1979). Sexual adjustment after radiation therapy for cervical carcinoma. *Medical Aspects of Human Sexuality, 13*, 87–88.

Langevin, R., Paitich, D., Freeman, R., Mann, K., & Handy, L. (1978). Personality characteristics and sexual anomalies in males. *Canadian Journal of Behavioral Science, 10*, 222–238.

Langevin, R., Paitich, D., Ramsay, A., Anderson, C., Kamrad, J., Pope, S., Geller, G., Pearl, L., & Newman, S. (1979). Experimental studies of the etiology of genital exhibitionism. *Archives of Sexual Behavior, 8*, 307–332.

Laws, D. R., & Holman, M. L. (1978). Sexual response faking by pedophiles. *Criminal Justice and Behavior, 5*, 343–356.

Laws, D. R. & Osborn, C. A. (1983). How to build and operate a behavioral laboratory to evaluate and treat sexual deviance. In J. G. Greer & I. R. Stuart (Eds.), *The sexual aggressor: Current perspectives on treatment* (pp. 293–362). New York: Van Nostrand Reinhold.

Lilius, H. G., Valtonen, E. J., & Wikström, J. (1976). Sexual problems in patients suffering from multiple sclerosis. *Journal of Chronic Diseases, 29*, 643–647.

LoPiccolo, J. (1977). Direct treatment of sexual dysfunction in the couple. In J. Money & H. Musaph (Eds.), *Handbook of sexology* (pp. 1227–1244). Amsterdam: Elsevier/North-Holland.

Lundeberg, P. D. (1977). Sexual dysfunction in patients with neurological disorders. In R. Gemme & C. C. Wheeler (Eds.), *Progress in sexology*. New York: Plenum Press.

Lundeberg, P. D. (1978). Sexual dysfunction in patients with multiple sclerosis. *Sexuality and Disability, 1*, 218–222.

MacDonald, J. M. (1971) *Rape: Offenders and their victims*. Springfield, IL: Charles C Thomas.

Mac Donald, J. M. (1973). *Indecent exposure*. Springfield, IL: Charles C Thomas.

MacNamara, D. E., & Sagarin, E. (1977). *Crime and the law*. New York: Free Press.

Marmor, J. (1980). Clinical aspects of male homosexuality. In J. Marmor (Ed.), *Homosexual behavior* (pp. 267–279). New York: Basic Books.

Maruta, T., Osborne, D., Swanson, D. W., & Halling, J. M. (1981). Chronic pain patients and spouses' marital and sexual adjustment. *Mayo Clinic Proceedings, 56*, 307–310.

Masters, W. H., & Johnson, V. E. (1970). *Human sexual inadequacy*. Boston: Little, Brown.

Masters, W. & Johnson, V. (1979). *Homosexuality in perspective*. Boston: Little, Brown.

Masters, W., Johnson, V., & Kolodny, R. (1982). *Human sexuality*. Boston: Little, Brown.

McCaghy, C. H. (1971). Child molesting. *Sexual Behavior, 1*, 16–24.

McCaghy, C. H. (1980). Child molesters' "explanations." *Medical Aspects of Human Sexuality, 14*, 105.

McCary, J. L. (1978). *McCary's human sexuality* (3rd ed.). New York: Van Nostrand Reinhold.

McCauley, C., & Swann, C. P. (1976). Male-female differences in sexual fantasy. *Journal of Research in Personality, 12*, 76–86.

McCauley, C., & Swann, C. P., (1980). Sex differences in the frequency and functions of fantasies during sexual activity. *Journal of Research in Personality, 14*, 400–411.

McCreary, C. P. (1975). Personality profiles of persons convicted of indecent exposure. *Journal of Clinical Psychology, 31*, 260–262.

McDermott, J. (1979). *Rape victimization in 26 American Cities*. Washington, DC: U.S. Department of Justice, Law Enforcement and Assistance Administration.

Mednick, R. A. (1977). Gender-specific variances in sexual fantasy. *Journal of Personality Assessment, 41*, 248–254.

Meiselman, K. (1978). *Incest*. San Francisco: Jossey-Bass.

Mohr, J. W., Turner, R. E., & Jerry, M. B. (1964). *Pedophilia and exhibitionism*. Toronto: University of Toronto Press.

Money, J. (1977). Determinants of human gender identity/role. In J. Money & H. Musaph (Eds.), *Handbook of sexology*. New York: Excerpta Medica.

Money, J., & Wiedeking, C. (1980). Gender identity/role: Normal differention and its transposition. In B. B. Wolman & J. Money (Eds.), *Handbook of human sexuality* (pp. 269–284). Englewood Cliffs, NJ: Prentice-Hall.

Money, J., Jobaris, R., & Furth, G. (1977). Apotemnophilia: Two cases of self-demand amputation as a paraphilia. *Journal of Sex Research, 13*, 1115–1125.

Moreault, D. & Fallingstad, D. R. (1978). Sexual fantasies of females as a function of sex guilt and experimental responses cues. *Journal of Consulting and Clinical Psychology, 46*, 1385–1393.

Morin, S. F. (1977). Heterosexual bias in psychological research on lesbianism and male homosexuality. *American Psychologist, 32*, 629–637.

Nadler, R. (1968). Approach to psychodynamics of obscene telephone calls. *New York Journal of Medicine, 68*, 521–526.

National Institute of Law Enforcement and Criminal Justice. (1978). *Forcible rape: Final project report*. Washington, DC: U.S. Government Printing Office.

Paitich, D., Langevin, R., Freeman, R., Mann, K., & Handy, L. (1977). The Clarke SHQ: A clinical sex history questionnaire for males. *Archives of Sexual Behavior, 6*, 421–436.

Perdue, W. C., & Lester, D. (1972). Personality characteristics of rapists. *Perceptual and Motor Skills, 37*, 1699–1712.

Phillips, D., Fischer, S. C., Groves, G. A., & Singh, R. (1976). Alternative behavioral approaches to the treatment of homosexuality. *Archives of Sexual Behavior, 5*, 223–228.

Podolsky, S. (1980). Sexual impotence in the aging diabetic male: Organic or psychogenic etiology? *The Gerontologist, 20*, 181.

Prince, V., & Bentler, P. M. (1972). Survey of 504 cases of transvestism. *Psychological Reports, 31*, 903–917.

Quinsey, V. L., & Carrigan, W. F. (1978). Penile responses to visual stimuli. *Criminal Justice and Behavior, 5*, 333–342.

Quinsey, V. L., & Marshall, W. L. (1983). Procedures for reducing inappropriate sexual arousal: An evaluation review. In J. G. Greer & I. R. Stuart (Eds.), *The sexual aggressor: Current perspectives on treatment* (pp. 267–289). New York: Van Nostrand Reinhold.

Quinsey, V. L., Steinman, C. M., Bergersen, S. G., & Holmes, T. F. (1975). Penile circumferences, skin conductance and ranking responses of child molesters and "normals" to sexual and nonsexual stimuli. *Behavior Therapy, 6*, 213–219.

Quinsey, V. L., Bergersen, S. G., & Steinman, C. M. (1976). Changes in physiological and verbal responses of child molesters during aversion therapy. *Canadian Journal of Behavioural Science, 8*, 202–212.

Quinsey, V. L., Chaplin, T. C., & Varney, G. (1981). A comparison of rapists' and non-sex offenders' sexual preferences for mutually consenting sex, rape, and physical abuse of women. *Behavioral Assessment, 3*, 127–135.

Rada, R. (1977). Commonly asked questions about the rapist. *Medical Aspects of Human Sexuality, 11*, 47–56.

Reiss, B. F. (1980). Psychological tests in homosexuality. In J. Marmor (Ed.), *Homosexual behavior*. New York: Basic Books.

Rosen, R. C., & Kopel, S. A. (1977). Penile plethysmography and biofeedback in the treatment of a transvestite-exhibitionist. *Journal of Consulting and Clinical Psychology, 45*, 908–916.

Ruff, C. F. Templar, D. I., & Ayers, J. L. (1976). The intelligence of rapists. *Archives of Sexual Behavior, 5*, 4.

Sagarin, E. (1973). Power to the peephole. *Sexual Behavior, 3*, 2–7.

Sagher, M. S. & Robins, E. (1973). *Male and female homosexuality*: Baltimore: Williams & Wilkins.

Sanders, D. S. (1980). A psychotherapeutic approach to homosexual men. In J. Marmor (Ed.), *Homosexual behavior*. New York: Basic Books.

Schiavi, R. C., Derogatis, L. R., Kuriansky, J., O'Connor, D., & Sharpe, L. (1979). The assessment of sexual function and marital interaction. *Journal of Sex and Marital Therapy, 5*, 169–224.

Siegelman, M. (1981). Parental backgrounds of homosexual and heterosexual women: A cross-national replication. *Archives of Sexual Behavior, 10*, 371–378.

Silny, A. (1980). Sexuality and aging. In B. Wolan (Ed.), *Handbook of human sexuality*. Englewood Cliffs, NJ: Prentice-Hall.

Smith, R. (1976). Voyeurism: A review of the literature. *Archives of Sexual Behavior, 5*, 585–609.

Smith, S., & Meyer, R. (1980). Working between the legal system and the therapist. In D. Cox & R. Daitzman (Eds.), *Exhibitionism*. New York: Garland.

Smithyman, S. D. (1979). Characteristics of "undetected" rapists. In W. H. Parsonage (Ed.), *Perspectives on victimology*. Beverly Hills, CA: Sage.

Smukler, A. J., & Schiebel, D. (1975). Personality characteristics of exhibitionists. *Diseases of the Nervous System, 36*, 600–603.

Socarides, C. W. (1970). Homosexuality and medicine. *Journal of the American Medical Association, 212*, 1199–1202.

Spengler, A. (1977). Manifest sadomasochism of males: Results of an empirical study. *Archives of Sexual Behavior, 6*, 441–456.

Stoller, R. J. (1971). The term "transvestism." *Archives of General Psychiatry, 24,* 230–232.
Stoller, R. J. (1977). Sexual deviations. In F. Beach (Ed.), *Human sexuality in four perspectives* (pp. 190–214). Baltimore; John Hopkins University Press.
Strassberg, D., Roback, H., Cunningham, J., McKee, E., & Larson, P. (1979). Psychopathology in self-identified female-to-male transsexuals, homosexuals, and heterosexuals. *Archives of Sexual Behavior, 8,* 491–496.
Sturgis, E. T., & Adams, H. E. (1978). The right to treatment: Issues in the treatment of homosexuality. *Journal of Consulting and Clinical Psychology, 46,* 165–169.
Sue, D. (1979). Erotic fantasies of college students during coitus. *Journal of Sex Research, 15,* 299–305.
Summit, R., & Kryso, J. (1978). Sexual abuse of children: A clinical spectrum. *American Journal of Orthopsychiatry, 48,* 237–251.
Templar, D. I., & Eberhardt, E. (1980). Necrophilia: A review. *Essence, 4,* 63–67.
Thompson, N. L., Jr., McCandless, B. R., & Strickland, B. R. (1971). Personal adjustment of male and female homosexuals and heterosexuals. *Journal of Abnormal Psychology, 78,* 237–240.
Tollison, C. D., & Adams, H. E. (1979). *Sexual disorders: Treatment, theory, research.* New York: Gardner Press.
Verba, H., Barnard, G. W., & Holzer, C. (1979). The intelligence of rapists, New data. *Archives of Sexual Behavior, 8,* 375–378.
Wabek, A. J., & Burchell, R. C. (1980). Male sexual dysfunction associated with coronary heart disease. *Archives of Sexual Behavior, 9,* 65–75.
Weinberg, M., & Williams, C. J. (1974). *Male homosexualities: Their problems and adaptations in three societies.* New York: Oxford University Press.
Wise, T. N., & Meyer, J. K. (1980). Transvestism: Previous findings and new areas for inquiry. *Journal of Sex and Marital Therapy, 6,* 116–128.
Wish, P. A. (1975). The use of imagery-based techniques in the treatment of sexual dysfunction. *The Counseling Psychologist, 5,* 52–55.
Wolfe, J., & Baker, V. (1980). Characteristics of imprisoned rapists and circumstances of the rape. In C. Warner (Ed.), *Rape and sexual assault* (pp. 265–278). Germantown, MD: Aspen Systems Corp.
Yalom, I. D. (1960). Aggression and forbiddenness in voyeurism. *Archives of General Psychiatry, 3,* 305–319.

Chapter 10

Eating Disorders

John P. Foreyt and Albert T. Kondo

Introduction

The *Diagnostic and Statistical Manual of Mental Disorders* (DSM-III) (American Psychiatric Association, 1980) includes four disturbances under the heading "Eating Disorders." They are anorexia nervosa, bulimia, rumination, and pica. The maladaptive eating that lead some to obesity was not included because obesity "is not generally associated with any distinct psychological or behavioral syndrome" (p. 67). However, our research and clinical observations have suggested that many afflicted with obesity have serious problems of eating. Therefore, it is included in this chapter as a major area for discussion.

  With our present state of knowledge, the diagnosis of eating disorders is characterized more by art than science and tentativeness rather than specific standards. This situation is reflective of our formative stage of development in understanding and treating these disorders. For all of them, we are just beginning to fully appreciate the multiple factors associated with their etiology and that they may interact in exceedingly complex ways (Foreyt & Kondo, in press, a). Illustrative of this complexity is Stunkard's (1981) speculation that restrained eating may have association with the number and condition of fat cells, or Wurtman *et al.*'s (Wurtman, Wurtman, Growdon, Henry, Lipscomb, & Zeisel, 1981) suggestion that carbohydrate craving is linked to an insufficient synthesis of the neurotransmitter serotonin.

JOHN P. FOREYT and ALBERT T. KONDO • Diet Modification Clinic, Baylor College of Medicine and The Methodist Hospital, Houston, Texas 77030.

This chapter will concentrate on three of the eating disorders: anorexia nervosa, bulimia, and those eating problems associated with obesity. This selection was made because of the severity, prevalance, and general concern shown for these disturbances.

Description of Conditions

Anorexia Nervosa

Of the three disorders described in this chapter, anorexia nervosa is the one most noted for its severe course and consequences. It is the eating disorder that can result in death, most often from the complications arising from the state of starvation.

Anorexia nervosa is a perplexing condition, for its most notable characteristic is self-imposed starvation in a country and culture blessed with an abundance of food. However, for anorectics, the apparent illogic of their actions is overridden by a psychological framework ruled by two powerful contingencies: the reward of weight loss and a morbid fear of fatness (Garner, Garfinkel, & Bemis, 1982).

The diagnostic criteria for anorexia nervosa are published in the DSM-III (APA, 1980) and are as follows:

- Weight loss of at least 25% of original body weight
- Disturbance of body image
- Intense fear of becoming obese
- Refusal to maintain body weight over a minimal normal weight for age and height
- No known physical illness that would account for the weight loss

In addition to these characteristics, others are frequently found in association with this condition. Besides the severe weight loss, the most consistent physical finding is amenorrhea among females. This symptom, like many of the others frequently observed, is the apparent physical manifestation of an organism's attempting to adapt to severe undernourishment. Additional symptomatology include low metabolic rate, low blood pressure, cold intolerance, insomnia, bradycardia, and pathological EEG patterns (Bemis, 1978).

Ninety-five percent of anorectics are female (APA, 1980). This disproportionate representation of females indicates the strong cultural influences in its etiology (Foreyt & Kondo, in press, b). In the United States and many of the other Western nations, slenderness has become synonymous with attractiveness, and it is apparent that the achievement of both is an expectation more of women than men (Al-Issa, 1980; Garner, Garfinkel, Schwartz, & Thompson, 1980).

A number of psychological traits characterize the anorectic, including shyness, anxiety, and obsessive-compulsive behaviors (Bemis, 1978). These characteristics, although the source of much inner turmoil, are frequently manifested in outward behaviors that are viewed positively by family and friends. In many families, the presymptomatic anorexic child is frequently perceived as the "pride and joy" of the brood, often characterized by parents as being well behaved, achieving, and perfectionistic (Halmi, Goldberg, Eckert, Casper, & Davis, 1977). Some (e.g., Bruch, 1978; Rosman, Minuchin, Baker, & Liebman, 1977), however, suggest that many of the anorectic traits are engendered by the particular interactional patterns and values of the families involved. Bruch (1977) noted that among anorectic families, parents tended to be overprotective, overconcerned, and overambitious. Within this setting, she noted that expectations of obedience and superior performance of the children were a concomitant observation.

Other psychological characteristics associated with anorexia included distorted thoughts and beliefs (Garner & Bemis, 1982), poor self-esteem (Garner, Garfinkel, & Bemis, 1982), distorted body image (Crisp & Kalucy, 1974), and fears over matters of self-control (Bruch, 1977). These characteristics, in combination with the familial setting, peer influences, particular experiences, and even the physiology of the child may lead to anorexia nervosa.

Bulimia

In recent years, bulimia has gained increasing attention as the extent of its occurrence and the severity of its symptomatology have become known. Although bulimia is literally translated to mean *ox hunger*, for most who have this condition, their eating has little association with the fulfillment of normal biologic hunger. The hunger is more frequently derived from inner needs, and for many this hunger is insatiable.

DSM-III (APA, 1980) lists the following criteria for bulimia:

- Recurrent episodes of binge eating.
- At least three of the following:
  1. Consumption of high caloric, easily ingested food during a binge.
  2. Inconspicuous eating during a binge.
  3. Termination of such eating episodes by abdominal pain, sleep, social interruption, or self-induced vomiting.
  4. Repeated attempts to lose weight by severely restrictive diets, self-induced vomiting, or use of cathartics or diuretics.
  5. Frequent weight fluctuations greater than 10 pounds due to alternating binges and fasts.

- Awareness that the eating pattern is abnormal and fear of not being able to stop eating voluntarily.
- Depressed mood and self-deprecating thoughts following eating binges.
- The bulimic episodes are not due to anorexia nervosa or any known physical disorder. (pp. 70–71)

Because of the media publicity given to this condition, bulimia has become largely known as the *binge–purge* syndrome. However, as the preceding criteria indicate, purging is not essential to fulfill the requirements of a diagnosis. Many consider "purging" to be inappropriate use of laxatives or diuretics; in a more general sense, "purging" is any action that is taken to reverse the effects of a binge and may include severely restrictive diets and/or excessive exercise. The latter is illustrated by a patient of ours who habitually "corrected" her binge episodes with 20-mile bike rides. The excursions were marked by their compulsive and urgent quality; they sometimes occurred at odd hours in the morning, during inclement weather, or even during the course of a social gathering.

Bulimia, like anorexia nervosa, is a problem primarily of young women. In this regard, it is probable that some of the sociocultural dynamics that result in anorexia operate to influence the onset of bulimia. White and Boskind-White (1981) theorized that this condition occurs because of the need for some women to fit into the role of "stereotyped femininity." In fulfilling this stereotype, they suggest that the basis for bulimia is also developed and reinforced; this includes a need to please others, tendencies toward passivity, and an excessive concern for appearance and thinness.

The physical toll taken by the practice of bulimia is not as great as the one experienced by the anorexic; however, it can be severe. Among the physical sequelae are esophageal rupture and hiatal hernias from frequent vomiting, urinary infections, impaired kidney function, irregular menstrual cycles, dental problems, and electrolyte disturbances (Neuman & Halvorson, 1983). Because many bulimics maintain a normal weight and appear healthy, the damage done by their compulsion often goes unrecognized, even by the closest of contacts, until medical intervention is required.

For most bulimics, there is a psychological cost of their practice that parallels the physical ones. Our society, as in many others, has standards of acceptable behavior concerning ingestion and elimination (including vomiting). Bulimic behavior with its sometimes prodigious consumption and forced elimination crosses the boundaries of acceptability. Most who engage in this practice are exceedingly aware of its unacceptability; some are even revulsed by it. This awareness is associated with the low self-esteem, feelings of inadequacy, and self-derogation ob-

served among many. The shame that accompanies this practice is probably the primary reason why this problem remained "in the closet" for so
long, and why it continues to remain there for many sufferers.

As in the other eating disorders, little is known of the causes of
bulimia. Many theories exist to explain its occurrence, ranging from the
psychoanalytic (Nemiah, 1950; Nogami & Yobana, 1977) and feminist
(White & Boskind-White, 1981), to physical explanations (Green & Rau,
1974; Russell, 1979). None of these theories has achieved widespread
acceptance. Hence, diagnosis and treatment of this disorder must proceed on a rather tenuous basis.

Obesity

From the outset, it should be noted that obesity is not an eating
disorder. It is a physical condition that may arise from an eating disorder. DSM-III made a similar distinction when it excluded obesity from its
eating disorder section because of its lack of consistent psychological
and behavioral characteristics (APA, 1980). When psychological factors
are associated with the cause and/or course of the condition, it is classified in the section entitled "Psychological Factors Affecting Physical
Condition."

The condition of obesity is usually defined as body weight 20% in
excess of ideal. Although this has become a widely used standard, it is
open to some error. Obesity is a state of excessive fat tissue, of which
weight is an indirect measure. It is possible, therefore, for an individual
to be overweight but not overfat; this is exemplified by the well-trained
football player or weight lifter. However, as few adult Americans
achieve such muscularity, the weight standard for obesity has broad
utility.

Obesity is a prevalent problem in the United States. Approximately
13% of adult males and 23% of adult females are obese (U.S. Department
of Health, Education, and Welfare, 1978). More than twice as many rate
themselves as obese, with two-thirds of that number trying to do something about it.

The problems associated with obesity are twofold—physical and
psychological. From the physical standpoint, obesity, especially in its
severe forms, increases the susceptibility for a number of conditions:
hypertension, hyperlipidemia, pulmonary and renal problems, diabetes
mellitus, and even early death (Brownell, 1982). Although the possibility
of acquiring these problems is of importance to most obese, it is our
observation that it is the psychological ramifications that cause the most
prevalent problems among this population. To be obese in this society

obsessed with slenderness is to be deviant, unattractive, and the target of moral judgment (Allon, 1975).

During the past two decades, the complexity of obesity has become better understood. Whereas it was once assumed that obesity was primarily the result of repetitive gluttony, it is now recognized that a number of influences are likely to be associated with its etiology: genetics, early feeding practices, family eating patterns and food preferences, exercise habits, and life-style (Stunkard, 1980). To underscore the assertion that excessive eating is not the sole cause of obesity, Wooley, Wooley, and Dyrenforth (1979) reported on 20 studies that indicated the obese eat no more than the lean.

For some obese, disordered eating is part of their difficulty. This may take many forms: night eating, excessive snacking, unconscious eating, and compulsive or binge eating. In our view, three factors are noteworthy in marking an act of disordered eating: the apparent precipitation of eating for emotionally laden reasons, the manner of eating, and the presence of guilt, self-recrimination, and/or self-loathing following the experience. A frequent accompaniment to these characteristics is an excessive concern over matters of body image and weight loss. For some, these become matters of desperation and chronic concern. In this way, they both precipitate and exacerbate their disordered eating. These characteristics form a common thread that serves to link anorexia nervosa, bulimia, and obesity as eating disorders, and as a baseline for diagnosing their presence.

Procedures for Information Gathering

The remainder of this chapter will concentrate on discussion of eating disorders in a general fashion without specific reference to each; however, each will be used to illustrate and clarify the concepts presented.

Accurate diagnosis is the cornerstone for the effective treatment of most, if not all, psychological difficulties; this is no less true for the eating disorders. Diagnosis serves the task of treatment: it guides and directs. In this regard, we do not circumscribe diagnosis by time, nor do we use it as separate from treatment; it is integral to the entire process.

Our procedure for gathering information is generally to incorporate this process into treatment as naturally and comfortably as possible. The initial meeting has more of the elements of an interview than subsequent ones; nevertheless, effort is made to reduce feelings of discomfort. It is not our general practice to use structured scales or questionnaires.

Their use at this time is considered unwarranted, as the eating disorders are yet without accepted theories of cause and course. Without this foundation, diagnosis of the factors important to an individual's problem is best characterized by tentativeness and experimentation. That is, issues suspected to have relevance to the client's eating problem are explored and investigated. Their validity is determined by the manner in which the client is affected; if they bring insight and/or change, then relevance is verified.

The multifactorial etiology of eating disorders often requires a multidisciplinary approach to treatment. In such cases, it is important for the therapist to be aware of the diagnoses of the others involved, as they may have relevance. For example, in anorexia nervosa, weight must be returned to a medically determined minimum before effective work can begin on the psychological issues (Bruch, 1973). In cases of bulimia, the client may seek psychotherapeutic help without prior consultation with a physician. It is incumbent upon the therapist to insist upon medical examination early in treatment as well as during its course if any form of purging is involved. As indicated previously, the continual practice of vomiting and abuse of diuretics or laxatives can lead to serious physical consequences. Our experience has been that the participation of a physician and dietitian is essential in the treatment of an eating disorder.

It is not our expectation that the initial diagnostic meeting (usually the first treatment session) will reveal much of the client's difficulties. Eating disorders and the associated practices (e.g., vomiting) are considered aberrant in our society, and most clients are acutely aware of this. Thus, it is common for information to be purposely withheld, "forgotten," or distorted in the early interviews. This is especially true for anorectics who frequently deny the existence of a problem and do not see the necessity of their presence in treatment. Obtaining accurate information is a *process* based on many of the factors that make for effective treatment: a good therapeutic relationship, trust, and a client's sense that the therapist is working with and for his or her benefit. We find that as our relationship with the client solidifies the diagnostic picture becomes concurrently richer.

Sensitivity is another important aspect of the process of diagnosis. The therapist needs to be aware of the sensitive areas of the client in probing for information and, at times, be willing to delay its receipt until readiness is apparent. A good example of this occurs with the use of food records. Although we find food records invaluable tools for diagnosis and treatment, some react to our use of them with considerable resistance. Food records require individuals to document patterns that they have frequently denied or suppressed. Their accurate utilization would be tantamount to a personal confrontation with their problem.

The therapist needs to be aware of the client's readiness for such confrontation in suggesting the use of food records.

A particularly sensitive area for many of the obese (and other individuals as well) is how their weight and weight loss affects their sexual relations. A recent patient of ours, Beth, had lost a substantial amount of weight in treatment and found that one of its concomitants was a deteriorating relationship with her husband. Symptomatic of this deterioration was his growing sexual impotence. This, needless to say, created stress in both parties. In terms of Beth and her eating disorder's treatment, these occurrences were viewed in terms of their possible utilization as rationale for returning to the prior state (i.e., overweight and disordered eating). From the standpoint of diagnosis, Beth revealed these problems and she saw their possible pertinence to treatment.

As implied in the example of Beth, we feel that diagnosis and treatment need to occur with the active involvement of both therapist and client. Clients often enter therapy with a perspective that they will be "treated" and that their role is essentially passive. Our approach is to emphasize the client's active role, that they can find the bases of their problems and make the necessary changes, and that the control is in their hands as much as it is in the therapist's hands. Bruch (1973) conveyed a similar thought when she noted:

> For effective treatment, it is decisive that a patient experience himself as an active participant in the therapeutic process. If there are things to be uncovered and interpreted, it is important that the patient makes the discovery on his own and has a chance to say it first. (p. 338)

If clients are to be participants in the diagnostic process, they need to be taught that they *can* do this, and they need to be shown *how*. Thus, we see part of our role in treatment as educators. Much treatment time is spent helping our clients understand their disorders, the many things that can influence their occurrence, and the importance of their collaborative involvement. This education is eclectic and is oriented to the disorder and individual. Some of the things we have used include bibliotherapy, modeling, role playing, and problem-solving methodologies.

Case Examples

Linda is a 32-year-old female employed at a temporary services agency. She is divorced and living with her current male friend, Bill, a 35-year-old real estate developer. When Linda came to her first session she weighed 164 pounds and stood 5 ft 5 in. tall. She said that she has always had a weight problem and had lost and regained excess pounds "countless times" over the past 10 years.

Two aspects of Linda's case had important diagnostic implications. One was her expectations for losing weight; the other was her lack of success in a behavior modification weight loss clinic.

THERAPIST: Linda, you mentioned over the telephone that you have the opportunity to be rehired by your former employer. Tell me more about that.

LINDA: I worked for 11 years as a stewardess for an airline that went bankrupt 2 years ago. That airline was my whole life. After it went under, I became depressed and have not worked regularly since that time. I am presently employed as a temporary, but my hours are very irregular. The airline has now begun flying again and because of my seniority I have the opportunity to be rehired. They told me last November that I would be called in June. The airline is enforcing a strict weight requirement and told me that I cannot weigh more than 140 pounds.

THERAPIST: Today is April 20. June 1 is 6 weeks away.

LINDA: I need to be at 140 pounds by then.

THERAPIST: To lose 24 pounds in 6 weeks you would have to lose an average of 4 pounds a week. You probably would not lose that much weight even if you starved yourself.

LINDA: I want to try.

THERAPIST: You are asking for trouble. On a realistic diet, you might lose around 12 pounds in the next 6 weeks, which would be very good, but you would be discouraged because you still would not make the weight you want by June 1. I think that the best thing for you to do is think of other alternatives for your future in addition to the airline.

LINDA: But losing the weight by June 1 and being rehired by the airline is the reason I came here.

THERAPIST: It is an unrealistic reason. Even if your lost the weight, what would happen after you were rehired? Would it be all right to regain your lost weight again?

LINDA: No. I want to be thin.

THERAPIST: It is sad that you do not have the time to lose 24 pounds by June 1, but it is a fact. You need to decide that you want to lose weight for *you*.

A second aspect of Linda's case was her failure to lose weight in a behavior modification weight loss clinic.

THERAPIST: Linda, tell me more about your experiences in the behavior modification clinic.

LINDA: The dietitian did not seem to know what she was doing. She told me that I had to eat all my food at the dining room table and that I could not watch television while I was eating, but she never told me why, and it did not really seem to help me lose any weight. I was still hungry all of the time.

THERAPIST: I mentioned over the telephone that much of our work together will include behavioral aspects. Have you thought about that?

LINDA: I think that is all right. You are supposed to know what you are doing.

THERAPIST: If your past experiences in that clinic are going to strongly affect your motivation, I think it might be best not to begin. It is very difficult to lose and maintain much weight without major life-style changes.

LINDA: I really want to try.

Reasons for wanting to lose weight and prior attempts have extremely important diagnostic implications. Without a clear understanding of the client's background, the therapeutic approach can easily lead to failure.

Karen is a 24-year-old female who came into treatment for bulimia. She had been married for 2 years to Dennis, a 27-year-old attorney. Her bulimia had become increasingly worse during the past year, and she had become frightened. Her husband called to make the appointment and accompanied her to the first session. Karen was later seen individually in therapy, and a pattern became increasingly clear. After graduating from college, Karen took a job as a filing clerk at a large Houston oil company at the insistence of her father. She was still in the same job when we began meeting. She was clearly overqualified, hated it, but she had not attempted to leave. Second, Karen had been a skilled organist at her local church where she was respected and in great demand on Sundays and for special occasions. She also had many close friends there. When she married, her husband insisted that she join his church, one of Houston's largest, where he was deacon and active on many church committees. Because the church had many talented organists, she had played only once there in almost 2 years. Third, Dennis' mother, who lived close by, called or visited daily. Her calls were frequently like "Put Channel 13 on right now. There's a program I want you to see," or "Look at the advertisement on page 6 of today's paper. There is a dress there you should buy."

THERAPIST: These examples we have been discussing over the past few sessions seem to be related.

KAREN: I have not seen the connection previously, but it is as if I do not have any control over my life anymore.

THERAPIST: Tell me more about that.

KAREN: Well, my father got me my job which I cannot stand, but I seem to be afraid to leave. I attend my husband's church and no longer play the organ which I love to do. My husband's mother tells me what I should watch, read, and wear. Who is running my life? About the only part of my life I control is my weight, by binging and purging.

Through problem solving and some assertive training, Karen decided to change jobs, attend her husband's church once a month with him and play the organ at her church the rest of the time, and take a more direct stance with her mother-in-law. By shifting the control to Karen, her bulimia decreased dramatically.

Information Important in Diagnosis

The diagnosis of an eating disorder is an imprecise endeavor. Without an acceptable theory, diagnosis and treatment become more a matter of clinical judgment and experience rather than the utilization of established procedures. Despite our present deficiencies, the considerable research conducted during the past several decades has provided a wealth of information and understanding by which we may proceed. Strong evidence suggests that the eating disorders are influenced by physiological factors, familial food habits, sociocultural influences, self-perception, familial interaction patterns, and emotional status. The following paragraphs highlight information that we, from our research and experience, consider important in the diagnosis of eating disorders. This information is applicable to all of the eating disorders, though the extent of applicability may differ with the disorder and individual.

Prior to an elaboration of *what* is required for diagnosis, a reiteration of the *how* of this process is important. For some patients, there is considerable shame, guilt, and pain associated with their problem. In this regard, the revelation of the particulars of their difficulty is often an emotionally trying task. Hence, we feel that sensitivity and tentativeness are essential in obtaining information. No information is worth risking the impairment of the therapeutic relationship. Information is most readily and comfortably obtained when it is achieved in the context of therapy, and not apart from it. That is, inquiries of behavior, interpersonal relationships, and feelings are made as part of a treatment session when appropriateness is obvious and the client is judged ready.

Medical and Physical Status

For almost all of the eating disorders, the point of departure for treatment is information concerning the state of the client's physical health. As noted earlier, the practices regularly conducted by some are causal of varying degrees of physical damage and even death. Therefore, medical assessment is a necessary first step to insure the physical welfare of the client. In cases where the disorder has severe physical ramifications, it is highly recommended that periodic medical evaluation be incorporated into the treatment plan. It should be noted that physical appearances of the individual may belie the physiological imbalances that are not always obvious. Many bulimics maintain a normal weight while in the throes of extensive purging practices. The electrolyte imbalances resulting from this behavior may not become observable until clients have achieved a severe state of distress.

In anorexia nervosa, the physical condition of the client is sometimes intimately associated with readiness for therapy. If the disorder
has progressed to its more advanced stages, the consequences of the
starvation will make any attempts at therapy fruitless. Such clients must
achieve a medically prescribed weight and strength before such efforts
can begin.

Because of the potentially severe consequences of anorexia, we suggest that treatment of a client begin even if all of the diagnostic criteria
have not been met. In particular, the criterion of 25% weight loss from
original (APA, 1980) must be viewed with flexibility. For some clients,
original body weight represents a degree of overweight; for others, normal or even underweight. In the latter cases, 15 or 20% weight loss may
yield severe emaciation.

Who Wants the Treatment?

"Who wants the treatment?" is an important question in processes
requiring personal change. When treatment has been sought *by* the
client, the motivation implied provides the basis for effective therapeutic
work. On the other hand, when the impetus for treatment derives from
another, greater difficulties can be expected. This is typified in anorexia
where it is frequently the case that the client is brought to treatment by
concerned parents. The client generally is unable to comprehend the
existence of a problem and is, therefore, disinclined to enter treatment.

The matter of "who wants the treatment?" is most variable in cases
of obesity. We occasionally find that a client has come for treatment
because of the insistence or at least strong encouragement of another.
The source of this encouragement is often the family physician, spouse,
or close relative. In such instances, the matter of client motivation is
explored in detail at the beginning of treatment. If it is apparent that the
client does not desire treatment, it is usually recommended that delay
occur until a more appropriate time.

Behavior

Behaviors are the external manifestation of the eating disorder; their
nature and frequency largely define the severity of the problem. Examples of these behaviors include binge eating, vomiting, limited food
intake, excessive exercise, and strange food-related rituals (e.g., order of
food consumption, insistence upon a specific place setting, and regular
departures to the bathroom after meals). It is helpful both for diagnosis
and treatment that such behaviors are quantified. By so doing, the client
and therapist have a baseline from which to compare later progress.

For the nonhospitalized client, self-report is the only practical way in which information on behavior may be obtained. This can be done either through use of food records or a short-term dietary and behavioral recall. It is our preference to use food records though both techniques have value. Because of the sensitive nature of these behaviors, we place no insistence upon these records if resistance to their completion is shown.

The behavioral patterns of the client may assist in the development of a more specific definition of the disorder and enhance the possibility of using appropriate interventions. This is exemplified by the bulimic and nonbulimic variations of anorexia. Some investigators defined a *bulimic anorectic* as an anorectic who purged. Strober (1981), however, studied the etiology of bulimia in anorexia nervosa and found significant differences. Primarily, his results indicated that the family life of the bulimic anorexic is more tumultuous, conflict ridden, and negative in comparison to that of the nonbulimic. Bulimics also seem to have greater tendencies to impulsive behaviors: drug use, alcoholism, stealing, and self-mutilation (Casper, Eckert, Halmi, Goldberg, & Davis, 1980; Garfinkel, Moldofsky, & Garner, 1980). In contrast to the typical view of the anorectic as introverted, the bulimic variation is likely to be more socially and sexually active (Casper et al., 1980; Johnson, 1982; Russell, 1979). From the symptom complexes that differentiate the bulimic and nonbulimic anorectic, disorders of substantially different etiological and psychological nature are suggested.

It has been our experience that the eating difficulties that plague the obese may also be divided into subgroups. Some of the ones we have recognized are emotionally laden (negative and positive affect), habitual, hearty, and social. If we diagnose the existence of a particular eating style/difficulty, our treatment orientation is in that direction.

Cognitive and Emotional Factors

Most, if not all, who suffer from an eating disorder have a structure of dysfunctional cognitions and affects that exist in association with their aberrant eating behaviors. It is our view that many of the emotional difficulties encountered by clients derive from distorted cognitive processes (Beck, 1976; Ellis, 1979). Thus, assessment of the predominant thought patterns and the factors that lead to their development is important in the understanding and subsequent treatment of the problem.

Body image in anorexia is one of the most powerful examples of how distorted cognitions can influence the cause and course of an eating disorder. The anorectic perceives her body as too large regardless of the degree of thinness achieved (Crisp & Kalucy, 1974; Garner, Garfinkel,

Stancer, & Moldofsky, 1976). Because this distortion does not diminish with weight loss, it maintains as a relentless incentive. Bruch (1973) noted that this disorder is not "cured" until the body image misperception has been corrected, even if substantial weight gain has been achieved in therapy.

Examples of cognitive distortions have been reported for anorexia nervosa (Garner et al., 1982), binge eating (Loro & Orleans, 1981), and obesity (Mahoney & Mahoney, 1976). We have found that certain of these distortions are present in all three disorders, indicating the possibility of a cultural pattern gone awry. In some obese, for example, staunch perfectionism is the cause of much distress and sometimes failure. These individuals proceed with substantial success on a diet until the first infraction occurs, no matter how minor. The inability to maintain a perfect record sends many into a binge that ends with self-recrimination and guilt. Perfectionism in the anorexic takes on an even more extreme form. Some carry this trait in all aspects of their life as well as in their anorexia. As indicated earlier, parents often characterize the ill child as the "perfect one."

We feel that cognitive distortions are often important in the development of the eating disorders and that their correction is an essential function of treatment. Therefore, accurate diagnosis of their nature is imperative.

Familial Factors

The eating disorders are the products of multiple influences. One of the most important of them is the family for it has impact on the individual's development of self-concept, values, food and eating patterns, and personal standards. Specific ways in which the family may have impact upon the eating disorders have been suggested by various clinicians and theorists (e.g., Bruch, 1973, 1977; Foreyt & Kondo, in press, a; Rosman, Minuchin, Baker, & Liebman, 1977; White & Boskind-White, 1981).

The therapist needs to find patterns of interactions and behaviors that appear to have relation to the client's difficulties. The works of Bruch (1973) and Rosman et al. (1977) provide insight into the characteristics of the obese and anorexic families. Of the two, the latter has been the subject of more research and, therefore, more is known. Similar to obesity, research of the familial factors associated with bulimia has been sparse. In a clinical investigation, Strober (1981) reported a number of significant differences between families of bulimic and nonbulimic anorectics. Families of bulimics, in comparison to nonbulimics, were found to have less structure, less cohesion, and more conflict and negativity.

In cases where the client remains in the care of the parents, diagnosis and treatment of the entire family is frequently necessary. A child or adolescent is little able to discern the familial complexities that have contributed to the problem, much less change them. For adults with an eating disorder, diagnosis of possible family contributions to causation is integral to treatment though their direct involvement is determined on an individual basis.

Social Factors

For many who have an eating disorder, social factors have association both to the etiology and perpetuation of their problem. From a sociocultural perspective, eating disorders are likely to be a product of contemporary American society (i.e., a society that places inordinate value on slimness while simultaneously emphasizing the consumption of our abundant food supply). At the personal level, these societal traits are translated into interpersonal transactions that lead the susceptible into an eating disorder. For many of the youthful, the most important social influence is the family, but others are important as well. In some cases of bulimia, for example, the idea of purging is obtained from an acquaintance or friend as an action to avoid the consequences of excessive eating. For the susceptible, it begins as a logical and apparently socially acceptable way to "have your cake and eat it too." Unfortunately, this rather innocent beginning can progress into a disturbing, all-encompassing compulsion. For anorectics, it is not unusual to find that their social activities and/or work have association to their disorder. Those involved in ballet, gymnastics, modeling, or cheerleading seem to have particular pressures to maintain sylphlike figures. A local high school has eligibility requirements for the cheerleading squad that include rather stringent height–weight standards.

One of the phenomena we frequently observe with individuals who suffer from an eating disorder is difficulty with interpersonal relationships. Among bulimics, problems in this area are the frequent cause of a binge. For obese young children, their self-imposed isolation impedes their social development. Lacking the rewards of social interaction, some seek solace in a way that only exacerbates their problem: eating.

The ways in which social factors may contribute to an eating disorder are varied and often complex. Their discernment is an important part of the diagnostic process.

Summary

It is difficult to cover all of the factors that need to be considered in the diagnoses of the eating disorders in a brief chapter. It is clear, however, that their diagnoses are far more complex than simply checking the criteria listed in the *Diagnostic and Statistical Manual of Mental Disorders* (DSM-III; APA, 1980). Their complicated nature, their multiple etiologies, and their highly refractory nature make them exceedingly challenging clinical problems. We hope that this chapter is a beginning step in the development of a better understanding of the many interacting factors involved in their proper diagnoses.

References

Al-Issa, I. (1980). *The psychopathology of women.* Englewood Cliffs, NJ: Prentice-Hall.

Allon, N. (1975). The stigma of overweight in everyday life. In G. A. Bray (Ed.), *Obesity in perspective* (Vol. 2, Part 2, pp. 83–102). Washington, DC: U.S. Government Printing Office.

American Psychiatric Association. (1980). *Diagnostic and statistical manual of mental disorders* (3rd ed.) (DSM-III). Washington, DC: Author.

Beck, A. T. (1976). *Cognitive therapy and the emotional disorders.* New York: International Universities Press.

Bemis, K. M. (1978). Current approaches to the etiology and treatment of anorexia nervosa. *Psychological Bulletin, 85,* 593–617.

Brownell, K. D. (1982). Obesity: Understanding and treating a serious, prevalent and refractory disorder. *Journal of Consulting and Clinical Psychology, 50,* 820–840.

Bruch, H. (1973). *Eating disorders.* New York: Basic Books.

Bruch, H. (1977). Psychological antecedents of anorexia nervosa. In R. A. Vigersky (Ed.), *Anorexia nervosa* (pp. 1–10). New York: Raven Press.

Bruch, H. (1978). *The golden cage.* Cambridge: Harvard University Press.

Casper, R. C., Eckert, E. D., Halmi, K. A., Goldberg, S. C., & Davis, J. M. (1980). Bulimia: Its incidence and clinical importance in patients with anorexia nervosa. *Archives of General Psychiatry, 37,* 1030–1035.

Crisp, A. H., & Kalucy, R. S. (1974). Aspects of the perceptual disorder in anorexia nervosa. *British Journal of Medical Psychology, 47,* 349–361.

Ellis, A. (1979). Rational emotive therapy, In R. J. Corsini (Ed.), *Current psychotherapies* (pp. 167–206). Itasca, IL: F. E. Peacock.

Foreyt, J. P., & Kondo, A. T. (in press, a). The family in weight loss: A behavioral perspective. In J. Storlie & H. Jordan (Eds.), *Obesity: Practical approaches to management* (Vol. V). New York: S. P. Medical and Scientific Books. (a)

Foreyt, J. P. & Kondo, A. T. (in press, b). Eating disorders. In P. Bornstein & A. Kazdin (Eds.), *Handbook of clinical and behavior therapy with children.* New York: Dorsey Press. (b)

Garfinkel, P. E., Moldofsky, H., & Garner, D. M. (1980). The heterogeneity of anorexia nervosa: Bulimia as a distinct subgroup. *Archives of General Psychiatry, 37,* 1036–1040.

Garner, D. M., & Bemis, K. M. (1982). A cognitive behavioral approach to anorexia nervosa. *Cognitive Therapy and Research, 6,* 123–150.

Garner, D. M., Garfinkel, P. E., Stancer, H. C., & Moldofsky, H. (1976). Body image disturbances in anorexia nervosa. *Psychosomatic Medicine, 38,* 327–337.

Garner, D. M., Garfinkel, P. E., Schwartz, D., & Thompson, M. (1980). Cultural expectations of thinness in women. *Psychological Reports, 47,* 483–491.

Garner, D. M., Garfinkel, P. E., & Bemis, K. M. (1982). A multidimensional psychotherapy for anorexia nervosa. *International Journal of Eating Disorders, 1,* 3–46.

Green, R. S., & Rau, J. H. (1974). Treatment of compulsive eating disturbances with anticonvulsant medication. *American Journal of Psychiatry, 131,* 428–432.

Halmi, K. A., Goldberg, S. C., Eckert, E., Casper, R., & Davis, J. P. (1977). Pretreatment evaluation in anorexia nervosa. In R. A. Vigersky (Ed.), *Anorexia nervosa* (pp. 43–54). New York: Raven Press.

Johnson, C. (1982). Anorexia nervosa and bulimia. In T. J. Coates, A. C. Petersen, & C. Perry (Eds.), *Promoting adolescent health: A dialog on research and practice* (pp. 397–412). New York: Academic Press.

Loro, A. D., & Orleans, C. S. (1981). Binge eating in obesity: Preliminary findings and guidelines for behavioral analysis and treatment. *Additive Behaviors, 6,* 155–166.

Mahoney, M. J., & Mahoney, K. (1976). *Permanent weight control.* New York: W. W. Norton.

Nemiah, J. C. (1950). Anorexia nervosa: A clinical psychiatric study. *Medicine, 29,* 225–268.

Neuman, P. A., & Halvorson, P. A. (1983). *Anorexia nervosa and bulimia: A handbook for counselors and therapists.* New York: Van Nostrand Reinhold.

Nogami, Y., & Yobana, F. (1977). On Kibarashi-gui (binge eating). *Folia Psychiatrica et Neurologica Japonica, 31,* 159–166.

Rosman, B. L., Minuchin, S., Baker, L., & Liebman, R. (1977). A family approach to anorexia nervosa: Study, treatment, and outcome. In R. A. Vigersky (Ed.), *Anorexia nervosa* (pp. 341–348). New York: Raven Press.

Russell, G. (1979). Bulimia nervosa: An ominous variant of anorexia nervosa. *Psychological Medicine, 9,* 429–448.

Strober, M. (1981). The significance of bulimia in juvenile anorexia nervosa: An exploration of possible etiological factors. *International Journal of Eating Disorders, 1,* 28–43.

Stunkard, A. J. (Ed.). (1980). *Obesity.* Philadelphia: Saunders.

Stunkard, A. J. (1981). "Restrained eating": What it is and a new scale to measure it. In L. A. Cioffi, W. P. T. James, & T. B. Van Itallie (Eds.), *The body weight regulatory systems: Normal and disturbed mechanisms* (pp. 243–251). New York: Raven Press.

U.S. Department of Health, Education and Welfare (1978). *Health: United States. 1976–1977.* Washington, DC: U.S. Government Printing Office.

White, W. C., & Boskind-White, M. (1981). An experiential-behavioral approach to the treatment of bulimarexia. *Psychotherapy: Theory, Research and Practice, 18,* 501–507.

Wooley, S. C., Wooley, O. W., & Dyrenforth, S. R. (1979). Theoretical, practical and social issues in behavioral treatments of obesity. *Journal of Applied Behavioral Analysis, 12,* 3–5.

Wurtman, J. J., Wurtman, R. J., Growdon, J. H., Henry, P., Lipscomb, A., &, Zeisel, S. H. (1981). Carbohydrate craving in obese people: Suppression by treatments affecting serotoninergic transmission. *International Journal of Eating Disorders, 1,* 2–15.

Chapter 11

Diagnostic Interviewing for Psychophysiological Disorders

Marcia M. Ward and Margaret A. Chesney

Introduction

Psychophysiological disorders bring many clients to their first interaction with mental health professionals—the diagnostic interview. More than for any subsequent interaction, the client is filled with trepidation, worrying about being labeled *crazy*, thereby forfeiting rights to serious medical evaluation in the future. The novice mental health professional may be filled with concern over blundering in front of a new client, and there is the potential of misdiagnosing the problem. The experienced mental health professional, however, often finds it a rewarding experience; sensitive detective work, deductive reasoning skills, and hypothesis testing can fit pieces of a complex puzzle into a comprehensive pattern.

The purpose of this chapter is to present guidelines for diagnostic interviewing of psychophysiological disorders. This is accomplished by first defining psychophysiological disorders. Next, the steps of the diagnostic interview are explained, and case illustrations for two common psychophysiological disorders are presented. Finally, the requirements for a diagnosis of psychophysiological disorder are discussed.

The professional who is interested in psychophysiological disorders

MARCIA M. WARD and MARGARET A. CHESNEY • SRI International (formerly Stanford Research Institute), Department of Behavioral Medicine, Menlo Park, California 94025.

is encouraged to read the chapter entitled "Behavioral Assessment of Psychophysiologic Disorders" (Blanchard, 1981), which presents an overview of other areas of assessment in addition to interviewing. Another chapter, "Psychophysiological Procedures" (Kallman & Feuerstein, 1977), presents techniques for measuring and assessing physiological responses. Other reference sources recommended for background reading are "Basic Interviewing Skills" (Johnson, 1981), "Behavioral Diagnosis" (Kanfer & Saslow, 1969),"Behavioral Interviewing" (Linehan, 1977; Morganstern, 1978), "Behavioral Assessment" (Roberts & LaGreca, 1981), "Assessment Strategies in Behavioral Medicine" (Keefe, 1979), and "Behavioral Assessment in Hypertension" (Chesney, Swan, & Rosenman, 1982).

Definition of Psychophysiological Disorders

In the second edition of the *Diagnostic and Statistical Manual of Mental Disorders* (DSM-II) (APA, 1968), psychophysiological disorders (Diagnostic Category 305) were given the following definition:

> This group of disorders is characterized by physical symptoms that are caused by emotional factors and involve a single organ system, usually under autonomic nervous system innervation. The physiological changes involved are those that normally accompany certain emotional states, but in these disorders the changes are more intense and sustained. The individual may not be consciously aware of his emotional state. (pp. 46–47)

In the third edition of the *Diagnostic and Statistical Manual of Mental Disorders* (DSM-III) (APA, 1980), psychophysiological disorders have been subsumed under "Psychological Factors Affecting Physical Conditions" (Diagnostic Category 316.00). The DSM-III presents the following diagnostic criteria for psychological factors affecting physical conditions:

1. Psychologically meaningful environmental stimuli are temporally related to the initiation or exacerbation of a physical condition (recorded on Axis III).
2. The physical condition has either demonstrable organic pathology (e.g., rheumatoid arthritis) or a known pathophysiological process (e.g., migraine headache, vomiting).
3. The condition is not due to a somatoform disorder.

Although the diagnostic criteria for psychological factors affecting physical conditions are among the briefest and most vague in the DSM-III, the following additional descriptive information is provided:

> This category enables a clinician to note that psychological factors contribute to the initiation or exacerbation of a physical condition. This category can be

used for any physical condition to which psychological factors are judged to be contributory. It can be used to describe disorders that in the past have been referred to as either "psychosomatic" or "psychophysiological. (p. 303)

This manual accepts the tradition of referring to certain factors as "psychological," although it is by no means easy to define what this phrase means. A limited but useful definition in this context is the meaning ascribed to environmental stimuli by the individual. Common examples of such stimuli are the sights and sounds arising in interpersonal transactions, such as arguments, and information that a loved one has died. The individual may not be aware of the meaning that he or she has given to such environmental stimuli or of the relationship between these stimuli and the initiation or exacerbation of the physical condition. The judgment that psychological factors are affecting the physical condition requires evidence of a temporal relationship between the environmental stimuli and the meaning ascribed to them and the initiation or exacerbation of the physical condition. Obviously, this judgment is more certain when there are repeated instances of a temporal relationship. (p. 303)

Common examples of physical conditions for which this category may be appropriate include, but are not limited to: obesity, tension headache, migraine headache, angina pectoris, painful menstruation , sacroiliac pain, neurodermatitis, acne, rheumatoid arthritis, asthma, tachycardia, arrhythmia, gastric ulcer, duodenal ulcer, cardiospasm, ulcerative colitis, and frequency of micturition. (p. 303)

This category should not be used for Conversion Disorders, which are regarded as disturbances in which the specific pathophysiological process involved in the disorder is not demonstrable by existing standard laboratory procedures and which are conceptualized with psychological constructs only. (p. 303)

A description of an ulcer case meeting the criteria for diagnosis as a Psychophysiological Disorder is presented in the *DSM-III Case Book* (Spitzer, Skodel, Gibbons, & Williams, 1981). The symptoms and disorders listed in Table 1 have been classified as possible psychophysiological disorders (APA, 1968; APA, 1980; Freedman, Kaplan, & Sadock, 1976; Sheehan & Hackett, 1978). It is imperative that the diagnostician understand that each of the disorders listed in Table 1 might occur as a result of a purely physiological reaction or disease, and thus would not qualify as a psychophysiological disorder. In order for one of these disorders to be defined as a psychophysiological disorder, there must be environmental factors that stimulate a psychological response innervating the autonomic nervous system. For example, a muscle contraction headache may occur in response to a noxious chemical or to muscle tension from squinting in an excessively bright environment. The headache is a result of an environmental stimuli, but there is no psychological interpretation mediating the physical response. Thus, these muscle contraction headaches do not meet the criteria of a psychophysiological disorder.

Environmental *antecedants* are critically important in psycho-

Table 1. Possible Psychophysiological Disorders

System	Examples
Skin	Neurodermatosis Rosacea Pruritus Acne Atopic dermatitis Hyperhydrosis Psoriasis
Musculoskeletal	Backache, muscle cramps, torticollis Myalgia Tension headache Arthritis
Respiratory	Bronchial asthma Hyperventilation syndrome Dyspnea Sighing Hiccups
Cardiovascular	Paroxysmal tachycardia Ectopic premature contractions Cardiac arrhythmia Essential hypertension Angina, vascular and cardiospasm Migraine headache Coronary heart disease
Gastrointestinal	Peptic, gastric, or duodenal ulcer Chronic gastritis Ulcerative or mucous colitis Constipation Hyperacidity Pylorospasm Heartburn Irritable bowel syndrome Nausea and vomiting
Genitourinary	Menstruation disturbance Micturition disturbance Dyspareunia Impotence
Endocrine	Hypopituitarism Hyperthyroidism, hypothyroidism Hypoglycemia Diabetes mellitus
Other	Posttraumatic headache Phantom limb pain Painful posttraumatic states

physiological disorders. Through classical conditioning, the *antecedants* acquire the power to elicit exaggerated or prolonged psychophysiological responses (Keefe, 1979). It has been suggested that classically conditioned physiological responses play a role, possibly major, in numerous diseases. Certain physiological changes occur naturally in response to external stimuli, but it is through classical conditioning that exaggerated responses, or symptoms, follow specific stressors. For example, a chronic conflict with a hostile co-worker may become associated with gastrointestinal distress, which over time is elicited by the work environment even when the antagonistic co-worker is absent. Often a classically conditioned response to one specific stimulus generalizes to other related stimuli. For example, an individual who experiences bronchospasms or asthma symptoms in a smoke-filled elevator, may experience similar symptoms in other confined spaces even when no smoke or air contaminants are present.

Environmental or social *consequences* are also important in psychophysiological disorders because, through operant conditioning, they may become powerful reinforcers of illness, complaints, or symptoms (Keefe, 1979). Social reinforcers have been shown to be important factors in pain syndromes (Fordyce, 1976; Fordyce, Fowler, Lehmann, & DeLateur, 1968). For example, pain associated with lower back strain may elicit extra attention from family members, pleasant massages from spouses, or pleas from concerned friends to lessen workload and "take it easy."

Procedures for Gathering Information

The major goals of the diagnostic interview for psychophysiological disorder are threefold: to identify the physical complaint: to determine that it is psychophysiological; and to rule out other disorders. To meet these goals the interviewer should (a) explore the presenting complaint thoroughly, in terms of symptomatic expression, physiological manifestations, and medical history; (b) ascertain that the symptom has been medically diagnosed and that medical treatment has been carefully considered; (c) quantitate the symptoms in terms of severity and frequency; and (d) determine the environmental and sociological antecedents and consequences of the symptom expression.

In the following sections, each of these steps is discussed. Examples are used to illustrate specific points in each step. Sample scripts of diagnostic interviews for two cases representing common psychophysiological disorders are then presented.

Define the Presenting Problem

The first important step in diagnostic interviewing is determining the parameters and nature of the presenting complaint. After gathering demographic information, such as the client's name, address, age, marital status, employment status, and referral source, ask the client what caused him or her to seek evaluation or treatment.

In order to gather enough information to make a correct diagnosis, the diagnostic interview must be structured, and the interviewer must direct the questioning. The interviewer may give the client some time to freely describe the presenting problem, but then must move toward a focused line of questioning (Keefe, 1979; Roberts & LaGreca, 1981), which covers the client's medical and psychiatric history and presenting symptoms.

Listen carefully to the individual's description of the presenting problem. Most individuals with physical complaints have previously consulted with medical professionals and will be quite direct about their symptoms and medical history. However, occasionally, a client will present a lengthy description covering many years of medical evaluations, and it will be necessary to direct the client to present only the most pertinent details.

It is important that the interviewer completely understand what the client is saying. If the client describes physical symptoms or medical diagnoses that are unclear or unfamiliar, then the interviewer must ask for clarification. In order to clearly understand the client's presenting problem and symptoms, it may be necessary for the interviewer to "be ignorant" about what the client means when using certain expressions (Keefe, 1979). For example, the client may complain of "constant pain." Yet upon further questioning, the client's description of the severity of the symptom may be much less than the interviewer presumed. In another case, the client may report feeling under "pressure" or "overstressed." The interviewer needs to understand what the client means specifically by these terms.

Document the History of Medical Evaluation and Treatment

Because all individuals with psychophysiological disorders present with a physical symptom, it is imperative that medical evaluation and treatment occur before or be concomitant with psychological evaluation and treatment. Many practitioners who evaluate or treat clients with psychophysiological disorders work in medical settings and/or require referral from a physician. It is unethical to apply psychological treatment

to a physical symptom that has not received appropriate medical attention. As Blanchard (1981) stresses,

> One must always keep in mind that with psychophysiologic disorders there
> is real pathophysiology; there are real lesions. . . . Thus, if there is a first rule
> in behavioral assessment of psychophysiological disorders, it is to have the
> patient seen by a competent physician first, or at least concurrently. (pp.
> 246–247)

For example, although many headaches and gastrointestinal symptoms
are stress related, some could be caused by a tumor.

Ask the client about all medical interventions. When did medical
interventions begin? What is the client's perception of their success?
Have all reasonable medical treatments been exhausted? If a medical
treatment is currently being prescribed, determine the client's perception of the role of psychological evaluation and treatment.

Whenever possible, obtain the client's signed consent on a request
for appropriate medical records. This enables the interviewer to speak
with any physicians or specialists, other than the referring professional,
who have treated the client. Professional etiquette suggests discussion
of the case with the source of the referral before the diagnostic interview
(Johnson, 1981). The referring professional can be a valuable source of
information about the client not only in terms of medical diagnosis and
reason for referral but also for judgments of the client as a possible
malingerer and as a candidate for psychological intervention.

While gathering the client's medical history, ask if the symptoms
run in the client's family. Do the client's parents or siblings have the
same symptoms? Certain psychophysiological disorders have evidence
of genetic determination, in particular, migraine headaches and cardiovascular disorders such as coronary heart disease and essential hypertension. Evidence that the symptom occurs in other family members
may help to confirm the diagnosis of psychophysiological disorder or
may help the interviewer to formulate hypotheses about environmental
antecedents that are present in the client's family life.

Quantitate the Severity and Frequency of Symptoms

It is helpful during the diagnostic interview to obtain a recent chronology of the disorder. If the symptoms occur on a daily basis, have the
client describe a typical day. If the symptoms occur less frequently but
on a predictable schedule, such as headaches that always start in the
afternoon, ask for a description of activities on a typical day when the
symptoms occur. Urge the individual to be specific about details leading
up to and following the onset of symptoms (see Keefe, 1979, for an
example of a typical day for an individual with torticollis).

This description of a typical day can then be supplemented with information from a symptom diary. A symptom diary lists each occurrence of the symptom, its start and end, its severity, any apparent environmental antecedents, and any medication taken. In behavioral assessment, the client is often directed to complete a symptom diary as "homework" after the first interview. Thus, the introduction of the symptom diary and instruction on how to complete it is appropriate to the diagnostic interview. An example of a symptom diary for migraine headache is presented later in the text. The symptom diary is useful in refining the therapist's hypotheses of environmental antecedents, planning behavioral interventions, and evaluating changes during treatment.

Next, ask the client how severe the symptom usually is. If the symptom is painful, how extensive is the pain, where specifically is it located, is the pain hot or cold, sharp or dull? It is particularly helpful to ask the individual to rate the pain on a 100-point scale with the lower end of the scale referring to no pain and the upper end of the scale referring to the most pain the client has ever experienced.

If the client uses vague symptom descriptions, it is recommended that the interviewer help him or her to describe the complaint in behavioral terms. For example, if the client complains of feeling tired all the time, the interviewer might ask which tasks are the most and the least difficult to accomplish. It is also helpful, especially for the depressed client, to discuss symptom-free periods.

Determine the Environmental and Sociological Antecedents and Consequences of the Symptom Expression

Now that the client has presented a history of the disorder and a description of a typical day, the interviewer should be formulating an idea of the environmental and sociological factors affecting the disorder. These hypotheses can be tested by asking specific questions about the effect of stressors on the symptom.

Some clients will come to the diagnostic interview believing that stress is an important factor in their condition, possibly the most important factor. These clients will probably present a list of episodes where a stressful occurrence has been followed by a symptom onset. This may be particularly true for clients whose symptoms frequently occur soon after a particularly stressful event, as with tension headaches (Blanchard, 1981). In these cases, additional precipitating stressful events that were not apparent to the client may be discovered during the course of therapy.

The client's perception that stress is linked to symptom onset is not sufficient to meet the criteria of a psychophysiological disorder. A frightened client may want to believe that the symptoms are "caused by stress" rather than that they are the result of serious pathology. In contrast to the clients who acknowledge that stress plays an etiological role in their condition, many clients will either be totally unaware of any connection or will deny any connection between stress and their symptom. For this reason, the idea that the symptom may be linked to stress or to environmental and sociological factors must be presented cautiously. If the client responds negatively, then the interviewer probably should not persist with this direct line of questionning but should explore relationships in a more indirect manner. In these cases, the interviewer must work as a detective, exploring relationships without arousing clients' misgivings.

Ultimately, the therapist tries to identify the learned physiological response or behavior pattern producing or exacerbating the physical symptom. However, this goal is rarely realized in the diagnostic interview. A more realistic goal for the diagnostic interview of psychophysiological disorders is ascertaining the extent of environmental and/or social factors in the symptom expression. The interviewer should be careful not to overinterpret during the diagnostic interview. Even knowing that environmental and sociological antecedants are playing an essential role in the development of the psychophysiological disorder, it is unwise to make interpretive statements to the client at this point. There is always a possibility that specific interpretations are incorrect or may produce concern in an individual who feels that the referral to a mental health professional was made because "the symptom is all in my head" (Johnson, 1981). Even for a client who is prepared to believe that the symptom is stress related, a specific interpretation may be startling and appear presumptuous.

It is a good idea to evaluate sociological factors influencing the disorder by asking about the client's living arrangements, quantity of social engagements, and social support system. The interviewer should specifically ask about the people the client lives with, about the client's family, about the client's friends who know about the symptom, and whether the client feels support from family, co-workers, and friends. In particular, ask about areas of conflict with others. Often, interpersonal conflicts precipitate symptom onset (Blanchard, 1981). The occurrence of interpersonal conflicts, especially unexpressed anger, should be explored.

Another reason for exploring the client's social support system is to identify any "secondary gains" that play a role in the symptom expression. The presence of secondary gains means that someone or something in the client's environment is reinforcing the "sick role."

These factors can be assessed by asking whether someone takes care of the individuals when they are ill, how their boss and co-workers respond when they need to take time off from work or leave work because they are ill, and what advice their family gives them for dealing with the symptom.

Any diagnostic interview should consider what factors induced the client to seek treatment at this time. Usually with physical complaints, the client has been seeking treatment for some time, often for years. Examine why the client is also seeking psychological evaluation and treatment at this time. Blanchard (1981) suggests that the Holmes and Rahe Life Events Scale be administered. These items, either used directly at the interview or given as a questionnaire, can help the diagnostician to understand stressful events in the client's recent past that may have precipitated a symptom episode or provoked the client to seek treatment.

The diagnostic interview is designed to gather data and to arrive at a diagnosis, not to provide therapy or treatment (Johnson, 1981). As a result of discussing the presenting problem with a concerned interviewer, however, the client may feel a sense of relief that someone understands, or at being able to get the problem "off my chest."

The skilled interviewer is able to convey to the client a sense of understanding and concern (Morganstern, 1976). It is usually very difficult for the client with a physical complaint to seek evaluation by a mental health professional. Clients often assume that this approach means that the physical symptom is "in their head." An interviewer who conveys understanding and concern can help dispel this belief and counteract the client's fears that the purpose of the interview is to evaluate his or her mind.

During the diagnostic interview, the client will carefully watch and listen to the interviewer and will sometimes seek out approval and signs of understanding. This gives the interviewer the ability to reinforce the client, to encourage him or her to be open and informative. However, because the interviewer is only beginning to understand the client during the first diagnostic interview, the interviewer must be prudent in the use of reinforcement (Keefe, 1979). Manipulative clients are very adept at creating situations where they win approval. Often, to give these clients any sign of approval in these situations is not therapeutic.

Case Examples

The steps of the diagnostic interview discussed in the previous section are illustrated in excerpted dialogue from two representative cases of psychophysiological disorders. Portions of a diagnostic interview with a 32-year-old female client reporting headache pain and a 58-year-old male client referred for behavioral intervention as an adjunct to pharmacologic treatment of hypertension are presented in this section. Because of space limitations, only portions of the diagnostic interviews that are of primary importance in assessment and diagnosis are included.

Migraine Headache Case

Headaches are among the most common painful ailments experienced by men and women. Psychological factors have long been implicated in migraine as well as other forms of headache. As with many psychophysiologic disorders, individuals presenting with headache pain must be carefully interviewed and evaluated to determine the appropriate diagnosis and treatment strategy. A number of organic disorders present as headache and necessitate a thorough medical and neurological examination to rule out the possibility that the headache pain is the result of disease, such as tumor. If the pain is determined to be "functional," several diagnostic options having different treatment implications are availiable: (a) vascular headache of the migraine type; (b) muscle contraction headache; (c) combined migraine and muscle contraction headache; and (d) delusional conversion of hypochondriacal headache. The following excerpts from the first two interviews with a 32-year-old female headache sufferer illustrate the types of questions asked during a proper diagnostic interview.

Initial Diagnostic Interview

I: When you called, you mentioned that you were interested in relaxation and biofeedback training for your headaches.

P: Yes, I really need some help with these headaches I get, and it's been getting worse.

I: For starters, please describe the pain you experience with your headache. There are different types of headache depending on the type of pain.

P: Well, it's a throbbing or stabbing pain that I get, and it's always on the right side of my head.

I: How long have you had these headaches?

P: They started in high school. I usually get one every couple weeks; sometimes more, sometimes less.

I: Have you seen a doctor or a counselor for these headaches before?

P: Yes, I talked with our family doctor, Dr. _____, about the headaches while I was in college, and I was given a prescription drug, Cafergot, for the headaches.

I: I would like to look over records regarding Dr. _____'s treatment of your headaches. Would that be okay with you? If so, I need your signature on this authorization for release of information.

P: Sure.

I: Did the Cafergot work?

P: Sometimes, if I took it early enough. If the headache got too far, then it didn't seem to have any effect, and it upset my stomach. I really don't want to take drugs for these headaches, though.

I: I understand. Let's see, as far as you know, has anyone else in your family had headaches like these?

P: Yes, my mother used to get bad headaches until she went through menopause. But she only got them occasionally.

I: How long does each of your headaches typically last?

P: Well, it varies. Usually it's about 6 to 8 hours, but I've had some that went on for days.

I: For days?

P: Yes, the pain will start on one morning and will stay with me all that day, all night, and throughout the next day.

I: Can you tell in advance that you may be getting one of these headaches; do you get any "warning signs"?

P: Not always. Sometimes they come out of the blue. Then there are times when I see a pattern of light, of shapes, diamonds that quiver. When I see these lights, I know I'm in for it.

I: While you are having the headache, aside from the pain, how do you feel?

P: Terrible. First of all, I can't keep working. I drop things, and I can't talk straight. I don't feel like I can do anything. Then, there are sometimes when the pain is so bad I feel nauseated, and I've vomited.

I: Have you noticed any pattern to your headache? For example, things that seem to trigger them?

P: I don't know. I've not been aware of anything in particular. Maybe when I've been really under pressure at work for some time, but other times that doesn't seem to make any difference.

I: OK, you've given me a good idea of what your headaches are like, and they certainly sound like the type of headaches for which biofeedback and relaxation training can help. But first, whenever a person has a persistent headache, it's best to have it checked out by a physician. So sometime during the next 2 weeks, while you are monitoring your headaches, I would like you to be seen by Dr. _____, a specialist in neurology. Dr. _____ will assist in the diagnosis of the pain and rule out the possibility that it is a symptom of an underlying problem.

P: What could it be?

I: Well, it is very rare, but sometimes headache pain can indicate potential problems with such things as blood pressure. As I said, it's very rare but important to check out, since you haven't seen a physician for this problem in about 10 years. This won't delay your treatment because during this time, while you're seeing the physician, you'll also be gathering important information that we will use in designing your treatment program. It will be important for us to see if there are any particular things that seem to precede or trigger your headaches. It's likely that there may be some headaches that don't fit any pattern. The best way to get a handle on this is for you to "monitor" your headaches on this form.

[Therapist explains how to fill out the self-monitoring form by recording the date and time of onset, any apparent antecedents, severity or intensity of pain, duration, medication taken, feelings, and consequences such as how the client and others behaved as a result of the pain.]

Follow-up Diagnostic Interview

Once organic causes of headache pain have been ruled out through a careful examination by a physician, the attention returns to psychological and behavioral factors. The headache pain needs to be placed into a context by identifying relevant environmental antecedents and their consequences. The diary or log kept by the client can be a valuable resource for the interview. However, it is common for clients to fail to recall environmental events in detail or to identify antecedent feelings in their first attempt at self-monitoring. The therapist should reinforce the client's attempts by building on what the client has noted, explaining the need for additional detail. Many clients will grow disinterested in detailed self-monitoring over time. Therefore, the therapist needs to capitalize on data collected in the first several weeks to obtain key information regarding the environmental context of the target behavior.

I: Dr. _____ has stated that your headaches do not appear to be caused by any specifically physical problems or diseases. So our focus turns to other causes. To do this, I'd like to turn to the diary you kept over the last 2 weeks to get a more specific, detailed picture of your headaches.

P: Well, here's my diary [see Figure 1]. I had two headaches over the last 2 weeks. The first one came on Friday after I saw you. Nothing special happened that day, so I don't see that there was anything that brought it on.

I: Well, let's look at the diary and see if we can use it to remind you of potentially important information. Let's look at that Friday.

P: Well, I got up and went to work.

I: For this first headache, let's be really detailed, as if we were detectives. What did you do when you woke up?

P: Well, I did my usual routine: shower, makeup, dress, and eat breakfast.

I: Sometimes food can trigger a headache. Do you remember what you ate?

P: Gee, it's hard to remember. Oh yeah, I was going to have a big lunch with my husband that day so I skipped breakfast. I just had some coffee.

I: After you finished getting dressed, what did you do?

P: I went to work, and then I did feel pressured because I wanted to get away early for lunch and things kept coming up.

I: Tell me about the things at work.

P: Well, I am a group leader, and I was trying to get some reports out, and I kept

Date	Time Symptoms Started & Ended	Rating of Severity	Medication Dose & Time	Causes	Consequences
FRIDAY 1-20	4 p.m. to 10 p.m.	PRETTY BAD	NONE	SOME WORK PRESSURE	LEFT WORK : WENT HOME TO BED
SATURDAY 1-28	3 am. to 6 p.m.	BAD	NONE	NONE	STAYED IN BED ALL DAY

Figure 1. Example of a symptom diary describing the occurrence of two migraine headaches.

being interrupted by my staff and by the phone. There was just so much more I wanted to get done and not enough time before I needed to leave.

I: Who decides how much you need to get done on a day-to-day basis, like on that Friday morning?

P: I guess ultimately I do, but my decisions are based on reality. I have too much to do.

I: Oh. It sounds like you've got quite a bit of responsibility. Tell me more about the phones.

P: My phone is always ringing. I would let my secretary get it, but then I'd just have to call the people back. By getting it myself, I get the phone calls out of the way.

I: Despite the pressures, were you able to make it to your lunch?

P: Yes, just in the nick of time.

I: Do you remember what you had for lunch?

P: We went to a little Italian place that serves a quick lunch. I had eggplant parmigiana and a small glass of Chianti.

I: Can you remember how they made the entrée?

P: The same as usual. The eggplant was breaded and fried and covered in tomato sauce with sauteed onions and melted parmesan cheese. And we had a cup of coffee before we left to go back to work.

I: The diary says that your headache started at 4 P.M. What did you notice?

P: Actually, I noticed a dull pain starting around 2:30 that afternoon, but I didn't really start paying attention to it until about 4:00.

I: Your diary shows that the headache lasted into the night. On a scale of 1 to 100 with 100 being the worst headache you've had, and 1 being free of headache pain, how would you rate the headache?

P: About a 50.

I: Last time you mentioned you sometimes have warning signs, did you have any this time?

P: No, not really. I did notice that my eyes were really sensitive to the light. Then the pain started.

I: The diary says that as a consequence of the headache you left work. Tell me about this.

P: I would have tried to work, but I know better, so I went home and went to bed. My husband is really sympathetic. He came home early and did everything he could to help me feel better.

I: What in particular did he do?

P: He fixed dinner and spent time with me. Otherwise he usually would be in his study working.

I: That gives me a good picture of that headache. On your diary you had some, but not all, of these details. For next week, when you are monitoring or tracking a headache, write down as much detail as you can; include what you are doing. If you're eating, write down what you ate. Also add what you and others, like your husband, do after the headache. Now, let's look at that other headache. When did it occur?

P: That headache came on over a week later, on Saturday. It was funny. I wasn't under any stress. It was the weekend, and I had earned it. I was worked extremely hard all week.

I: What were you working on?

P: I was preparing for a big briefing that we had all day Friday.

I: You said in the dairy that the headache started at 3 A.M. What happened?

P: I woke up Saturday about 3:00 A.M. and knew I was going to get a headache. The lights were there.

I: Tell me about the lights.

P: Well, there was a bright point of light right in the middle of my field of vision. I could see things on either side but nothing in the middle. Then it got bigger and became a crescent-shaped zigzagged line of diamond shapes flashing on and off like neon lights. After about 15 minutes they faded away.

I: After the lights, what happened?

P: Well, I was really looking forward to Saturday, doing nothing, to just taking time off to relax. What happened? I spent the day in bed, in pain.

I: Using the scale of 1 to 100, how would you rate the pain of this headache?

P: About 65. It was bad, but I've had ones that were worse.

I: Besides going to bed what did you do?

P: Not much. I just rested. I couldn't watch TV or read. My husband stayed with me. We talked off and on. He worked in the bedroom. He's very supportive.

Case Summary. These excerpts highlight diagnostic issues in the assessment of headache pain, including the need to rule out organic causes and to distinguish among the types of headaches. This client's symptoms follow most closely the pattern of migraine headaches.

The interviews also reflect the importance of environmental antecedents and consequences. Specifically, several of the classic migraine triggers were present prior to the client's first headache. These triggers included skipping a meal (i.e., breakfast), psychological stress (on the job), and several foods high in tyramine, a substance thought to play a role in migraine. If the headache had occurred in the absence of the stress, in other words the only causal factors were diet related, then the headache would not have been considered under the rubric of *psychophysiological disorder*. It is common, however, for such disorders to result from multiple causes with psychological stress exacerbating other causal factors.

The second headache also follows a typical migraine pattern; that is, it came after, rather than during, a stressful period. The sequence is thought to be related to the proposed two-step physiological mechanism underlying migraine: a period of prolonged constriction of the intra- and extracranial arteries followed by a rebound dilation associated with the onset of pain.

The excerpts also indicate the potential importance of environmental consequences of psychophysiologic disorders. The husband's supportive behavior may be reinforcing the client's headaches.

Essential Hypertension Case

Over twenty-three million Americans between 18 and 74 years of age have hypertension or high blood pressure. Of these, approximately 5% have elevated blood pressure as a result of specific endocrine or renal disorders. The remaining 95% have essential hypertension, that is, elevated blood pressure not due to a specific cause. The absence of a definitive causal factor has led investigators to explore behavioral and environmental influences, such as stress, on blood pressure. Epidemiologic, laboratory, and applied research have consistently shown a link between various forms of stress and transient blood pressure responses (Henry & Stephens, 1977; Kaplan, 1980). Such associations have led to suggestions that nonpharmacologic approaches including relaxation, biofeedback, and stress management may be used as an alternative to pharmacologic interventions in mild hypertension or as an adjunct in more elevated hypertension. However, the proposed association between blood pressure and either transient or chronic stress remains open for study. The excerpts presented next are from a diagnostic interview with a 58-year-old male client with hypertension referred to a psychologist by his cardiologist.

Initial Diagnostic Interview

I: From your call, I understand that Dr. _____ referred you to me for stress management to assist you in controlling you blood pressure.

P: Yes, that's about it. But I'm not sure why he suggested I come here. I don't feel tense and nervous, so I don't know what you can do for me.

I: Well that's the purpose of this meeting—to see if there is anything I can do for you. First of all, it would be helpful if you would tell me about your blood pressure history. When did a doctor first mention to you that you might have high blood pressure?

P: Let's see. It was 5 years ago at my first executive physical. I had just been promoted and got company physicals as a "perk." The company physician told me to see my private doctor, which I did.

I: What did Dr. _____ say?

P: Well, he said that my pressure wasn't in the serious range and had me come back to have it checked several times. When it still stayed high, he put me on Dyazide. That seemed to work for a while. Then my blood pressure started jumping around. Sometimes it would be okay, and then other times it would be higher than ever.

I: Did you ever skip your medication?

P: [Laughs] Dr. _____ thought that was the reason. But I take my medication "religiously," and even so, my wife reminds me at least once a day.

I: Has your weight changed by 5 or more pounds over the last several years?

P: No. I really watch that. I'm proud to say that I can still fit into the tux I wore in 1947 when we were married. We also have cut out salt. We use one of those salt substitutes at home.

I: By any chance, do you remember when it was that your blood pressure became more erratic?

P: Let me think. That was a couple years ago in the spring.

I: Do you remember if there were any major changes in your daily activities or work situation around that time?

P: Changes? Well, yes, it was then that we got this large contract, and I was promoted to a management position. I guess I should've been glad about the promotion—the pay is good, but I enjoyed my work as an engineer more.

I: How does your position as a manager differ from your position as an engineer?

P: Well, as an engineer I had specific jobs to do, and I always knew that if I applied myself, I would succeed in getting the job done on time and done well.

I: And now?

P: Now I'm responsible for seeing that entire projects are completed within time and budget constraints. This isn't so difficult by itself. It's only that I have to depend on everyone else to do their part of the job. If they fail, then I get "blasted."

I: Have they ever failed to meet a deadline?

P: Sure. The tough part for me is that I can't go in there, roll up my sleeves, and help to get the work done on time. I'm responsible, and yet I'm forced to rely on others to meet that responsibility. I have to sit back and watch us miss the mark, and then I pay the price!

I: That's quite a load to carry. About the time of the promotion did anything else happen?

P: No, not really. We've lived in the same house for over 5 years. The wife and kids are fine. As far as my family and home goes, that's what I really live for!

I: Some people have home blood pressure kits. Have you taken your blood pressure at home with one of these?

P: I bought one of those from a discount store once, but the readings were really inconsistent—I think I got a lemon.

I: Why do you think that?

P: Because my readings at home didn't agree with the readings that the company nurse took.

I: It is possible that your blood pressure at home is considerably different from your blood pressure at work. In fact, blood pressure tends to be responsive to different environmental situations. For example, it may be higher at work when you are under pressure in your position as a manager and lower at home when you are enjoying time with your family.

To get a better picture of what may be related to your blood pressure fluctuations, would you be willing to take your blood pressure each morning and evening at home and to have the company nurse take it each day at work?*

P: For how long?

I: If you get several readings a day and fill out the log, then just for 1 week.

P: When should I have it taken at work?

I: Well, you could have the company nurse take it twice a day, once in the morning and once each afternoon. Another alternative is that you can take it yourself with your own unit several times during the day at work in addition to the readings you'd be getting in the morning and evening at home. Of course, you'll need to stop by to have your unit checked for accuracy before we can trust the readings you get.

Fill out this diary or log each time you take a blood pressure. This is really important because we'll use the log to examine how your blood pressure responds to specific activities while you are at work and at home. Also, it would be helpful for me to review your medical records. To do that, I would need you to sign this form to authorize Dr. _____ to release his records to me.

P: No problem.

Follow-up Diagnostic Interview

I: Well, how did it go with measuring your blood pressure?

P: It was okay. I was out of the office all day Tuesday so I didn't get any measurements, but I got at least two on the other days, and I think I got it at some good times.

I: Let's look at the blood pressures to check for patterns [see Figure 2].

---

*In the case of the hypertensive man, it is recommended that the client have his blood pressure taken at work by the company nurse and at home with a home blood pressure kit that has been professionally calibrated. This technique for measuring blood pressure levels and variability across settings and situations is often quite helpful in developing diagnoses and treatment plans. Other alternative measurement techniques are available. The best of these is to have the client wear an ambulatory blood pressure monitor for a day. Such devices pump up the cuff and take measurements on a set interval schedule. Thus, more representative blood pressure values are obtained than when the individual chooses when to have a measurement taken. A more economical alternative is for the interviewer to purchase a reliable home blood pressure kit to lend to the client for a week at a time periodically throughout treatment.

BLOOD PRESSURE RECORD				
Date	Time	Blood Pressure		Activity
		Systolic	Diastolic	
Monday	7 p.m.	126	76	home — watching TV
Tuesday	8 a.m.	128	78	ready to leave for work
	8 p.m.	130	82	after eating dinner
Wed.	9 a.m.	146	94	working at desk
	11 a.m.	152	98	working at desk
	2 p.m.	180	104	meeting about supplies
	6 p.m.	136	88	helping to get dinner
Thurs.	7:30 a.m.	122	74	getting dressed
	10 a.m.	136	88	back from staff review
	1:30 p.m.	140	92	back from business lunch
	9 p.m.	132	80	reading newspaper
Friday	9:30 a.m.	165	98	back from Director's meeting
	2 p.m.	140	92	reviewing bids
	10:30 p.m.	136	84	home from dinner out
Sat.	11 a.m.	136	82	break from raking yard
	3:20 p.m.	128	70	after nap
Sunday	2 p.m.	132	86	back from brunch
	8 p.m.	136	78	after watching the news

Figure 2. One week blood pressure and activity record.

One thing that is readily apparent is that your blood pressure does vary quite a bit. This is normal; most people's blood pressures vary throughout the day. Let's look at your diary to see if we can find anything that raises your blood pressure.

Looking over this list one clear pattern is that your blood pressure is lower at home.

P: My family will like that.

I: I remember that you said last week that you enjoy your family and home life.

Let's contrast your blood pressures at home with those at work. The home blood pressures range around 120 to 136 over 70 to 90. The work blood pressures range around 130 all the way up to 180 over the high 80s, to 90s, and up to 104.

P: That's really something. Maybe I should consider retiring. [Laughs]

I: This pattern of higher pressures at work is pretty typical. From the perspective of blood pressure management these patterns provide just the information we need. If your blood pressure was going up and down without any relationship to your activities, then we wouldn't know where to focus to identify specifically what situations are pulling your blood pressure up. Well, looking at the list, let's start with that high reading at 2 o'clock on Wednesday.

P: I don't even need to look at the diary. I remember what was happening. I was talking to Jim _____, the task leader on one of our most important projects. He was telling me that some equipment wasn't ordered despite the fact that we requested it weeks ago and had a "RUSH" on it. Now, when we really need that equipment, it's not here! Just incompetence! Anyway, the upshot of the whole thing is that we're going to be late in delivering on the contract.

I: What did you say?

P: Not much. What could I say? It wasn't Jim's fault directly.

I: How did you feel?

P: Utterly frustated and furious. But what good would it have done to get mad at Jim? This is exactly the thing about my work that really gets to me. Things go wrong; people just don't give their all to the work; they don't care. I care because as the saying goes, the buck stops here. It's my neck on the line.

I: You feel responsible, yet so much is outside your direct control.

P: That's it.

I: Looking back at the list, what do you remember about what was going on at 9:30 on Friday? That was the highest blood pressure in the morning.

P: Let's see. That was after the director's meeting where we were supposed to deal with budgets. I stayed up into the night working on the budget forecast. To be honest, budgets are something I loathe. I asked my secretary to come in early, so at 7:00 A.M. we were both in the office preparing the budget. Then I raced to the meeting, budget in hand, only to learn that the other directors didn't get theirs done! The VP said, "Oh well, there's no critical rush, we'll discuss it next week!"

I: How did you feel?

P: I was really burned up. This happens *all* the time! I do my part. It is supposed
   to be important to get things done right and on time—it is with everyting else
   in the business—but then the other directors can get by with missed
   deadlines.
I: What did you do?
P: Nothing. What could I do? Make a scene? I didn't want the other directors to
   think that I thought I was superior or something. So I just shoved the budget
   back into my folder for next week. I didn't want anyone to know it, but I was
   burning up inside!

Case Summary. These excerpts highlight diagnostic issues in evaluating a
hypertension case. This case illustrated the fact that some individuals will deny a
relationship between stress and their health problem when indeed such a relationship may exist. In these instances, sensitive detective work by the interviewer or therapist is instrumental in diagnosing the problem and developing a
treatment plan. Periodic blood pressure measurements, in conjunction with the
diary of activities corresponding to measurements, are essential in such investigations.

The foregoing excerpts also demonstrate how the interviewer or therapist
"rules out" other possible behavioral factors such as sodium intake and weight
gain that are known to affect blood pressure. The client's report of job-related
stress (i.e., his recent promotion) coincident with his blood pressure increase
supports the diagnosis of psychophysiological disorder. This is further indicated
by his report that he is frustrated and angered by this stress but does not express
his irritation. Such unexpressed anger responses have recently been related to
elevated blood pressure (Harrell, 1980) and have implications for behavioral
treatments for essential hypertension.

Critical Information Required to Make the Diagnosis

As demonstrated in the two case studies in the previous section, the
diagnostic interview takes the form of questions that test out various
diagnostic hypotheses (Johnson, 1981). Usually, it starts with hypotheses of diagnoses based on the client's presenting problem, but often
other hypotheses must be tested, and alternative diagnoses must be
ruled out. The following section reviews the criteria for making a diagnosis of psychophysiological disorder.

To review, according to the DSM-III (APA, 1980), the diagnosis of
psychophysiological disorder is made if three conditions are met:

1. Psychologically meaningful environmental stimuli are temporally related to the initiation or exacerbation of a physical
   condition.

2. The physical condition has either demonstrable organic pathology or a known pathophysiological process.
3. The condition is not due to a somatoform disorder.

In the following sections, the criteria for each of these three conditions
are described. Additional information on how psychophysiological disorders differ from other mental disorders can be gained through a thorough understanding of the diagnostic criteria described in the DSM-III.

Establish a Temporal Relationship between Psychologically Meaningful Stimuli and Physical Condition

Psychophysiological disorders include any physical complaint for
which psychological factors are judged to be contributory. Psychological
factors may contribute either to the initiation of the complaint by producing a physiological response that is intense and sustained or exacerbation of the physical complaint. In psychophysiological disorders, psychological factors and physical conditions have a temporal relationship.

Often the temporal relationship between psychological factors and
physical symptoms is obvious, as in the case of muscle-contraction
headaches or ulcer symptoms that follow a stressful episode. In the
hypertension case described in the previous section, the two highest
blood pressure readings occurred soon after an interpersonal conflict.
Occasionally, the temporal relationship is present but appears delayed,
as in the headache case when the second migraine occurred on Saturday
during the "let-down" period after a stressful work week.

For psychophysiological disorder to be diagnosed, the interviewer
must ascertain that the symptom results from psychologically meaningful environmental stimuli. In particular, it is critical that the interviewer rule out physical conditions that are provoked by environmental
stimuli that are not psychologically meaningful. Examples of these are
environmental toxins and allergens that produce headaches or skin disorders, caffeine intake that produces tachycardia or ectopic premature
contractions, air conditioning drafts that exacerbate backaches, and
medications that produce side effects in the form of asthma, nausea, and
impotence.

Demonstate Organic Pathology or a Known Pathophysiological Process

In psychophysiological disorders, the major presenting complaint is
physical. The physical complaint may be a single symptom, but it is
often a physical disorder. The physical complaint is anatomically correct, of realistic proportion, and has documented organic pathology.

Most often, the symptom or disorder involves the autonomic nervous system such as the cardiovascular, respiratory, or gastrointestinal systems.

For psychophysiological disorder to be diagnosed, the interviewer must ascertain that the physical condition has either demonstrable organic pathology or a known pathophysiological process. This conclusion is reached by obtaining a clear medical history from the client. If the client expresses vague, generalized complaints, then the interviewer must persist in asking for clarification. If the description remains vague or unclear, the interviewer should consider diagnoses other than psychophysiologic disorders.

Beyond the diagnostic interview, obtaining medical records pertaining to the client's physical complaint will determine whether the physical condition results from organic pathology. If medical records do not suggest the presence of organic pathology but are inconclusive, then the interviewer should refer the client for further medical evaluation. If the medical records are exhaustive and indicate that no known pathology is producing the symptoms, then the interviewer should consider an alternative diagnosis such as somatoform disorder (see following section for description of five somatoform disorders).

Rule Out Somatoform Disorder

Somatoform disorders differ from psychophysiological disorders in that they have no demonstrable physiological mechanism though they do have a strong link to psychological factors or conflicts. Somatoform disorders include somatization disorders, conversion disorders, psychogenic pain disorders, hypochondriasis, and atypical somatoform disorders. Each of these disorders is defined next.

Somatization disorders consist of recurrent and multiple somatic complaints that are not related to any physical disorder (APA, 1980, p. 241). Their onset is usually before age 30. Medical attention is repeatedly sought.

Conversion disorders involve a loss or alteration in physical functioning that cannot be explained by any physical disorder or known pathophysiological mechanism and that is not under voluntary control (APA, 1980, p. 244). This loss or alteration in physical functioning is an expression of psychological conflict or need. Conversion disorders are usually of quick onset and resolution, appearing during extreme psychological stress. The physical symptom enables the individual to either avoid some activity that involves conflict or to get support from others.

Psychogenic pain disorders involve a complaint of severe and prolonged pain that cannot be explained by any physical disorder and that has evidence of etiological psychological factors (APA, 1980, p. 247). The pain enables the individual either to avoid some activity that involves conflict or to get support from others.

Hypochondriasis involves an unrealistic interpretation of physical signs or sensations and unrealistic fears and beliefs that are not supported by a medical diagnosis and are not resolved by medical reassurance.

Atypical Somatoform disorders involve the presentation of physical symptoms or complaints that are "blown out of proportion," are not supported by demonstrable organic findings or known pathophysiological mechanisms, and that are linked to psychological factors (APA, 1980, p. 251).

Somatoform disorders must be ruled out at the time that the medical history is taken. This is sometimes difficult to do within the diagnostic interview. However, the individual should be questioned about past diagnostic laboratory procedures and findings. If the client responds that the cause of the condition could never be determined, the interviewer should suspect somatoform disorders. Of course, the easiest way to confirm suspected somatoform disorders is to obtain the client's consent to contact any physician who previously evaluated him or her.

Summary

The material presented in this chapter is designed to serve as a guideline for diagnostic interviewing when a client presents with a physical complaint. The process of gathering information, formulating and testing hypotheses, and finally arriving at a diagnosis of psychophysiological disorder is discussed. Descriptions of related disorders, such as somatoform disorder, are also presented so that the interviewer will be aware of these related disorders and can make a correct diagnosis. The presentation of material from two case summaries is intended to provide examples of some of the principles of diagnostic interviewing. A well-conducted initial interview not only will lead to accurate diagnosis but also to the development of an effective treatment plan.

ACKNOWLEDGMENTS

The authors thank Gary Swan , Nanette Frautschi, and Cori Welch for their helpful comments on an earlier version of this chapter.

References

American Psychiatric Association, (1968). *Diagnostic and statistical manual of mental disorders* (2d ed.). Washington, D.C.: Author.

American Psychiatric Association, (1980). *Diagnostic and statistical manual of mental disorders* (3d ed.). Washington, DC: Author.

Blanchard, E. B. (1981). Behavioral assessment of psychophysiologic disorders. In D. H. Barlow (Ed.), *Behavioral assessment of adult disorders* (pp. 239–269). New York: Guilford Press.

Chesney, M. A., Swan, G. E., & Rosenman, R. H. (1982). Assessment of hypertension. In F. J. Keefe & J. A. Blumenthal (Eds.), *Assessment strategies in behavioral medicine* (pp. 19–36). New York: Grune & Stratton.

Fordyce, W. E. (1976). *Behavioral methods in chronic pain and illness.* St Louis: C. V. Mosby.

Fordyce, W. E., Fowler, R. S., Lehmann, J. F., & DeLateur, B. J. (1968). Some implications of learning in problems of chronic pain. *Journal of Chronic Diseases, 21,* 179–190.

Freedman, A. M., Kaplan, H. I., & Sadock, B. J. (1976). *Modern synopsis of psychiatry II.* Baltimore: Williams & Wilkins.

Harrell, J. P. (1980). Psychological factors and hypertension: A status report. *Psychological Bulletin, 87,* 482–501.

Henry, J. P., & Stephens, P. M. (1977). *Stress, health, and the social environment: A sociobiologic approach to medicine.* New York: Springer-Verlag.

Johnson, W. R. (1981). Basic interviewing skills. In C. E. Walker (Ed.), *Clinical practice in psychology* (pp. 83–128). New York: Pergamon Press.

Kallman, W. M., & Feuerstein, M. (1977). Psychophysiological procedures. In A. R. Ciminero, K. S. Calhoun, & H. E. Adams (Eds.), *Handbook of behavioral assessment* (pp. 329–364). New York: Wiley.

Kanfer, F. H., & Saslow, G. (1969). Behavioral diagnosis. In C. M. Franks (Ed.), *Behavior therapy: Appraisal and status* (pp. 417–444). New York: McGraw-Hill.

Kaplan, N. (1980). *Clinical hypertension* (2d ed.). Baltimore: Williams & Wilkins.

Keefe, F. J. (1979). Assessment strategies in behavioral medicine. In J. R. McNamara (Ed.), *Behavioral approaches to medicine, application and analysis* (pp. 101–129). New York: Plenum Press.

Linehan, M. M. (1977). Issues in behavioral interviewing. In J. D. Cone & R. P. Hawkins (Eds.), *Behavioral assessment: New directions in clinical psychology* (pp. 30–51). New York: Brunner/Mazel.

Morganstern, K. P. (1976). Behavioral interviewing: The initial stages of assessment. In M. Hersen & A. S. Bellack (Eds.), *Behavioral assessment, a practical handbook* (pp. 51–76). New York: Pergamon Press.

Roberts, M. C., & LaGreca, A. M. (1981). Behavioral assessment. In C. E. Walker (Ed.), *Clinical practice of psychology* (pp. 293–346). New York: Pergamon Press.

Sheehan, D. V. & Hackett, T. P. (1978). Psychosomatic disorders. In A. M. Nicholi, Jr. (Ed.), *Harvard guide to modern psychiatry* (pp. 319–353). Cambridge: Belknap Press, 1978.

Spitzer, R. L., Skodol, A. E., Gibbons, M., & Williams, J. B. W. (1981). *DSM-III case book* (1st ed.). Washington: American Psychiatric Association.

Part **III**

Special Populations

Chapter 12

Families

Susan Stewart

Introduction

Family therapy is not merely another way to approach problems presented by individuals. To the contrary, it is a radically different way of understanding behavior. Although families usually present one of their members as symptomatic, family therapists are interested in understanding symptomatic behavior in the context in which it occurs rather than understanding it as the product of a biological or psychological process occurring within one person. This does not mean that individual biological or psychological processes are not considered but rather that the clinician expands his or her field of consideration from the individual patient to the interactional context in which his or her symptoms appear. Because most people live in families, the clinician's field of consideration becomes the patient and his or her family.

Population

Because family therapy is not a specific approach to a specific problem, it is appropriate for a wide range of problems, from patients with affective and cognitive disorders to so-called "problems in living." Although this approach can and frequently does incorporate interventions

SUSAN STEWART • Department of Psychiatry, Western Psychiatric Institute and Clinic, University of Pittsburgh School of Medicines, Pittsburgh, Pennsylvannia 15213.

on the individual level, such as medication, most interventions are aimed at changing the relationships between family members so that symptomatic behavior is decreased or disappears.

Family therapy is a diverse rather than a unified approach to psychotherapy. Schools of family therapy range from those that base themselves in the psychoanalytic and behavioral traditions to those that see themselves as revolutionary approaches owing little to any forms of psychotherapy that existed before them.

The issue with which the clinician must deal is usually not whether family therapy is appropriate, but which form of family therapy is appropriate for which family with which problem. Behavioral orientations are quite effective in resolving discipline problems in families with small children if the parents are able to work together to carry out the therapist's program (Gurman & Kniskern, 1981). If they cannot, some intervention on the marital/parental level will be necessary. If the presenting problem is a cognitive disorder, a supportive, educational model of family intervention might be most effective (Anderson, Hogarty, & Reiss, 1980). Structural family therapy has been used successfully in treating psychosomatic disorders (Minuchin, 1978) and drug and alcohol problems (Stanton & Todd, 1976). Families with a severely intractable symptomatic member, particularly one who has not responded to other forms of family treatment, may respond to approaches utilizing paradox, such as those described as *systemic* (Weeks & L'Abate, 1981) or *strategic* (Madanes, 1981). Therefore, it is important for the clinician to have a good understanding of the nature of the presenting problem and of any previous treatment in order to adjust his or her approach to that most likely to be successful.

The Question of Diagnosis

The purpose of diagnosis is to discover how family interaction contributes to the maintenance or exacerbation of symptoms in one or more members. This may be a question of how family factors affect a member with a biologically based psychiatric syndrome, such as schizophrenia or clinical depression. Or, it may be a question of how one family member's symptomatic behavior stabilizes an otherwise potentially disruptive situation. Diagnosis largely depends on both the problem presented by the family and the theoretical orientation of the family therapist.

The family therapy movement is both young and greatly divided in its theoretical approach to diagnosis. So-called "pure systems thinkers" rarely address themselves to processes that are limited to one individual, whether they are psychological or biological. Other approaches begin with the diagnosis of one family member as their starting point and structure interventions accordingly. However, even when the symptoms of one family member are clearly recognized in the diagnosis, terms such as *schizophrenic family* or *psychosomatic family* are not useful. This is because they generally describe the symptoms of one family member rather than indicate with any specificity what factors in a family may be contributing to the maintenance or exacerbation of those symptoms. Therefore, although the work of some researchers provides hope for the future (Cromwell, Olsen, & Fournier, 1976; Olsen, Sprenkle, & Russell 1979; Tseng, Arensdorf, McDermott, Jr., Hansen, & Fukunaga, 1976), at this time there is no such thing as family diagnosis in the conventional sense. As Hoffman (1981) has pointed out, "the family therapy movement has done better in the area of how-to-change-it than what-to-change" (p. 176).

However, for the clinician willing to take a flexible, pragmatic approach, there are some universal considerations that, taken together, can guide the clinician to an understanding of the context in which symptoms exist. These considerations are the family life cycle, child, adolescent, and adult developmental issues, the individual needs, desires, and pathology of family members, and the patterns of family behavior that promote or prevent the family's meeting needs and solving problems.

Procedures for Gathering Information: A Pragmatic Approach to Family Diagnosis

Families are small, complexly organized social systems that have certain functions to carry out. These functions change as family members grow and change over time. Families pass through stages that have been variously identified. For our purposes we will use an adaptation of Fleck's (1966) scheme of five functions families perform: (a) produce a marital/parental coalition; (b) nurturant tasks; (c) enculturation of the younger generation; (d) emancipation of offspring from the family; and (e) solve family crisis. The clinician must keep in mind that the family life cycle is a theoretical construct for help in thinking about families and needs to be adjusted for any given family, particularly one-parent families and remarried parents.

Briefly, the first task of the newly married couple is to negotiate a relationship that both find satisfactory in terms of their needs for affection and autonomy. If they fail at this early stage, the marriage may dissolve, or dissatisfactions may become a permanent part of their relationship. The major task of the next stage of family life is the nurturing of children. This involves a major shift in that both parents are required to change their relationship to accommodate the needs of infants and young children, and one parent may have to give up, at least temporarily, a job or career important to her. The third stage in the life cycle is a broadening of the nurturance stage to include the enculturation of the children. Disagreements between parents as to how this ought to be done may arise, be resolved, or become a permanent part of how the family functions. Unresolved covert conflict between parents at this stage may not make itself operational until the next stage of family functioning is reached: that of emancipation of offspring from the parental family. During this stage, the needs of the adolescent for a strong parental coalition against which to test his or her needs for autonomy and self-definition can cause years of unresolved tensions to erupt between parents.

A major function of the family during all stages of the life cycle is to cope with stress. Some stresses are unavoidable, such as those presented by the changing needs of family members. However, stress on a family system is not always the product of the internal developmental needs of its members. It may come in the form of problems produced by sources outside the control of the family, such as prolonged unemployment due to recession or the development of physical illness in one family member. The important thing is to understand the sources of stress in a family and the ways in which the behavior of family members fails to deal with the stress in a satisfactory fashion.

The following is an example of how one family moves through its life cycle, and how failure to successfully carry out functions at one stage leads to subsequent family dysfunction:

Forming the Marital Coalition

John and Mary were married after knowing each other for over a year. Each thought he or she knew the other well and knew what to expect from the relationship. However, John soon found that Mary was complaining about things that had never bothered her before, particularly his two nights per week out with the boys, playing sports, and his habit of spending whatever money he had on pleasure with no thought to saving. In response to her complaints, John began staying out later and later, and when Mary complained even more, he responded with angry, defensive arguments. Their arguments escalated from the subject of John's nights out and his spending habits to accusations on Mary's part that he did not love her. Unsure of his confused feelings, John would withdraw into a sullen silence. Their relationship became characterized by stormy sessions followed by days of not speaking to each other.

John and Mary began their marriage thinking they knew each other well. However, family therapists have learned that people evaluate the behaviors, attitudes, and role performances of their spouses and other family members on the basis of assumptions about life that are subliminally learned during childhood and that are largely beyond awareness (Reiss & Oliveri, 1980). Because Mary's family valued closeness and emphasized all family members being together every evening, she felt rejected when John chose to spend time with his friends. Such behavior was acceptable before marriage because she had not cast John in the role of husband with all her expectations of what that meant. John's easy spending habits represented a confirmation of his rejection of responsibilities toward her and the future. John may well have responded to her complaints as he did because he perceived her complaints, consciously or unconsciously, as an effort to control his behavior.

Although clashes between the conscious and unconscious wishes, expectations, and assumptoms of newlyweds are perhaps inevitable, the outcome is not. Had Mary brought up her objections in a different way, John might have responded differently, and they might have developed a workable means of resolving differences. As it was, they failed to develop a method to solve their problems. It is not a matter of "who started it," as the blame could be put on John for staying out later, or for responding defensively; on Mary for escalating from a specific complaint to a general assumption about the meaning of his behavior; or on John for withdrawing into a sullen silence. The important information for the therapist to note is that they established a dysfunctional pattern that resulted in escalation of conflict and therefore distress, rather than a resolution of the problem. The pattern itself then becomes the problem, as more and more disagreements are deadlocked.

Should John and Mary seek professional help at this early stage in their marriage, their problems could probably be resolved with a minimum of help. However, let us follow them through the various stages of the family life cycle to see what problems could arise as a result of their failure to deal constructively with their problems.

Nurturance and Enculturation

As more and more of John's friends got married, his outside activities lessened with a consequent decrease in opportunities to spend money on his own pursuits. Although Mary's complaints decreased, she retained suspicion that John was not as committed to the marriage as she. Also, on some level she had learned that complaining to John brought about negative results, so she kept most complaints to herself. However, when they did have a fight, she dredged up all the complaints she had kept to herself and flung them at John, who characteristically withdrew, sometimes leaving the house. However, both considered their marriage normal and not particularly unhappy.

Like most young couples they wanted children and were happy when Mary became pregnant. They experienced a lessening in conflict during the pregnancy and the early months of their son's life. John dismissed his feelings of having been displaced in Mary's life as unworthy, and took advantage of how busy she was to increase the hours he spent managing his business. Mary was content with her role of caretaker and only occasionally complained of his absences. When she did, he flatly stated he was doing it for her and their son and refused to discuss it.

John and Mary continued their pattern of having sporadic and un-expectedly bitter disagreements throughout the births of two more children. In between fights they got on well enough, and both enjoyed their children. However, as the years passed John began to feel that Mary was too easy with the children and that they would grow up without the self-discipline they would need to be successful. Rather than risk a direct confrontation, he began to criticize their behavior and to set strict rules that he expected Mary to uphold. Mary, noticing his sternness, reacted by becoming even more permissive, frequently contradicting his rules.

This family was developing a distinct and not uncommon structure that has its roots in the failure by John and Mary to resolve their early marital differences. Because they never learned to recognize just what those differences were and how to resolve them constructively, every major issue became a potential source of bitter conflict. Their pattern of avoiding such issues extended to their parenting. John got most of his needs met through his business, and when he was acting as a parent he allowed himself to become polarized into the role of disciplinarian. Mary got most of her emotional needs met through the children, but in pro-tecting them set up an escalating circular pattern in which she under-controlled to compensate for what she perceived to be John's over-control. The message to the children on an unconscious level was, "You don't have to pay attention to your father."

Given children with normal developmental problems and no severe pathology, a family structure such as this would probably support the needs of all family members, despite the difficulties. However, should some stress appear, such as severe business difficulties, or should one of the children present a problem, the family could be unable to deal with it. For example, a hyperactive child would have great difficulty integrat-ing the mixed messages from these parents. A clinician examining only the child might fail to recognize the effect of the parental power struggle.

Emancipation

Despite their parents' differences, all three children did well in school and formed healthy relationships with their peers. However, as the children grew older and spent more and more time with their peers, Mary began to feel less and less needed by them. She began to suffer from feelings of depression and discontent. She focused this discontent on the amount of time John spent managing his business as well as on the amount of time the children spent with their friends and other aspects of their behavior. She became critical, subtlely undermining her children's sometimes clumsy efforts to make decisions for themselves. The children responded by spending more and more time away from home, as did John, which contributed to an escalation in Mary's feelings of discontent. The situation finally came to a head when their oldest son, Peter, was caught breaking into a house to steal some liquor for him and his friends. John's response was to severely curtail their son's freedom, grounding him for a month and revoking his driving and telephone privileges. Mary blamed their son's behavior on John's frequent absences, and behind John's back allowed their son to use the telephone and to see his friends.

Emancipation in our culture requires that children gradually divest themselves emotionally and behaviorally from their dependence on their parents. This requires that parents go through a reciprocal process, supporting their children's efforts to make decisions for themselves while providing enough guidance to insure that they do not hurt themselves while they learn to take responsibility for their own behavior. This process puts considerable pressure on the parental relationship, often causing previously ignored problems to surface. In this case, John and Mary's early failures to resolve their differences constructively, their methods of coping with conflict through nagging and withdrawal, and their pattern of overcontrol and undercontrol of their children all contributed to their son's crisis. If the pattern were to continue, their son might fail to learn responsibility for his own behavior, becoming a chronic offender.

So far we have understood Peter's actions in terms of the behavior of family members that contribute to or maintain his symptomatic behavior. However, his behavior can also be said to have a function in stabilizing the family system. Adolescents frequently act out behaviorally as a response to dimly perceived problems in their families. Peter's antisocial act might well have been a response to Mary's depression. Should his antisocial behavior continue, it would divert the attention of all family members from his mother's depression as well as providing her a good reason to become overly involved with him. This would restore her previously satisfying role of parent and presumably restore the balance the family had achieved before Peter became an adolescent, albeit in a pathological way.

At this point in the family's life cycle, Peter's acting out can also be seen as serving the function of receiving outside intervention, even though this was the last thing he intended. In small social systems such as families, it is useful to separate motivation from the function any behavior serves. Because we all experience life from our own perspective, which includes our internal reasons for doing something, we are familiar with the notion of motivation. However, because the function of any behavior in a system can only be discerned from outside the system, we are usually not aware of the function of our behavior in our own families. Yet, it is the function of any behaviors in a family system that forms the heart of family diagnosis.

Let us assume that at this point John and Mary consult with friends who have had similar problems and are given the name of a family therapist. The clinician then has the problem of getting the family into treatment and finding out what family problems might be contributing to Peter's antisocial behavior.

Getting Families into Treatment

Getting families into treatment is often harder than engaging individuals. First, family therapy often does not make sense to people. After all, you do not take the whole family to the doctor when one person has a broken arm. Therefore, family members are likely to be suspicious of the request that they all appear for sessions. They may fear the therapist will blame them for their relative's problem, or that upsetting feelings will get out of control, causing further distress.

Second, family therapy is a relatively new form of treatment, and professionals who refer families for treatment may have an unclear idea of its purpose, practice, and usefulness. The way a referral is made is very important. The referring source must convey the message that family therapy is the very best form of treatment for this family's problem, or they are not likely to follow through. Professionals who are unclear or unconvinced about the usefulness of family therapy will not be able to overcome the natural hesistance a family might feel about this form of treatment. In fact, institutions and agencies that focus on the individual as the "patient" or "client" during an evaluation period may reinforce the family's notion that one of their members is the problem and only he or she should be seen.

Institutions and agencies that engage in prolonged evaluation processes may also make the job of engaging families more difficult because they increase the time between the initial request for help and the initial family interview. Families tend to call for help during a crisis. The crisis itself provides motivation and an inclination to cooperate with what perceived helpers suggest they do. If they are not seen quickly, the crisis may resolve itself in some less than ideal way. For example, a woman called the juvenile authorities to complain that her 15-year-old son had attacked her and had verbally abused his stepfather. The juvenile authorities removed the boy from his home on an emergency basis and conducted an evaluation. They concluded that the boy was not out of control, as his mother had alleged, but was reacting to stresses within the family. They recommended family therapy. But by the time the clinician received the referral, the other family members were convinced that the boy was the entire problem, and that as long as he was in placement the family was calm. The unfortunate result was that the boy became permanently separated from his family, and the stresses that produced the crisis in the first place remained unresolved. To the clinician involved it seemed evident that the next child to reach adolescence would trigger another crisis.

Under whatever circumstances the clinician receives the referral, his or her next task is to form a connection with a member of the family in a position to make a decision about therapy, usually a parent. The therapist needs to be prepared to encourage and answer questions, particularly questions about his or her own competency to deal with the problem. People are usually responsive to explanations that are simple and forthright and delivered in a confident tone of voice. If they are not responsive, the clinician must be prepared to spend some time gently exploring the roots of the resistance. If all other forms of persuasion fail, the therapist can ask that the family come in for one visit to see for themselves what it is like. Because family therapy may be difficult to understand in the abstract, but makes so much sense in the actual experience, one visit is usually all the therapist will need to convince the family of the efficacy of this form of treatment.

A crucial factor in the step of getting the family into treatment is that the clinician must form a connection with a powerful member of the family without allowing himself or herself to be drawn into an alliance that may impede his or her objectivity. Family members frequently try to assure themselves that the therapist will be on their side by complaining about the behavior of other family members or by offering to tell the clinician "a secret" about another member. The clinician should decline to hear "secret" information and should listen politely to complaints about other members only until the family member accepts the message that these matters are better discussed at a family session.

The Diagnostic Interview

In one sense, all family therapy sessions are diagnostic in that the therapist is always evaluating the system's response to events that occur both in sessions and between sessions. However, for the purposes of this chapter, I will limit myself to the process of diagnosis that occurs in either the first interview or the first few interviews. The number of interviews it takes to accomplish the process is dependent on both the skill of the therapist and the openness of the family to outside intervention. This process can be divided, for the sake of discussion, into three phases, although the phases overlap.

The first phase is universal to all forms of psychotherapy and consists of making a connection with the family. This process is more complicated than that of establishing a therapeutic relationship with an individual patient, not just because there are more people, but because the family is a system and as such has rules about sharing private information with outsiders. Such rules are commonly referred to as *boundary* rules. The job of the therapist is to establish himself or herself within the family boundaries as a person who can not only be trusted with intimate information but who is given the status of an authority within the system.

The speed with which a family allows a therapist within its boundary is to some degree diagnostic of how firm or loose its boundaries with the outside world are, and to some degree diagnostic of how willing family members wish to cooperate with each other to resolve anxiety-producing problems. Some families maintain a rigid boundary, essentially shutting the therapist out, refusing to share any meaningful information, and refusing to allow him or her any authority within the family. Fortunately, this is a relatively rare occurrence, as most families this resistant fail to accept a referral for family therapy in the first place. Some families seem to have no boundaries at all, overwhelming the therapist with information about their problem and expecting the therapist to take full responsibility for "fixing" all of them.

Most families, however, cooperate with the therapist to the degree that he or she manages to allay their anxiety about the new situation and demonstrate his or her usefulness to them. The first step is to conduct introductions and to gather information about ages, schools, and jobs.

This step is not for the therapist's information, because he or she probably already has this information on the intake form. But it is to establish an atmosphere of cooperation and to give family members a chance to establish at the onset that they are competent in certain areas of their lives, even if they do have problems that require that they consult a therapist. The therapist can use this stage to "win over" members who have been previously labeled as *very resistant*. For example, a young woman was referred with her parents after being discharged from a psychiatric hospital. The inpatient family therapist passed along the information that her father was very skeptical about the efficacy of any kind of psychotherapy. During the opening stage of the initial interview the therapist learned that the father worked for an electrical power company as a linesman. She quickly confessed to a fear of electricity, including anxiety while just plugging in appliances. A full 20 minutes was taken up with the father's explanations about how electrical power is transmitted, but he was cooperative with the therapist thereafter.

The second phase is to focus on the problem as the family sees it. This usually means focusing on the behavior of one member, which implies that the therapist agrees with the family that one member is the problem. The therapist with a systems orientation obviously does not believe this, but it is not necessary to convince family members that they all are part of the problem. In fact, such a move would be counterproductive, as it would embroil the therapist in a struggle over the definition of the problem.

Therapists can either choose a specific family member to ask to describe the problem, such as the family member with whom they have already established contact by phone or can "throw the question up for grabs" to see who assumes the role of spokesperson for the family. For example, the therapist might say, "Well, Mrs. Beals, I spoke to you on the phone, and we discussed the problems you folks have been having, so why don't you fill everyone in on what we talked about?" Or, the therapist might say, "Who wants to tell me what brings you here today," while focusing his or her eyes somewhere between the family members so as not to inadvertently select someone. The information as to who acts as spokesperson is useful mostly in observing how easily the role is shared with other family members. For example, if a mother takes the lead, explains the problem, but then answers questions that the therapist has directed to other family members, the therapist can hypothesize that she is overly intrusive into the psychological space of her family. The therapist is not interested in why she is overly intrusive, but rather, what are the implications of her intrusiveness regarding the function of the symptom in the system at this particular time? If the symptomatic person is her husband, and if he is depressed, the therapist might hypothesize that he has little room to be a parent in a family dominated by his wife. If the symptomatic person is an adolescent, the therapist might hypothesize that the youngster's need to take over more and more responsibility for his or her behavior and have increasing freedom and privacy is being overwhelmed by the mother's intrusiveness. If the symptomatic person is the mother, the therapist might hypothesize that she takes too much responsibility for everyone, presumably thinking it is her job to do so.

At this stage in the diagnostic interview, the therapist must function as a combination of detective and computer while always paying attention to how the family members are perceiving him or her and responding to questions and comments. Building the therapeutic alliance is the first order of business because if the family does not return for more sessions, the diagnosis is meaningless. However, unless the therapist can make some meaningful interventions, the family is likely to leave feeling that they have not been helped. The therapist, therefore, should be sure to ask each person his or her perception of the problem and how it affects him or her personally. This establishes a bond with all members of the family while at the same time providing useful information.

As stated earlier, the therapist is trying to understand the function of the symptom at this point in the family's life cycle. While the therapist is gathering information about the family's perception of the problem, he or she is looking for patterns of behavior that repeat themselves. From these patterns the therapist will deduce the rules that govern the family's structure and functioning. In the earlier example of the mother who interrupted everyone to give her definition of the problem, a possible rule might be that all family members deferred to her. This rule might have been quite functional when the children were younger, but it has become a problem when the family reached the stage where it had to emancipate its children.

Typically, families either maintain a rigid focus on the identified patient (IP), maintaining that he or she is the only problem in the family, or they wander from subject to subject or make random attacks on each other. The most important thing for the family therapist to realize is that he or she must be in charge of the session. If the family maintains a rigid focus on the IP, he or she must finds ways to loosen that focus. If the family wanders from one subject to another, the therapist must tighten the focus so that a workable problem emerges.

The third stage of the interview is to formulate a definition of the problem that is acceptable to the family and to define some attainable goals. This does not mean that the therapist has to apprise the family of all of the possible problems he or she sees or suspects, but that the family must be convinced that he or she understands the problem in a way they can all agree with. For example, in the case of John and Mary and their son Peter, some indication of the parental disagreement about discipline is likely to emerge. The therapist, knowing that it is usually better to focus on the presenting problem until others emerge, may suspect underlying marital problems but instead focus on Peter, but in a supportive way. He or she might sum up the problem in the following way:

> So, Peter, it seems that you are saying that your parents do not always agree on the rules for you and your sisters. And you, Melissa and Connie, you're not so ready to say they disagree, but you do say that maybe they do. At least, sometimes you're confused about what's o.k. and what isn't. And John and Mary, you think that might be a problem. I think at his age Peter is trying to find out what's right and wrong for him, and I think he's made a mistake. I think he still needs your help, so perhaps we could start by working on the two of you agreeing on what's right for him, with him here to tell us what he thinks, of course. That's important too.

Because family therapy operates on many levels, all family problems do not have to be directly discussed for the situation to improve. For example, in the case of John and Mary, the therapist could hypothesize that the underlying marital problems might or might not emerge overtly as they struggled to set rules for Peter. If resentments did not run deep, they might be able to use the help the therapist provided in resolving the problem of rules for Peter to resolve other differences, and hence the marital relationship might improve without direct intervention.

A Diagnostic Interview

The following is an example of a diagnostic interview. The therapist has already chatted with all family members. The family consists of two white middle-class parents and their 14-year-old daughter and 12-year-old son. The presenting problem is uncontrolled vomiting spells by the daughter. The problem is serious, as the daughter has diabetes and has required hospitalization several times after these episodes to restore her insulin balance. During the opening introductory chat, the therapist notices that the daughter smiles frequently at her mother but ignores her father and brother.

THERAPIST: So, Jeannie, I understand you've had some problems with your diabetes. I've talked to your doctor, who seems quite fond of you, by the way. I understand you've been working together for sometime to get your illness under control.

JEANNIE: He's O.K. I guess, except he wories too much. He's always bugging me about my blood tests and insulin levels . . . you know. . .

FATHER: He wouldn't have to bug you if you took better care of yourself. All you're interested in is buying more tight jeans and makeup. You don't . . .

JEANNIE: Speaking of people who bug me, you're really the one. You're always after me about everything! And money, money, money is all I hear from you all the time. I'm sick of it! And I'm sick of you.

MOTHER: Now, now. Don't you two start [smiling at Jeannie]. We're here to discuss Jeannie's problem.

THERAPIST: Mrs. Beals, you sound like this happens a lot. Does it?

BOBBY: Oh, all the time. She's really a big mouth [indicating Jeannie].

JEANNIE: Oh yeah, you little snot. Why don't you tell her [indicating therapist] about how you get teased and beat up on your way to the bus everyday.

THERAPIST: Hold on, now everybody, you're going way too fast for me [holding out her hand toward Jeannie as if to restrain her] O.K. Now that peace is restored, for a moment anyway, let me get in a quick question. Mrs. Beals, I was asking if your husband and your daughter have these, uh, disagreements a lot.

MOTHER: Well, they do. But they've always been that way. I've tried . . . [smiles again, first at therapist and then at Jeannie].

THERAPIST: And how about you and Jeannie. Do you have these disagreements too?

MOTHER: Oh, every once in awhile. But we're very close. You know how mothers and daughters are.

The therapist in this case had noticed the frequent smiles between mother and daughter, the lack of eye contact between daughter and father unless they were fighting, and the way Bobby had quickly interrupted when she had asked a direct question about the fighting between father and daughter. She interpreted this sequence to mean that her question had caused Bobby some anxiety, and that by attacking his sister he was diverting attention away from the issue. His sister's counterattack seemed to indicate that Bobby might be protecting his father in a way that was habitual in the family. The tone of disrespect in Jeannie's voice indicated that she felt as safe attacking her father as she did her sibling, and the fact that her mother intervened as if her father and she were siblings rather than father and daughter, her failure to support her husband, and her smiles toward her daughter *all* indicated covert support for her daughter rather than her husband. The therapist then took charge, stopped the sequence, and asked a question about the process she had observed, focusing on the conflict between father and daughter. She then asked a direct question to confirm her hypothesis about the relationship between mother and daughter. She next attempted to establish a temporal relationship between Jeannie's attacks and her arguments with her father. Failing, she switched to explore the relationship between Bobby and his father.

THERAPIST: Oh, yes. I know about mothers and daughters. And I know how hard it is [looks directly at father] to be the head of the household and have to worry about making ends meet. Tell me, Mr. Beals, have you ever noticed any relationship between your arguments with Jeannie and her vomiting attacks. I mean, does she ever vomit after you two have had a disagreement?

FATHER: I'd have to think about it, but I wouldn't say so. She brings those things on herself, if you ask me.

THERAPIST: Jeannie, what do you think. Do you ever get so upset after an argument with your father that you get sick?

JEANNIE: It's got nothing to do with him. I don't care about him. I'm not sick in the head. They don't have to bring me to a shrink [looking at father]. You'd just love to have me be mentally ill, like all those names you call me.

FATHER: Jeannie, I'm just trying to help you, bringing you here. I just . . .

THERAPIST: O.K. I'm not married to the idea that the vomiting spells have anything to do with your fights. It was just an idea. And, Jeannie, nobody thinks you're mentally ill or crazy or anything like that. Now, Bobby, we know your sister fights with your father. How about you, do you fight with your father?

BOBBY: Nah. He teaches me to do all kind of things. Like about the car and how to fix things. And he helps me practice my judo.

THERAPIST: [With raised eyebrows] Judo?

FATHER Yeah. I'm giving him judo lessens to toughen him up. So he won't keep getting beat up.

THERAPIST: And you practice with your father, Bobby? He's so much bigger than you. Don't you get hurt?

BOBBY: [Giggling] Oh, sometimes he hits a little hard. But it's just to toughen me up.

Notice that the therapist is careful to give the father some support regarding his role as head of the household before mentioning the possibility of a link between the symptom and the interaction between him and his daughter. The therapist must always be careful that family members do not feel blamed for the problems of their symptomatic members. The therapist must be quite active in sessions, establishing a focus so that family members do not diffuse anxiety in their usual ways. In this case the father–daughter fighting seems to operate to diffuse all tension in the family, so the therapist acts to stop the fighting so that other issues can emerge. In this sequence, the therapist sensed the anxiety around the issue of linking the symptom to the fighting and backed away from the issue, reassuring the patient that she was not crazy, and changing the focus. By this time she is impressed by the amount of anger both the patient and the father have shown and is trying to see if anger is also operative in the father–son relationship. The questioning of the appropriateness of Bobby's practicing judo with his father was an attempt to give him or other family members a chance to comment.

MOTHER: Oh, Bobby, tell the truth now. You're always complaining behind his back [again smiling broadly]. I've told you to tell him directly when he hits too hard.

FATHER: I don't hit him too hard. He needs to toughen up anyway [turns to therapist]. You see, he goes to a special school for smart kids, and the kids in the neighborhood are jealous.

JEANNIE: They are not. He's just such a punk they can't stand him.

FATHER: And you stand there and do nothing to protect him. Your own brother . . . [practically shouting].

THERAPIST: O.K., let me get in here a minute, Mrs. Beals. Where are you when all the action is going on?

MOTHER: Oh, I try to stop it. But I'm afraid my husband has quite a temper [smiling again]. I just try to separate them, you know, send Jeannie to her room. Or take her out shopping. We love to go shopping together.

THERAPIST: I see. So you try to be the peacemaker?

MOTHER: Yes, that's me alright. The peacemaker.

By this time the therapist has hypothesized that Jeannie acts as a conduit for family tensions, particularly for those between her parents. She notes, for example, that the mother actually rewards Jeannie for fighting with her father by taking her out shopping, presumably for all those tight jeans her husband complains about having to pay for. She also notes that the mother smiles inappropriately while talking about the fighting. This could indicate that she does not take it seriously, or that the subject makes her anxious. She may be afraid that her husband will explode in the session as he does at home. It is important that the therapist maintain a tight control over the situation, while exploring it gently, and keeping some of her more anxiety-producing hypotheses to herself.

THERAPIST: O.K. So now I understand that there is a lot of, uh, disagreements in the house, and that mother tries to keep the peace. Now, Mr. Beals, I know you only want what's best for your daughter. So your fights with her must be your way of trying to convince her what's best. Do you get any help from your wife in convincing your daughter what's best?

FATHER: [Obviously reluctant to answer] Oh, sometimes.

THERAPIST: But maybe not as often as you'd like?

FATHER: [Bitterly] Those two just keep me around to pay the bills.

THERAPIST: I see. So maybe you feel left out sometimes?

FATHER: I just go to the garage and work on the car.

THERAPIST: Oh yes, you told me earlier you were a master mechanic. Boy, I wish I had a master mechanic around.

MOTHER: Oh yes. He saves us a lot of money. And he works on all his family's cars, too. Saves everybody a lot of money.

The therapist relabels the father's fighting as his way of being a good parent. Such relabeling of behavior that may be considered negative often avoids one family member's feeling picked on by the therapist and allows for exploration of potentially painful areas: in this case the obvious lack of agreement between parents and the mother's obvious alliance with her daughter. When the father bitterly announces his feeling of being used by his wife and daughter, the therapist colludes with the mother to allow everyone to focus on one of father's positive attributes. The therapist stores away the information about the lack of an effective parental coalition and speculates that many unresolved marital difficulties lie at the heart of the problem.

The therapist is now aware that the family has shared more information than might have been intended. Her hypothesis is that Jeannie has been acting as a stabilizing force in the marital relationship for a long time. She has provided her mother with the companionship missing in the marriage, and has detoured the anger (which might threaten the continuation of the marriage) into her relationship with her father. The source of the father's anger is unknown at this point, but he appears isolated in the family except for his relationship with his son, and even that appears somewhat tenuous. The appearance of symptoms in Jeannie can be explained by her developmental need to separate and individuate from a tight and very volatile family system whose stability has depended on her remaining overly close with her mother. The therapist's job is to present a definition of the problem and some goals that will be satisfactory to all family members so that they will cooperate with the therapeutic process.

THERAPIST: So, Mr. Beals, while your ending up in the garage is good for the family pocketbook, I'm thinking maybe it's not so good for you. I know it's not good for a father to feel left out, especially for one who is trying so hard to be a good father that he is even willing to come to family therapy. I think maybe one of the things we could work on would be to find other ways of your being a good father. Teenagers can be tough on their parents and . . .

JEANNIE: Parents can be tough on their teenagers too!

THERAPIST: That's sometimes true too, Jeannie. But my guess is that your father can get some help from your mother in terms of learning how to negotiate with you rather than fight. You know, we all learn to get along with men by learning to get along with our fathers. And that means sons, too, Bobby.

BOBBIE: Ah, we get along.

THERAPIST: I'm sure you do. But there are lots of things a father can teach a son besides judo and how to fix cars. Like how to get along with women.

BOBBY: [Blushing] Ah . . . .

THERAPIST: And Mrs. Beals, I'm sure you would like it if there were less fighting around the house. Do you think you could help your husband learn how to avoid fights with Jeannie and still be a good father?

MOTHER: [Looking doubtful] Well, I can try. But they've been fighting for a long time . . .

THERAPIST: Yes. Well, maybe it's high time for a change.

FATHER: What's this got to do with Jeannie throwing up.

THERAPIST: I'm not exactly sure right now, but we'll keep a close eye on the vomiting as well. Do you think you can go along with my idea about lessening the fighting?

FATHER: I'll do anything if it will help.

THERAPIST: I know you will.

The therapist has just made an informal treatment contract with the family. Her main thrust was to the father because she perceived him as being the most resistant. However, she was careful to include some gain for everyone. Although she did not mention the notion that Jeannie's symptoms might be related to fights with her father, she was relying on the process of making covert family tensions overt to relieve the need for such a symptom. The symptom did, in fact, disappear immediately, even though the fighting did not.

Summary

The question of diagnosing families in any conventional sense remains open. The important issue is for the therapist to understand the ways in which family members contribute to the maintenance or exacerbation of symptoms in a family member, and/or the function symptomatic behavior may be serving to stabilize the family system. The therapist must be able to recognize recurring patterns of family behavior and use those patterns to understand how a particular family fails to resolve its problems.

The most important initial consideration is to establish a working relationship with all family members. The initial phone call and interview are crucial to establishing such a relationship. The therapist must be prepared to spend time answering questions about family therapy and about his or her professional and personal qualifications. The therapist must also be prepared to take responsibility for maintaining a coherent focus so that anxiety-producing issues can be discussed without undue stress on any family member. The therapist must also formulate an initial definition of the problem acceptable to all family members in order to form an initial treatment contract. This contract may or may not overtly address itself to all the problems the therapist sees or suspects, depending upon the family's readiness to acknowledge such problems.

To a larger extent than in other forms of therapy, family therapy assumes health and strength rather than pathology. The therapist seeks to mobilize whatever strengths exist in the system to solve the problems. The assumption of health rather than pathology helps establish a cooperative, hopeful attitude on both the part of the therapist and the family. In fact, perhaps the primary job of the therapist is to establish such a climate of hope. Families, like individuals, change slowly, and with many ups and downs. If the therapist has established, early on, a good working relationship and an atmosphere of hope, a family becomes much more willing to reveal and deal with failures in problem solving.

References

Anderson, C. M., Hogarty, G. E., & Reiss, D. J. (1980). Family treatment of adult schizophrenic patients: A psychoeducational approach. *Schizophrenia Bulletin, 6,* 490–505.

Cromwell, R. E., Olsen, D. H. L., & Fournier, D. G. (1976). Tools and techniques for diagnosis and evaluation in marital and family therapy. *Family Process, 15,* 1–49.

Fleck, S. (1966). An approach to family pathology. *Comprehensive Psychiatry, 5,* 307–320.

Gurman, A. S., & Kniskern, D. P. (1981). Family therapy outcome research: Knowns and unknowns. In A. S. Gurman & D. P. Kniskern (Eds.), *Handbook of family therapy.* (pp. 742–775). New York: Brunner/Mazel. .

Hoffman, L. (1981). *Foundations of family therapy.* New York: Basic Books.

Madanes, C. (1981). *Strategic family therapy.* San Francisco: Jossey-Bass.

Minuchin, S., Rosman, B. L., & Baker, L. (1978). *Psychosomatic families: Anorexia nervosa in context.* Cambridge: Harvard University Press.

Olsen, D. H. L., Sprenkle, D. H., & Russell, C. S. (1979). Circumplex model of marital and family systems: 1. Cohesion and adaptability dimensions, family types, and clinical applications. *Family Process, 18,* 3–25.

Reiss, D., & Oliveri, M. D. (1980). Family paradigm and family coping: A proposal for linking the family's intrinsic adaptive capacities to its responses to stress. *Family Relations, 29,* 431–444.

Stanton, M. D., & Todd, T. (1976). *Structural family therapy with heroin addicts: Some outcome data.* Paper presented at the meeting of the Society for Psychotherapy Research, San Diego.

Tseng, W. S., Arensdorf, A. M., McDermott, Jr., J. F., Hansen, M. J., & Fukunaga, C. S. (1974). *Family diagnosis and classification.* Paper presented at the annual meeting of the American Academy of Child Psychiatry, San Francisco.

Weeks, G. R., & L'Abate, L. (1982). *Paradoxical psychotherapy: Theory and practice with individuals, couples and families.* New York: Brunner/Mazel.

Chapter 13

Children

Alan M. Gross

Introduction

Few issues in child psychopathology have been the object of as much controversy as diagnosis. Extant diagnostic systems have been criticized for a variety of reasons. Empirical clinicians and researchers point out that present taxonomies of childhood disorders violate many of the scientific criteria for an acceptable classification system (Quay, 1979). In addition, these taxonomies are based on a disease model of abnormal behavior, and many question whether this is an appropriate model for the study of human behavior (Ciminero & Drabman, 1977).

Another problem associated with current diagnostic systems for children is their failure to yield high levels of interrater reliability in clinical practice (Wells, 1981). The new *Diagnostic and Statistical Manual of Mental Disorders*, third edition (DSM-III) has attempted to improve upon this situation. In contrast to the second edition, DSM-II, there is an increase in use of empirically derived and operationally defined criteria to describe each diagnostic category (Nathan, 1981). Recent studies of diagnostic reliability of the childhood disorder categories (e.g., Cantwell, Russell, Mattison, & Will, 1979) using DSM-III found improved reliability over levels obtained using DSM-II. However, reliability levels were still extremely low (Taylor, 1983).

Portions of this chapter are taken from "Behavioral Interviewing" by Alan M. Gross. In *Child Behavioral Assessment*, T. H. Ollendick & M. Hersen (Eds.), 1983. New York: Pergamon Press. Copyright 1983 by Pergamon Press. Used by permission.

ALAN M. GROSS • Department of Psychology, Emory University, Atlanta, Georgia 30322.

The usefulness of current diagnostic systems in treatment planning has also been the subject of debate. Hobbs (1975) has suggested that the generality of the diagnostic categories and the absence of attention to situational influences on behavior greatly reduce the value of diagnosis in the development of an effective intervention. Regardless of diagnosis, the therapist must still conduct an individual assessment of the situational factors that must be altered in order to effect the desired behavior change.

Despite the problems associated with child diagnosis, there is growing recognition of the important place it holds in the study and treatment of child psychopathology (Achenbach, 1974). Diagnosis offers an accepted method of organizing data and communicating about abnormal behavior (Evans & Nelson, 1977). Although there is no doubt that treatment planning requires a systematic analysis of a child's environment, diagnosis can greatly contribute to this process. Diagnosis can put the therapist in touch with a wealth of clinical and research data related to a youngster's problem. Because behavior problems do not always occur in isolation but rather covary with other maladaptive responses, diagnosis can alert the clinician to behaviors to be assessed, indicate potential controlling variables, and suggest possible treatments. Moreover, research on psychopathology is facilitated by the delineation of differential characteristics of diagnostic subtypes.

It is clear that there are a number of limitations as well as benefits associated with current systems of diagnosis of psychopathology in children. The problems have led some clinicians generally to avoid using diagnosis (Wells, 1981). The benefits have led others to minimize the system's drawbacks. Attempting to eliminate the flaws and capitalize on the benefits of an empirically derived taxonomy of childhood psychopathology is the obvious solution toward which professionals should work. Unfortunately, this is a difficult problem with no simple solutions.

Regardless of one's feelings about diagnosis and abnormal child behavior, there is little doubt that it has become an inescapable aspect of clinical work with children. As more insurance companies expand their coverage to include psychological services, clinicians will be regularly confronted with having to label a child in order for the youngster's family to qualify for insurance reimbursement. More important, however, is the fact that numerous state and federal agencies require that a child be diagnosed as having a specific disorder in order to qualify for services. Moreover, the type of service, funds, and/or treatment placement will be determined by the diagnostic label.

The purpose of the present chapter is to discuss the major issues involved in diagnostic interviewing with children. Rather than describing the various diagnostic categories and the criteria that comprise them, the focus will be on the practical aspects of diagnostic assessment of children's behavior problems. Included in the chapter will be a discussion of the differences in diagnostic interviewing with adults and children. This will be followed by a discussion of the applied aspects of interviewing children. Case descriptions also will be provided to illustrate the methodology.

Child versus Adult Diagnostic Interviewing

The diagnostic interview serves a number of functions. At the most simplistic level of analysis, diagnosis might be considered the process by which an individual is assigned to an accepted classification scheme. In practice, however, diagnosis is much more of an ongoing process. It initially functions as a screening device helpful in determining whether there is a problem; and if one exists, what is the nature and extent of the difficulty (Mash & Terdal, 1981)? To this end, the diagnostic interview provides data specifying target behaviors and situational variables associated with their occurrence. Recognizing clusters of behavioral covariation that are relatively constant across a group of individuals (that are at times differentially associated with etiology and prognosis) also provides important information for use when selecting an initial intervention strategy.

The process just described leads to the generation of hypotheses upon which assessment and treatment decisions are made. Although diagnosis provides a starting point for intervention, it is clear that each contact with a patient produces new information. This information contributes to the refinement of treatment hypotheses making diagnosis a continuous process.

Although the goals of the diagnostic interview are the same regardless of the target population, there are a number of aspects of diagnostic interviewing with children that differentiate it from interviewing individuals with adult disorders. Unlike most adult patients who attend therapy after identifying themselves as having behavorial difficulties, a child usually appears at the therapist's office because an adult (parents or teacher) has determined that a behavior problem exists (Gross, 1983). As such, it is not uncommon for the child and adult to disagree over the existence of the problem as well as over the specifics of the problem area. When differences in opinion exist, the therapist must exhibit great sensitivity to both the child and his or her family if efficient and effective data collection is to occur. Failure to address the disparity in perceptions may inhibit the development of cooperation between parents, child, and therapist during the treatment intervention.

A number of investigators have also noted that the factors leading to children being referred to a psychological clinic often are related more to parent and environmental variables than the child's behavior. Harris (1974) reported that referral rates are associated with socioeconomic status, with middle-class families being the most frequent users of these services. Oltmanns, Broderick, and O'Leary (1977) suggest that marital discord can be a major factor in a parent's perception of child deviance. And, Rickard, Forehand, Wells, Griest, and McMahon (1980) argue that the presence of parental depression may affect whether a child's behavior is viewed by her or his parents as deviant. These findings indicate that interviewers cannot simply assume that because a child is referred for treatment that he or she in fact exhibits behavior problems. Parent perceptions of child behavior can be affected by a variety of personal factors; and therefore the clinician must obtain multiple sources of information. Moreover, an assessment of parental adjustment and or expectations regarding the behavior of children may be necessary before any determination of child deviance can be made.

Children also differ from adults in that frequently they are under stronger and more obvious sources of social control. This necessitates that serious consideration be given to the child's environment during the diagnostic assessment. Interviews should be conducted with significant others (e.g., parents, teachers, peers) from the child's environment. This is especially important because generally children have experienced, or are experiencing, some type of intervention (e.g., parent-designed treatment) at the time they are referred. Failure to interview individuals who are likely to be involved in daily attempts to control the youngster's behavior may result in an inaccurate understanding of the youth. Moreover, it is important to obtain information from various adult sources because the child may not have the verbal skills necessary to describe the problem adequately.

Clinicians working with children must also consider cognitive skills and abilities in the diagnostic process. Frequently, a youngster's behavioral problems are related to learning difficulties. This may necessitate the evaluation of the child's intellectual abilities and academic skills.

Another major characteristic of diagnosis with children is the importance of considering developmental variables. Youngsters exhibit uneven developmental change. The social significance and meaning of problem behaviors may vary with age (Prugh, Engel, & Morse, 1975). The diagnostician of children must have a strong background in developmental psychology in order to completely comprehend the nature and significance of the responses observed. Finally, uneven developmental change carries implications regarding the stability of diagnostic information (Mash & Terdal, 1981). Conduct at one age may not be predictive of later behavior. Reevaluation should be the norm in child diagnosis.

DSM-III and Diagnosis of Childhood Psychopathology

The DSM-III divides the disorders of childhood into five broad classes: *intellectual, behavioral, emotional, physical,* and *developmental.* These general categories were created on the basis of the predominant area of disturbance. The intellectual category consists of problems of mental retardation. The behavioral category consists of overt behavioral problems such as attention-deficit disorder and conduct disorder. Anxiety disorders and difficulties such as elective mutism and oppositional disorder are included in the emotional grouping. The physical class of childhood disorders includes eating disturbances, stereotyped movement disorders (tics), and problems with physical manifestations (enuresis). Lastly, autism and specific developmental disorders (language development) are grouped in the developmental category.

The individual diagnostic categories listed under each broad class of disorders are accompanied by a large amount of descriptive information provided to assist the clinician in making diagnoses. The most important aspect of this information is the section on essential features. *Essential features* are the behaviors that must generally be present in order to make the diagnosis. For each diagnostic category the essential features are clearly defined. Associated features of the disorder, which include behaviors that are often, but not invariably present, are also described.

The presentation of essential and associated features accompanying each diagnostic category clearly defines the behaviors the clinician must observe in order to make a particular diagnosis. General knowledge of these features will indicate certain directions to be followed when gathering information during the diagnostic assessment. Unfortunately, it is rarely the case that a child will present all of the problem behaviors, or only problem responses, particular to one disorder. To assist the clinician further in the decision-making process, each diagnostic category also includes information concerning age of onset, impairment, predisposing factors, sex ratio, familial pattern, and possible disorders from which it should be differentiated. Using this information, clinicians can direct their questions toward obtaining data that will help clarify whether the behavior problem displayed fits the pattern associated with a given disorder.

As previously stated, children exhibiting psychopathology frequently display problem responses that may be found in more than one diagnostic category. For example, a youngster who demonstrates the essential features of a conduct disorder also may display many of the essential features of a developmental reading disorder. The DSM-III allows for all of this information to be coded into each diagnosis by recommending the use of a multiaxial evaluation system.

In the multiaxial system, diagnostic information can be presented on five axes. Axis I indicates the major clinical syndrome, whereas Axis II refers to personality disorders and specific developmental disorders. Physical conditions are coded on Axis III. Axes IV and V present supplemental data regarding severity of psychosocial stress and the child's highest level of functioning in the previous year. This information is indicated by a numerical rating that has defined reference points. The latter two axes may be most relevant for treatment planning. Moreover, when a child meets the criteria for more than one diagnosis, an indication of principal diagnosis can be included to indicate the condition most responsible for the request for treatment.

A demonstration of how the multiaxial system can be used is illustrated by the following case. Six months after her divorce, a woman brings her son to the clinic because of a recent increase in noncompliant behavior. The diagnostic interview reveals that since his parents' divorce the youth has begun to bedwet and display a response pattern typical of a conduct disorder. This information could be summarized in diagnosis as follows:

- Axis I: 312.23 Conduct disorder, socialized, nonaggressive
- Axis II: V71.09 No evidence of a disorder
- Axis III: 307.60 Functional enuresis
- Axis IV: 5 Severe
- Axis V: 2 Very good

The diagnostic system that characterizes the DSM-III provides the clinician with a means of summarizing a large amount of descriptive diagnostic data. Guidelines are provided for delineating specific major syndromes and associated developmental and physical disorders. Indication of present stressors and previous levels of adaptive functioning can also be suggested. As with the use of any classification system, the accuracy and quality of diagnostic information delivered will be a function of the clinician's skill in using this system. In order to be able to effectively diagnose childhood psychopathology, clinicians must be well acquainted with the diagnostic criteria for each disorder. Moreover, they must possess interview skills so that they may seek the information necessary to determine if a child's behavior is representative of a particular disorder.

The Interview

In the assessment and diagnostic process with children, a variety of individuals may be interviewed. In order to determine which adults are significant to the child's situation and should be included in the assessment process, the behavior problem must first be defined. As such, diagnostic assessment is usually initiated with both the child and his or her parents being seen during the first interview (Ollendick & Cerny, 1981). Therapists differ in their approach to structuring the first session, but it is generally agreed that the child and his or her parents should be seen alone and together. With children under 6 years of age, the parents are usually seen first, followed by the child alone, and finally with all three together. With older children the order of interview may be altered.

Whether interviewing the parents (teacher) or child, the interviewer is attempting to gather considerable information. Although some might argue that the primary purpose of a diagnostic interview is to identify the target behaviors, the focus of the interview should be much broader. In addition to defining the problem behavior(s), the clinician should attempt to discover the associated antecedent and consequent stimuli, to assess the parents' mediational potential, to evaluate the youngster's potential strengths, and to identify potential rewarding and aversive stimuli that might prove helpful in treatment planning. A developmental history should also be obtained. This information will put the child's behavior in perspective and contribute to determining the significance of the difficulty.

Interview: Meeting with Parents

The therapist begins the first interview by gathering demographic information about the child (e.g., age, grade in school). This is followed by an attempt to obtain a description of the problem. General questions from the interviewer such as "What prompted you to come to the clinic?" or "Can you tell me what problems you are having with your child?" can be used to initiate this process. Because the therapist is also interested in gaining insight as to what variables may be cuing and maintaining the child's behavior, specific questions regarding details of the response and the situation in which it occurs should be asked "Exactly what does he do?" "What do you do when he does that?" "Does it always occur at dinner time?" Additionally, information concerning frequency and duration of problem responses is collected.

The questions described serve to initiate the interview process, define the problem, and determine possible environmental stimuli related to its occurrence. Subsequent questions will be determined by the nature of the presenting complaint. Questions addressed to the parents and child presenting with attention-deficit disorder will differ from those directed to the family of a depressed youth. The interviewer's questions still are intended to describe behaviors and identify associated stimuli. Familiarity with the essential and associated features of the various child syndromes is imperative for this process. Awareness of which behaviors typically covary with others will determine the direction of the interview. For example, parents whose primary concern is their son's apparent inability to stay on task should be questioned regarding the occurrence of other behaviors known to covary with attention problems. This approach will help delineate the child's full range of responses in need of treatment, differentiate the disorder from similar childhood disorders, and yield useful data for determining the severity of the problem and suitability of potential treatments.

Following this stage of data collection, the interviewer may begin to assess the youngster's behavioral assets. Asking parents what behaviors they would like to see their child perform may result in this information (e.g., "What would you like him to do when that occurs?"). This line of questioning will lead to the determination of appropriate alternative responses to teach the child. It also will help assess parental expectation of child behaviors.

Although not imperative to the development of a diagnosis, information concerning rewarding and aversive stimuli for use in the treatment program should be obtained. The majority of child therapy programs involve the reinforcement of appropriate responding and the extinction or punishment of inappropriate responding. As such, discovering which events in the youngster's life may be effective reinforcers and punishers should prove useful during treatment planning. Asking parents about their child's likes and dislikes (What does she or he do after school?; Does she/he like TV?) is often an efficient technique for gathering this information.

A nonspecific variable that therapists also attempt to assess during the diagnostic interview is the parents' mediation potential i.e., whether the therapist assesses the probability that the parents will successfully complete the treatment intervention). This potential is inferred from a number of variables: degree of behavioral insight, degree of distress, value of contingencies for successful behavior change, reliability of the parent, and degree of interference from competing problems in parents' lives (Haynes, 1978). The interviewer must use the behavior sample provided by observing the parents in the interview to evaluate some of the variables mentioned. However, the ability of parents to comply with instructions over time will also provide objective data regarding mediation potential.

Interview: Meeting with the Child

The purposes of interviewing the youngster are similar to those of interviewing parents. An attempt is made to hear the child's definition of the problem situations, to assess behavioral strengths, and to identify potential consequent stimuli. With children under 5 years of age, however, the therapist can expect that this tactic will lead to little useful content information, although such is not necessarily the case with older children. This interview generally begins with the therapist asking the child why she or he thinks she or he has been brought to the clinic. Following the youth's response, the therapist usually shares his or her opinion about this issue with the youngster. The clinician's reply conveys to the child that the entire family would like to work to make things more pleasant for everyone at home. The therapist may also ask about family and peer interactions as well as about preferred activities (e.g., "What do you like to do with your friends?"). These questions help the therapist to determine events that may serve as rewards in the treatment program. Although some practical information can be obtained in interview with the child, the major goal of this phase of the interview process is to convey to the youth that the family and not the child is going to be the focus of treatment, and that the child's thoughts and feelings will be important factors in the formulation of the intervention strategy.

In addition to descriptive data, interviewing the child and his or her parents also provide other very useful diagnostic information. This procedure affords the clinician the opportunity to directly observe how the parents and child behave during the interview. For example, observing the child's response to questions may give an indication of the youth's social skills development. Moreover, the clinician can arrange the interview environment so that firsthand observation of the target behaviors may occur (e.g., attention deficit to a reading task, motor activity level, noncompliance). Observing the child and parents together may allow the interviewer to see how the parents respond to inappropriate and appropriate child behavior. Despite the novelty of the interview situation and the possibility that the family is attempting to present itself at its best, or worst, the interview with the child and his or her family is the first direct observation provided to the therapist. The information gotten as a result should be used to generate and evaluate diagnostic questions.

After interviewing the child, the initial interview is generally closed with a brief summary discussion with the youngster's parents. During this time the therapist presents his or her conceptualization of the problem(s) to the parents. Suggestions as to which problem area should be targeted immediately are also discussed. This summary provides parents with a framework with which to redefine and view the problem. When additional information is desired, this is also a good time for the therapist to give parents homework assignments (e.g., "Please write down each time you have a problem getting Seymour to finish eating. Also briefly describe the situation").

Interview: Meeting with the Teacher

After parents, children generally spend more time with their teacher than any other adult. Frequently, it is a youngster's teacher who calls attention to the youth's behavioral difficulties. As such, the teacher is an important person to consider during the assessment process. Additionally, interviewing teachers at times may provide corroboration of parental reports of child behavior.

Similar to the parent interview, teachers are asked to provide a description of the problem responses, the setting in which they occur, and possible controlling variables. Here again, interviewers should tailor their questions to evaluate their hypothesis regarding potential behavioral syndromes.

Interviewing the teacher may lead to identification of areas of behavioral assets and deficits that are not easily obtained from parents. Social skills may be assessed by inquiring about the child's interactions with peers (e.g., Does he have many friends?" "Does she interact with boys and girls" "Do the other children include him when they are selecting team players?"). Teachers are frequently very accurate in identifying children with a high likelihood of developing school problems (Ciminero & Drabman, 1977; Keefe, Kopel, & Gordon, 1978).

Questions regarding academic performance may also delineate important areas for intervention. A good set of questions to ask in this area includes: Does she or he do her/his work? Are assignments completed on time? Relative to classmates how would you evaluate his or her performance in math, science, etc.? and "Does she or he have difficulties staying on task?"

Finally, the interview with the teacher should result in an assessment of the willingness of the teacher to assist in the intervention program. Generally, teachers are very interested in the performance of their students. An interviewer who consults with a child's teacher and exhibits a sincere appreciation of his or her observations and comments is likely to readily elicit a cooperative response.

Interview Structure

Although there is general agreement regarding the types of material to obtain during a diagnostic interview, there is some disagreement regarding whether the interview format used to gather this information should be structured or unstructured (Maloney & Ward, 1976).

Unstructured interviews impose minimal constraints on the topics discussed. The therapist has great flexibility and may follow the cues of parents in choosing the sequence of topics. This may be a good approach when confronted with a case in which there appear to be a number of behavior problems (Haynes, 1978). However, even in the unstructured interview there is a certain degree of structure. The therapist asks questions that will meet the goals of the interview. The major characteristic of unstructured interviews is that the sequence of topics discussed may vary across interviewers.

In structured interviews, the topics discussed follow a prearranged format. The interviewer directs the conversation of the parents, and the likelihood of following up on a tangential topic frequently is a function of whether there is time remaining in the session after the predetermined questions have been addressed. A number of structured diagnostic interview scales have been developed. The more commonly used instruments are the Child Behavior Checklist (Achenbach, 1978; Achenbach & Edelbrock, 1979), the Kiddie-SADS (Puig-Antich & Chambers, 1978), and the Diagnostic Interview for Children and Adults (Herjanic, Herjanic, Brown, & Wheatt, 1975).

The Child Behavior Checklist (CBCL) is comprised of both social competence and behavior problem items. The scale can be completed by parents, or children aged 4 to 16. Items assess involvement in activities such as job, sports, and chores, and social relations with peers. Information regarding school performance and academic behavior is also assessed. The CBCL consists of 118 items that are scored on a 3-point scale (e.g., not true, somewhat true, and very true). Factor analyses have revealed a number of response clusters that differ with sex and age of the child. They include somatic complaints, depression, social withdrawal, hyperactivity, aggression, and delinquent behavior. Moreover, this instrument has been shown to differentiate clinic from nonclinic children (Achenbach & Edelbrock, 1979).

The Kiddie-SADS is designed to assess depression and its concommitant symptoms as well as other diagnostic categories in children. This instrument is based on Endicott and Spitzer's (1978) Schizophrenic and Affective Disorders Schedule (SADS), and a DSM-III diagnosis is obtainable from this interview. The Kiddie-SADS is appropriate for children aged 6 to 16. Various symptoms are rated for occurrence and degree of severity. Moreover, the interview is designed to provide information on both present and past psychopathology. Although adequate work regarding the reliability of this measure has been performed, few validity data have been presented.

The Diagnostic Interview for Children and Adolescents (DICA) was developed for use with youngsters aged 6 to 16. This structured interview consists of 207 questions. Many of these questions only require a *yes* or *no* response. Items assess four major content areas: factual information (e.g., age, address), behavior (e.g., at home, with peers), psychiatric symptoms (e.g., phobias, compulsions), and mental status (e.g., orientation, judgment). The DICA has been shown to have adequate reliability and that child interview responses are capable of distinguishing psychiatric and control children.

Structured interviews have a number of appealing aspects. They increase the probability that interviewers will cover the same material in a similar manner with all families. This method may be valuable in terms of providing a list of content areas that should be addressed during the diagnostic process. It is also conceivable that conducting very structured interviews will help the clinician develop a frame of reference from which to view child behavior problems. However, aside from the CBCL, few normative data exist for these instruments. There also may be times when the diagnostic situation requires more flexibility than is allowed when using a structured format. Finally, these instruments were primarily designed to identify symptoms. As such, they may not provide adequate information upon which to begin developing a treatment plan.

Because diagnostic interviewing should encompass more than identifying a behavioral syndrome, it may be more useful to utilize the best aspects of structured and unstructured formats. The therapist might begin the process with minimal structure, using open-ended questions designed to identify the problem. After establishing the nature of the difficulty, the clinician might begin to increase the structure of the interview. At this point the interviewer might assess whether responses that typically covary with the problem behavior described are also occurring. This could lead to hypothesis testing concerning whether the youngster is exhibiting a response pattern that approximates a specific behavioral syndrome. Moreover, following identification of target behaviors, questions aimed at identifying environmental variables associated with the problem responses would be appropriate.

Interview Behavior

A number of interviewer behaviors have been suggested as important to the facilitation of the interview process (Haynes & Wilson, 1979).

Scheiderer (1977) has suggested that the efficiency and effectiveness of interviews can be improved by preparing patients for the interview. He has demonstrated that providing detailed instructions to patients to be open and specific regarding their responses to interview questions significantly increases personal self-disclosure and reduces impersonal discussion.

The therapist's use of reinforcement can also contribute to the effectiveness of the interview (Morganstern & Tevlin, 1981). The function of reinforcement in the interview is to establish the interviewer as a dispenser of social rewards (e.g., praise), to increase the likelihood that the patient returns for additional sessions, and to raise the frequency of desirable types of speech (e.g., problem specifics) (Haynes, 1978). Reinforcing behaviors may include eye contact, body posture, verbal praise, and affective comments (i.e., remarks that communicate to the patient that the therapist has been listening and that may be reinforcing) (Morganstern & Tevlin, 1981). These behaviors can be used with adults and children. Primary reinforcers such as food can also be employed to reward children for their good interview performance. As with all stimuli used as rewards, each may not be an effective stimulus for all patients. As such, the interviewer needs to be aware of the parameters involved in the effective use of reinforcers.

Finally, Maloney and Ward (1976) suggest that therapists use open-ended questions when interviewing (e.g., "Describe what happens when you ask Jerome to pick up his toys"). They state that this type of question prevents patients from assuming a passive responder role. Although a closed question (e.g., "Is it difficult to get Jerome to pick up his toys?") can be responded to with a *yes* or *no* response, open-ended questions require the patient to decide what is pertinent, where to start, and what to include in his or her response. Not only does this type of question provide the therapist with an opportunity to listen to the subject's perspective on the problem, but it also affords the opportunity to see how parents and children handle themselves in a relatively unstructured situation. Moreover, the phrasing of open-ended questions may be less biased and therefore result in more valid information (Haynes, 1978).

Case Illustrations

Having described a general diagnostic interviewing strategy for use with children, it seems appropriate to provide case illustrations of the application of these procedures. Clinical examples of diagnostic interviews with two children are provided. Although only two diagnostic categories are represented, they will illustrate how diagnostic assessments with children involve the use of a general interview strategy, and how the specifics of the interview process are shaped by the nature of the youth's disorder and the clinician's familiarity with childhood diagnostic categories.

Attention-Deficit Disorder (ADD) with Hyperactivity (DSM-III 3M.01). The essential features of ADD with hyperactivity are signs of developmental inappropriate inattention, impulsivity, and hyperactivity (APA, 1980). Associated aspects of the disorder include obstinacy, bossiness, emotional liability, low frustration tolerance, temper outbursts, and lack of responsiveness to discipline. Children usually begin to evidence the disorder by the age of 3, and symptoms frequently disappear with the onset of puberty. These youngsters usually demonstrate academic and social functioning impairment as a result of the disorder. Moreover, boys are 10 times more likely than girls to develop this problem.

Rex is a 6 year-old Caucasian male brought to the outpatient clinic because of problems at home and school. His parents reported that he has difficulty sustaining attention, and he fails to comply with parental commands. At the initial interview, the therapist first met with Mr. and Mrs. A. while Rex remained in the waiting room. The therapist began the session by explaining the purpose of the first meeting and emphasizing the importance of Mr. and Mrs. A. describing the difficulties in detail.

THERAPIST: Please tell me what prompted you to make an appointment.

MRS. A.: We are having a terrible time with Rex. He has always been an active boy. But now it seems as if he is always on the go. He doesn't seem able to sit still. He goes from one activity to another and never seems to finish what he starts. Also, his constant movement results in my having to discipline him because he is always getting into things he's not supposed to. When I discipline him he doesn't listen.

THERAPIST: Please give me an example.

MRS. A.: Yesterday after school I took him with me to the grocery store. I spent most of my time trying to keep him from destroying the store. He kept pulling things off the shelves, climbing in and out of the grocery cart, and running up and down the aisles. I tried asking him to sit quietly in the cart and that didn't work. I yelled and even spanked him and that didn't work. He just doesn't seem able to sit still. I think he actually tries to do what we ask but just gets distracted so easily.

THERAPIST: Does he have trouble sitting still in other situations?

MRS. A.: I can't really think of many times when it's not a problem for him.

THERAPIST: Does his teacher report that he has trouble paying attention and sitting still in class?

MR. A.: She says he is always fidgeting in his chair, leaving his seat, or talking out in class. She also says he doesn't seem able to stick to an assignment and work continuously on it until it is completed. The only way he gets his work done is if she sits and works with him on an individual basis.

THERAPIST: Does he have trouble sticking with activities at home.

MRS. A.: He comes into the house for 5 minutes, and it looks like a disaster area. He'll start playing with a toy. That will last a minute before he gives that up and starts playing with something else. And he never puts one toy away before he starts to use another.

THERAPIST: Is he like that if you play with him in a one to one interaction?

MR. A.: I suppose he's a bit better, but he still needs to be reminded pretty regularly about what he's supposed to be doing.

The therapist has identified a number of characteristics of Rex's behavior that suggest attentional deficits and a high activity level. Continuing with this line of questioning, the therapist begins to investigate whether other responses known to covary with the behaviors (that are associated with ADD) are also occurring.

THERAPIST: You've said he has a difficult time finishing what he starts. Is he very easily distracted.

MRS. A.: Yes. If I send him off to do something, the least little thing can turn him in a different direction.

THERAPIST: When he is engaged in a preferred activity like watching TV does he sit quietly?

MR. A.: No! He's constantly fidgeting, moving, and talking. It drives me crazy when we are all together trying to watch TV.

THERAPIST: How does he get along with peers.

MRS. A.: I think he intimidates the neighborhood kids. He's very bossy and can really throw tantrums or fuss when he doesn't get his way. He also is very physical with other children. I don't think he means to hurt anyone, but he does seem to bang into or knock the other kids down more than his share.

THERAPIST: Has Rex always been very active?

MRS. A.: Yes, it almost seems as if he went from crawling to running. I initially thought he was just an active little boy. It's hard to judge. Watching him on the playground with other kids his age, he doesn't appear so unusually active. I guess around the time he started kindergarten we became more concerned. His teacher commented that he was difficult to control. It seems that it has gotten worse since then.

The initial part of the interview was concerned with defining the child's problem. An attempt was also made to evaluate whether the child exhibited behaviors that frequently covary with attentional problems and meet the general guidelines for ADD. Upon determining the nature of the problem, the therapist began to seek specifics of parent–child interactions in order to possibly identify environmental variables related to the problem responses.

THERAPIST: You stated he is easily distracted, and as such, it is difficult to get him to follow instructions. Please give me an example and tell me how you typically handle it.

MRS. A.: As you might guess, it is really difficult to get him to do schoolwork. He's only in first grade, but he still is supposed to practice his letters and do little assignments. I'll tell him to sit at the dining room table where it is quiet and do his work. He sits for a second, and then he's up on his way to see what he heard his Dad doing, or to see where I am. Sometimes, I'll check on him, and he's drawing or playing with his pencil, or even exploring under the table.

THERAPIST: What do you do?

MRS. A.: I tell him to go back to work. He usually responds, but then is off 30 seconds later.

THERAPIST: What do you do then?

MRS. A.: I have yelled and spanked to no avail. Now, I frequently sit with him and watch him or help him until it's completed.

THERAPIST: Is it the same with you.

MR. A.: Pretty much. I holler louder so he might listen a few seconds longer.

The therapist's line of questioning identified some likely variables that may be contributing to the maintenance of the problem responses. Rex's failure to stay on task results in a large amount of attention. Once target behaviors and potential controlling variables had been described, questioning then proceeded to identify the youngster's desirable behaviors and potential rewards.

THERAPIST: Describe some situations in which Rex behaves very appropriately.

MRS. A.: Oddly enough, he is really good if it is just the two of us, and we are doing a task together. He is good at helping me with some housework if it's not too repetitious. He is also really good if we sit and read a story together.

THERAPIST: Do you want him to be able to sit and work on a task for a reasonable length of time?

MR. A.: Yes, and that he listen better when he is told to do something.

THERAPIST: Tell me some things that Rex really likes.

MRS. A.: Well, he likes certain food treats, and there are a few TV shows he seems to enjoy. He also loves to wrestle with his dad or play ball.

After obtaining information regarding target behavior, situational variables, alternative responses, and potential rewarding stimuli the therapist met alone with Rex. The therapist attempted to assess the youngster's knowledge of why he was in the clinic as well as note the occurrence of any of the behavior problems reported.

THERAPIST: Do you know why you are here, Rex?

REX: No, maybe 'cause I get in trouble at home.

THERAPIST: Your mom and dad want to learn how you and they can get along without yelling. Would you like that?

REX: Yeah.

THERAPIST: Do you like to play sports?

REX: Yeah. Me and my dad play football.

THERAPIST: Do you like to play with your dad?

REX: Yeah.

THERAPIST: What do you like to do after school?

REX: I like to watch cartoons and play.

THERAPIST: Rex, in that box in the corner there are some toys. Why don't you take them out and place them on the floor. You can pick one for us to play with. [This procedure was done to create the opportunity for the therapist to observe whether Rex could attend to a task when he is confronted with desirable competing stimuli.]

At the conclusion of his interview with Rex, the therapist met with Rex's parents and presented a brief summary of his observations.

THERAPIST: Your description of the problem situations was very detailed and clearly presented. Rex is displaying a number of problem behaviors. In particular, an unusually high activity level, impulsivity, and distractibility. These difficulties seem to be affecting him at home and at school. I will probably want to talk to his teacher to get more details about classroom performance. We can discuss that later. He also seems to be at a point where he may be starting to develop social problems with peers. You said some of the kids are beginning to show signs of being intimidated by Rex.

It also appears that there are a number of aspects of your behavior that may be affecting his responding. For example, his inattention and high activity level presently produce a great deal of one-to-one attention whether it is in the form of lectures, yelling, or simply sitting with him and working on a task together. There are a number of things you can do that may help him become less inattentive and more compliant.

MRS. A.: We will be happy to do most anything that is needed.

THERAPIST: The difficulties Rex is displaying fit a pattern of behavior that is commonly referred to as *attention deficit disorder with hyperactivity*. That is only important to us in that sometimes the youngsters who exhibit this behavior pattern respond to medication that reduces their activity level and increases attention span. So I think in the future we will talk about obtaining a consultation with your pediatrician. However, beyond medication purposes it is best not to think in terms of ADD, but rather view the situation in reference to specific response situations that are problematic. I want you simply to write down in detail the events surrounding two difficulties you have with Rex this coming week. Specify the situation, what he did, and what you did. I also would like permission to call Rex's teacher. Please call him and tell him I will be calling. You did an excellent job today of clearly presenting a picture of what has been going on. Keep up the good work.

The results of the initial assessment revealed that Rex was displaying a behavior pattern that met a large number of the criteria of ADD with hyperactivity. After defining the problem, the therapist collected information designed to identify situational variables that would be useful in treatment planning. He also interviewed Rex's teacher via telephone to determine the extent of Rex's difficulty at school. Treatment consisted of medication obtained by means of a pediatric consultation. Rex's parents were taught behavior management skills and instructed in how to develop a program to reward task-appropriate behavior and extinguish inappropriate behavior. Rex's parents worked with Rex's teacher to develop a behavioral intervention at school. A total of 25 weekly therapy sessions were required to effectively alter Rex's and his parents behaviors.

Infantile Autism (DSM-III 299.0X). The essential features of infantile autism are lack of responsiveness to other people, gross impairment in communication skills, and bizarre responses to various environmental stimuli (American Psychiatric Association, 1980). Symptom onset occurs within the first 30 months of life. More specifically, these youngsters fail to develop normal attachment behaviors. In infancy, these deficiencies may be manifested by a failure to cuddle and indifference or aversion to physical contact. Communication deficits involve both verbal and nonverbal behaviors. Language may be absent. When language does develop, it is often characterized by echolalia and immature gramatical structure. Bizarre responses to the environment include violent reactions to minor changes in it. Associated aspects of the disorder include labile mood, underresponsiveness or overresponsiveness to sensory stimuli, and self-stimulatory or self-injurious behavior. Autism appears to be chronic and affects boys three times more often than girls. The disorder is extremely incapacitating and special education is almost always required.

Otis is a 2-year-old male Caucasian referred for psychological evaluation. His parents reported that Otis displayed a variety of bizarre behaviors and appeared to be behind his peers in the development of language. At the initial interview, the therapist first met with Otis' parents while he remained in the waiting room under the supervision of his aunt. Before beginning the interview, the therapist instructed Mr. and Mrs. B. to be very detailed in their responses to his questioning.

THERAPIST: Please tell me what prompted you to make an appointment.
MRS. B.: Our pediatrician suggested we come see you. We have talked to her about Otis, and she thinks he is showing signs of what she called autistic behavior.
THERAPIST: Tell me about the behaviors you discussed with your pediatrician.

MRS. B.: Well, there are a few things he does that scare us. He just doesn't seem interested in anyone. He doesn't like to be touched or held. He doesn't even play with us or other kids. He sits and rocks or will spend long periods of time spinning a toy top he has.

THERAPIST: Has he always been unaffectionate?

MRS. B.: Pretty much. Even as a small baby he never seemed to like to be held. At first, I thought that maybe it had to do with feeding. But it became more clear that it occurred anytime we tried to have any contact with him.

THERAPIST: What occurs?

MR. B.: He just struggles to get free. He may scream and twist and turn in your arms until you let him go.

THERAPIST: When you set him down and leave him alone, is this when he starts rocking?

MR. B.: Not necessarily. He does that frequently when we aren't interacting with him.

THERAPIST: Please describe that.

MRS. B.: He sits cross-legged and moves his body forward and back like this. He rocks and just stares off into space.

The therapist has identified a number of Otis's problem responses. Noticing that these behaviors are associated with a group of responses that comprise the criteria of infantile autism, the therapist directs his subsequent questions toward determining whether Otis is also performing those other behaviors.

THERAPIST: You said that Otis doesn't play with people. Tell me about that.

MRS. B.: He just doesn't show any interest in people or kids. If you try to get him to play he just fusses.

THERAPIST: If you attempt to alter what he is doing by trying to get him to play or simply change the situation he is in, does he also fuss?

MR. B.: Yes. He screams and hollers and will sometimes start rocking really hard or biting himself.

THERAPIST: Please describe this.

MRS. B.: He usually will bite the back of his hand or his arm.

THERAPIST: Does he exhibit other self-injurious behavior?

MRS. B.: No, just the biting.

THERAPIST: You've said that when you attempt to alter what he's doing he screams. This is clearly one form of communicative response. Does he communicate with you verbally?

MRS. B.: He doesn't really use any words. He has a couple of sounds that appear to indicate displeasure and happiness. One is a fairly high-pitched scream. He does this when he is excited. When he is mad he sort of screams and whimpers.

The initial part of the interview was concerned with problem identification and attempting to determine how closely Otis's behavior met the response criteria for infantile autism. Subsequent questioning began to search for environmental variables related to the occurrence of the child's unusual behavior.

THERAPIST: When you try to get Otis involved in an activity, or if you want to get him to stop rocking or spinning his top, what happens specifically?

MRS. B.: As I said, he pitches a fit. He screams and cries. He will try and wrestle free. Sometimes he starts to bite himself.

THERAPIST: Then what happens?

MR. B.: We used to yell at him to stop or spank him, but that doesn't seem to work very well. So I guess we mostly hold his hands away from his mouth and then leave him alone after he calms down.

THERAPIST: If everytime you try to interact with him one of these tantrums occurs, it must make it very little fun for you to try to have contact with Otis.

MRS. B.: Yes, that's true, its very hard. I guess that's partly why I'm here. I feel myself starting to have minimal involvement with my son beyond meeting general daily care requirements.

The therapist's questions discovered some possible environmental factors associated with the occurrence of Otis's problematic behavior. Once target behaviors had been described, the therapist attempted to identify the youth's response strengths and potential reinforcers.

THERAPIST: So far we have talked about Otis's difficulties. What do you see as his strengths?

MRS. B.: For a child he seems to have really good coordination. Watching him play with his top, it surprises me how dexterous he is.

THERAPIST: What things seem to be a treat for him?

MRS. B.: Its hard to say since he really seems to like being left alone.

THERAPIST: Are there any foods that he enjoys?

MR. B.: The kid is crazy for raisins and potato chips.

After obtaining information about the characteristics of target behaviors, situational variables, and potential reinforcers, the therapist was ready to meet with Otis. However, because of the child's age and the nature of Otis's problem the therapist instead chose to observe Otis and his parents interacting. They met in the therapist's office and were instructed to attempt to engage Otis in play behavior. Mr. and Mrs. B. were also asked to alter Otis's activity three times during the brief observation in order to increase the likelihood of prompting target behaviors.

The interview was concluded with the therapist presenting Otis's parents with a brief summary of his impressions.

THERAPIST: You did a really good job giving me a clear picture of what's going on with Otis. He appears to be exhibiting some problem behaviors including self-stimulation and self-injurious behavior. And, as you noted, he is also behind where he should be in the development of social and verbal skills.

You mentioned that your pediatrician stated that Otis has displayed signs of autism. A number of the problems we discussed today fall into a behavior pattern that is sometimes called *infantile autism*. What causes the behavior pattern is not known. For our purposes, however, we are going to be more concerned with the specific difficulties he exhibits. This is because your behavior can affect these responses. For example, right now it appears that Otis's tantrums and biting results in his getting you to leave him alone. We will begin working on how to control those difficulties without having to limit your contact with him. Clearly, he needs to interact if he is to develop social and verbal skills. This week I want you to note two occurrences in which Otis displays self-injurious behavior. Monitor what was going on, what happened, what you did, etc. You might even jot it down so it will be easier to remember. That will provide us with a good starting point next week when we begin talking about treatment.

MRS. B.: That will be no problem.

THERAPIST: I also want to discuss briefly another aspect of possible treatment. Otis is rapidly approaching preschool age. There are a number of social developmental benefits associated with preschool. Obviously, there are some special considerations regarding sending Otis to preschool. However, there are many good programs designed for children who exhibit behavioral difficulties similar to Otis. A moment ago, I said we weren't going to be very concerned with the term *autism*. However, that label may be important in choosing a preschool special education facility. That is, many programs will identify themselves as being designed specifically for children displaying autistic behavior. It may be necessary to label Otis as autistic for the purposes of enrolling him in a special education program. However, I prefer you to think in terms of problem behaviors and consider *autism* solely as a summary term that will be helpful in qualifying Otis for certain treatments.

The results of the assessment revealed that Otis was exhibiting a behavior pattern that met a large number of the criteria for infantile autism. After defining target behaviors, information was collected regarding environmental variables that might prove useful in treatment planning. Treatment consisted of training Otis's parents in behavior management skills. Otis also was enrolled in an appropriate special education center. Otis's parents met with the therapist on 15 occasions, and subsequent training was conducted by the school staff in order to combine classroom and home treatment efforts.

Practical Problems

The methods described provide a systematic approach to diagnostic interviewing that is relatively successful. It emphasizes the importance of developing interview skills as well as knowledge of the behavior patterns that characterize the various childhood disorders. Effective diagnostic interviewing also requires the ability to recognize and handle some of the common problems that occur during the diagnostic process.

Parent reports often serve as the primary source of data during a diagnostic interview. A number of investigators have suggested that parents may not be accurate data sources. Yarrow, Campbell, and Burton (1970) found that parental retrospective reports of their children's behavior did not reflect actual behavioral development. Parents tend to present a more socially desirable picture of their children. This distorted information may make it difficult to clarify present complaints. This would be particularly bothersome in a situation where developmental data were necessary for a differential diagnosis.

In contrast to these findings, however, Herjanic and Campbell (1977) found that parents can be reliable reporters. They interviewed children and then parents, using the same set of interview questions. A comparison of parents and child responses showed an overall agreement level of 80%. Higher agreement (84%) was obtained when only factual questions were considered. These findings suggest that to maximize the accuracy of parent reports an attempt should be made to ask specific questions that require very little subjective evaluation. Moreover, seeking independent corroboration from additional significant others may also help to minimize invalid data.

The diagnostic process can also be hampered by the behavior of the child and his or her parents during the interview. The interview is a novel situation, and it is possible that the behavior displayed may not be representative of the family's behavior in general. Parents may attempt to present a good picture of the family. Schopler (1974) has suggested that parents may feel guilty and responsible for their child's inappropriate responding and attempt to minimize the seriousness of the problem. Moreover, with younger children, being interviewed by an unfamiliar adult in a "doctor's" office may prompt a rare display of appropriate behavior. To minimize these potential problems, the clinician should attempt to develop good rapport with the family before pursuing sensitive issues in depth. Explaining to parents your appreciation for the responsibility they are taking in attempting to help their youngster with his or her problems may also help decrease any guilt feelings that might color the accuracy of their reports.

Another problem often encountered in diagnostic work with children is the failure of a child to clearly meet the criteria of one particular disorder. It is common for youngsters to display a variety of inappropriate behaviors that cut across a number of diagnostic categories. Moreover, developmental considerations may further hinder the assignment of a child to a particular category. In these cases, the best solution is to defer a diagnosis until more information can be obtained. The clinician and patient would best be served by using the diagnostic code that indicates there is not enough data upon which to make a diagnosis (DSM-799.90), and then presenting descriptive information regarding the problem behaviors observed.

Parents frequently want to begin to discuss treatment plans before the interviewer has completed the diagnostic assessment. After describing their current situation, they may react with surprise to further questions regarding history and developmental factors. Explaining the structure of the diagnostic assessment process at the onset of the initial session may help prevent this problem from occurring.

Although generally not a problem with young children, confidentiality can create difficulties for the clinician interviewing preadolescents and adolescents. Youngsters may be reluctant to discuss various areas of behavior (e.g., sex, alcohol, suicide) for fear that this information may be given to their parents. This results in an inaccurate representation of their responding as well as distrust between the child and therapist. There are no specific formulas for dealing with this dilemma, and to a degree the clinician must exercise his or her own personal judgment regarding revealing information to parents. However, one approach is to explain to the child and his or her parents that in most instances you will respect each individual's right to privacy, but information concerning behavior you feel may result in serious harm (e.g., suicide) to the youngster will be passed on to parents. Moreover, the youth should also be forewarned when the clinician plans to share something with his or her parents.

Finally, starting the diagnostic interview can be problematic if the youngster reacts to the therapist with fear and crying. Parents often fail to explain to their children why they are being taken to a therapist's office. Many parents simply tell their children they are going to see a doctor. Some children also react negatively to the suggestion that they are to be left alone in the waiting room while their parents are interviewed. Having toys in the waiting room is frequently all that is required to entertain children while their parents are being interviewed. Spending a few moments engaged in a pleasant activity in the waiting room with the youth and his or her parents before taking the child into your office may also result in the elimination of the child's being afraid of being alone with the therapist.

The potential problems described are frequently encountered by clinicians involved in diagnostic assessments. Undoubtedly, additional difficulties will arise during this process. The clinician must remain flexible in dealing with these unanticipated situations. Remaining calm will allow the therapist to think through alternative strategies such that the ultimate goal of the diagnostic process can be achieved.

Special Considerations

A diagnosis summarizes observations, in a global manner suggests possible treatments, and puts therapists in touch with a wealth of preexisting experimental and clinical data. However, a diagnosis also results in a label being affixed to a youngster, and labels can affect how people react to children.

Neisworth, Kurtz, Jones, and Madle (1974) had observers monitor the behavior of a hyperactive and a nonhyperactive child. One group of subjects was told that one child was hyperactive and the other was not hyperactive. The remaining subjects were given no diagnostic information about the children. It was reported that when observers were told a child was hyperactive, they reported significantly more hyperactive behavior than if they were uninformed or told the child was not hyperactive. Similar findings have also been reported by Foster, Ysseldyke, and Reese (1975).

It has also been reported that diagnostic labels may influence adult tolerance of children's inappropriate behaviors. Stevens-Long (1973) has parents rate videotapes of an overactive, average-active, and underactive child interacting with an adult. The adult in the film repeatedly attempted to join the child in play. The youth responded to the adult's overtures by saying *no* and hitting the adult. Over the course of the film raters were given 10 opportunities to rate how they felt about the child and indicate how they would discipline the youngster. One-half of the raters were told the youth was emotionally disturbed. The others were given no diagnostic information. It was observed that labels tended to reduce the severity of the adult's reactions to the child's behavior. Children labeled emotionally disturbed received less negative affect ratings and less strict discipline ratings than nonlabeled children. Similar findings have been reported by Algozzine, Mereer, and Countermine (1977).

It appears that labels may bias the manner in which adults react to children. The child may receive attention more readily for inappropriate rather than desirable responses. It is also possible that adults may display greater tolerance for aberrant behavior if a youth carries a diagnostic label. The end result of these labeling biases may be that expectations and demands on the youngster may be reduced. This would make it more difficult for a child to learn to perform the appropriate adaptive responses. Moreover, labels may also affect a child's perceptions of himself or herself and his or her personal responsibility for his or her inappropriate behavior (Whalen & Henker, 1976).

Despite the beneficial aspects of diagnosis, there appear to be a number of negative consequences associated with labeling children. Considering these potential problems is important in treatment planning. In circumstances where there is no requirement that a child be assigned to a diagnostic category, it may be most useful not to make a summary diagnosis but rather to describe specific target behaviors. When a diagnosis is required, clinicians should explain to parents its purpose. They should also stress that it will be more useful for treatment to think of the child's difficulties in terms of response-environmental variables rather than global diagnostic categories.

It is clear that being a good diagnostician of childhood disorders involves more than interviewing skills and an understanding of the definitions of childhood psychopathology. Developmental considerations are of paramount importance in determining the significance of problem behaviors. Adult expectations can greatly affect the process of determining whether a youngster's responding is considered deviant. Moreover, diagnostic labels can influence adult reactions to children and their behavior.

The child clinician must be sensitive to a variety of factors that extend beyond identifying a cluster of target behaviors if he or she is to benefit from the diagnostic process. Careful consideration of the variables that distinguish children from adults, although keeping in focus that the goal of the diagnostic interview is to determine the child's problem such that an effective and efficient treatment program can be constructed, should help the clinician obtain maximum return on his or her investments in developing diagnostic interviewing skills.

References

Achenbach, T. M. (1974). *Developmental psychopathology*. New York: Ronald Press.

Achenbach, T. M. (1978). The Child Behavior Profile I. Boys aged 6–11. *Journal of Consulting and Clinical Psychology, 46*, 476–488.

Achenbach, T. M., & Edelbrock, C. S. (1979). The Child Behavior Profile II. Boys aged 12–16 and girls aged 6–11 and 12–16. *Journal of Consulting and Clinical Psychology, 47*, 223–233.

Algozzine, B., Mereer, C. D., & Countermine, T. (1979). The effects of labels and behavior on teacher expectations. *Exceptional Children, 44*, 131–132.

American Psychiatric Association. (1968). *Diagnostic and statistical manual of mental disorders* (2d ed.). Washington, DC: Author.

American Psychiatric Association. (1980). *Diagnostic and statistical manual of mental disorders* (3rd ed.). Washington, DC: Author.

Cantwell, D. P., Russell, A. T., Mattison, R., & Will, I. (1979). A comparison of DSM-II and DSM-III in the diagnoses of childhood psychiatric disorders: I. Agreement with expected diagnosis. *Archives of General Psychiatry, 36*, 1208–1213.

Ciminero, A. R., & Drabman, R. S. (1977). Current developments in the behavioral assessment of children. In B. B. Lahey & A. E. Kazdin (Eds.), *Advances in clinical child psychology* (Vol. 1) (pp. 47–82). New York: Plenum Press.

Endicott, J., & Spitzer, R. L. (1978). A diagnostic interview. *Archives of General Psychiatry,* *35,* 837–844.

Evans, M., & Nelson, R. O. (1977). Assessment of child behavior problems. In A. R. Ciminero, K. S. Calhoun, & H. E. Adams (Eds.), *Handbook of behavioral assessment* (603–682). New York: Wiley.

Foster, G. G., Ysseldyke, J. E., & Reese, J. H. (1975). I wouldn't have seen it if I hadn't believed it. *Exceptional Children, 41,* 469–473.

Gross, A. M. (1983). Behavioral Interviewing. In T. H. Ollendick & M. Hersen (Eds.), *Child Behavioral Assessment* (pp. 61–79). New York: Pergamon Press.

Harris, S. L. (1974). The relationship between family income and number of parent-perceived problems. *International Journal of Social Psychiatry, 20,* 109–112.

Harris, S. L. (1979). DSM-III—Its implications for children. *Child Behavior Therapy, 1,* 37–46.

Haynes, S. N. (1978). *Principles of behavioral assessment.* New York: Gardner Press.

Haynes, S. N., & Wilson, C. C. (1979). *Behavioral assessment.* San Francisco: Jossey-Bass.

Herjanic, B., & Campbell, W. (1977). Differentiating psychiatrically disturbed children on the basis of a structured interview. *Journal of Abnormal Child Psychology, 5,* 127–133.

Herjanic, B., Herjanic, M., Brown, F., & Wheatt, T. (1975). Are children reliable reporters? *Journal of Abnormal Child Psychology, 3,* 41–48.

Hobbs, N. (1975). *Issues in the classification of children.* San Francisco: Jossey-Bass.

Keefe, F. J., Kopel, S. A., & S. B. Gordon. (1978). *A practical guide to behavioral assessment.* New York: Springer.

Maloney, M. P., & Ward, M. P. (1976). *Psychological assessment: A conceptual approach.* New York: Oxford University Press.

Mash, E. J., & Terdal, L. G. (1981). Behavioral assessment of childhood disturbance. In E. J. Mash & L. G. Terdal (Eds.), *Behavioral assessment of childhood disorder* (pp. 3–76). New York: Guilford Press.

Morganstern, K. P., & Tevlin, H. E. (1981). In M. Hersen, & A. S. Bellack (Eds.), *Behavioral assessment: A practical handbook* (pp. 71–100). New York: Pergamon Press.

Nathan, P. E. (1981). Symptomatic diagnosis and behavioral assessment: A synthesis. In D. H. Barlow (Ed.), *Behavioral assessment of adult disorders* (pp. 1–11). New York: Guilford Press.

Neisworth, J. T., Kurtz, P. D., Jones, R. T., & Madle, R. A. (1974). Biasing of hyperkinetic behavior ratings by diagnostic reports. *Journal of Abnormal Child Psychology, 2,* 323–330.

Ollendick, T. H., & Cerny, S. A. (1981). *Clinical behavior therapy with children.* New York: Plenum Press.

Oltmanns, T. F., Broderick, J. E., & O'Leary, K. D. (1977). Marital adjustment and the efficiency of behavior therapy with children. *Journal of Consulting and Clinical Psychology, 45,* 724–729.

Prugh, P. G., Engel, M., & Morse, W. C. (1975). Emotional disturbance in children. In N. Hobbs, (Ed.), *Issues in the classification of children* (Vol. 1, pp. 261–299). San Francisco: Jossey-Bass.

Puig-Antich, J., & Chambers, W. (1978). *Schedule for affective disorders and schizophrenia for school-aged children (6–16 years)—Kiddie-SADS.* New York: New York State Psychiatric Institute.

Quay, H. C. Classification. (1979). In H. C. Quay & J. S. Werry (Eds.), *Psychopathological disorders of childhood* (2d ed., pp. 1–42), New York: Wiley.

Rickard, K. M., Forehand, R., Wells, K. C., Griest, D. L., & McMahon, R. J. (1980). *A comparison of mothers of clinic referred deviant, clinic referred non-deviant, and non-clinic children.* Unpublished manuscript, University of Georgia.

Scheiderer, E. G. (1977). Effects of instructions and modeling in producing self-disclosure in the initial clinical interview. *Journal of Consulting and Clinical Psychology, 45,* 378–384.

Schopler, E. (1974). Change of direction with psychotic children. In D. A. Davids (Ed.), *Child personality and psychopathology: Current topics* (Vol. 1, pp. 205–236). New York: Wiley.

Stevens-Long, J. (1973). The effect of behavioral context on some aspects of adult disciplinary practice and effect. *Child Development, 44,* 476–484.

Taylor, C. B. (1983). DSM-III and behavioral assessment. *Behavioral Assessment, 5,* 5–14.

Wells, K. C. (1981). Assessment of children in outpatient settings. In M. Hersen & A. S. Bellack (Eds.), *Behavioral assessment: A practical handbook* (pp. 484–533). New York: Pergamon Press.

Whalen, C. K., & Henker, B. (1976). Psychostimulants and children: A review and analysis. *Psychological Bulletin, 83,* 113–1130.

Yarrow, M. R., Campbell, J. D., & Burton, R. V. (1970). Recollections of childhood: A study of the retrospective method. *Monographs of the Society for Research for Child Development, 35*(5).

Chapter 14

Assessing Deficits and Supports in the Elderly

Larry W. Dupree and Roger L. Patterson

Introduction

This chapter is based upon the view that the "aging process" and its associated behaviors reflect interaction between the individual and often changing environmental events and consequences. For these reasons, a practical and less biased approach to assessing the behavior of aged individuals is through a behavioral interview that taps person–situation interaction. Also, the interview/assessment approaches presented in this chapter presume that the professional (a) will view the elderly from a perspective larger than that defined by his or her specific training; (b) will see major areas needing evaluation other than physical problems; (c) will see aging as a developmental rather than pathological process (with change not necessarily occurring across all areas); (d) will not view the elderly as rigid, slow to change, or hopeless; and (e) will seek other than custodial or limited intervention.

Older people are subject to the same problems as younger people. However, a large number of problems of the elderly may be said to be related to major losses that tend to occur more frequently in later life. The following section offers general descriptive information of this at-risk population.

LARRY W. DUPREE • Florida Mental Health Institute, University of South Florida, Tampa, Florida 33612.   ROGER L. PATTERSON • Veterans Administration Medical Center, Tuskegee, Alabama 36083.

The Elderly as an At-Risk Population

Because of the rapid accumulation of changes and the consequent accumulation of stress, the aged are a high-risk group in the area of mental health (Ingersoll & Silverman, 1978). An estimated 15 to 25% of the elderly have significant mental health problems (U.S. President's Commission on Mental Health, 1978). However, this estimate may be substantially low in that there has been a growing trend in recent years to transfer patients out of costly state hospitals (where many of them previously resided) into other less expensive boarding situations, which are typically excluded from prevalence studies of mental disorders among the elderly. The Health Care Financing Administration (HCFA, 1981) reports that in 1979, $17.8 billion were spent on nursing home care.

The aged (i.e., 65 and above) population increased by approximately 680% between 1900 and 1977, whereas the total United States population increased by approximately 290% (U.S. Department of Commerce, Bureau of the Census, 1978). Between 1970 and 1977 the aged, as a category, increased approximately 18%, whereas the under age 65 group increased by about 5%. During the 1970–1977 period the total population increased by approximately 6%. The Health Care Financing Administration (HCFA, 1981) notes that the elderly as a category are expected to more than double by the year 2030; the population age 85 and older is expected to triple; and the total population will increase by only 40%. Thus, the elderly are increasing both in terms of number and proportion.

Approximately 5% of all persons age 65 and over (or over 1 million Americans) are in long-term-care facilities (Reisberg & Ferris, 1982). A large number (58%) of these are diagnosed as senile, experiencing a chronic brain syndrome or some related disorder. Thus, one form of "mental disorder" alone is the most frequently diagnosed condition among institutionalized elderly. Yet, even though these disorders are noted among the institutionalized, HCFA (1981) reports that in 1979 the major reason for institutionalization in long-term-care facilities was the lack of self-care. These facilities (such as nursing homes) are becoming our repository of elderly "mentally ill." Institutionalization seems more to be a result of person–environment incongruence (deficits without supports) than the diagnosed disorder.

Of the 95% of the elderly residing in the community, Reisberg and Ferris (1982) report that approximately 10 to 15% are cognitively impaired, and an equal number experience significant affective disorders. Butler (1975) also notes that the incidence of psychopathology increases with age. He reports that functional disorders (especially depressions and paranoid states) increase steadily with each decade. This also occurs with organic brain diseases after age 60. Suicide also increases with age (particularly among elderly white men), with approximately 25% of all recorded suicides being committed by the elderly—a group representing only approximately 10% of the total population. Unfortunately, the vast majority of the elderly having mental health problems do not receive help.

Problems in Identifying and Investigating Elderly Behavioral Problems

The Influence of Ageism

Many mental health specialists share their culture's negative attitudes toward the elderly. Butler and Lewis (1977) refer to "professional ageism," which represents the negative attitudes of mental health professionals toward the elderly. Old people are seen as "different," discriminated against because they are old, and categorized in unfavorable terms (e.g., senile, rigid, demanding, old fashioned, etc.).

Even though professional ageism is often not verbalized, it usually manifests itself behaviorally in the assessment, treatment planning, and hope for change expected of older clients (Butler, 1969, 1980; Caplovitz & Rodin, cited in Rodin & Langer, 1980; Dupree, O'Sullivan, & Patterson, 1982; Palmore, 1973). Views noting that mental illness in old age is inevitable, untreatable, disabling, and irreversible become a self-fulfilling prophecy, often leading to partial assessment and/or incomplete intervention. This, in turn, then confirms the original beliefs regarding the older client.

Conceptualizing Problems of the Elderly

Hoyer (1973) states that "the way in which the aging process is conceptualized will to a large extent indicate the use of a particular intervention approach" (p. 18). It also affects the quality and extent of assessment. Three models used in conceptualizing the problems of the elderly and offering explanations as to why some people cease to perform competently with increasing age are the social, behavioral, and medical models. The social model attributes changes in behavior, or differences in behavior between the elderly and younger adults, to different roles permitted each of these groups by their culture/society. We tend to expect less responsibility and decreased functional ability on the part of our society's older members. Miller (1979) notes that we accept lesser levels of functioning in these specific areas: self-care behavior, task behavior, and relationship behavior.

The medical model considers deviations from normal functioning as due to illnesses or disease: most notably, improper physiological functioning that purportedly occurs as a natural (and expected) consequence of aging.

The behavioral model sees behavior as the product of learning; and learning is a result of environmental events occurring immediately before a behavior (antecedent events) and immediately after a behavior (consequence of the behavior, or reinforcers). As one ages, both the antecedent and consequent events associated with behavior change. Thus, behaviors change (Baltes & Barton, 1977; Patterson & Jackson, 1980a, 1980b). Some appropriate behaviors are gradually lost due to changes in antecedent and reinforcing conditions, and other (perhaps inappropriate) behaviors appear in response to newer environmental antecedents and consequences.

The three models have been viewed as being in conflict, but it is obvious that changes in all three classes of variables occur throughout the life span. All three, therefore, may be considered as causes of changes associated with aging (Patterson, in press). It is necessary to have knowledge of the deficits and excesses within all three classes of variables in order to fully understand the behavior of any older person. Each class of variables contributes to the individual's level of environmental competence. To concentrate solely upon any single class of variables results in assessing the individual poorly and not recognizing all contributors to lowered levels of competency. Thus, restoration of adaptive behavior is not likely to be complete.

Consequences Associated with the Assessment Approach Used

Marcer (1979) has argued that orthodox methods of assessment of the elderly (e.g., as reviewed by Miller, 1980) are largely irrelevant and that techniques need to be developed that measure changes in everyday, relevant behavior. Kendrick (1982) believes that not only are most of the established, traditional methods irrelevant to the elderly's everyday behavior but that also they are irrelevant to the subjects. This position is also supported by Schaie (1974, 1976, 1978) relative to traditional measures of intelligence as applied to the elderly. In summary, then, it appears that psychological/psychiatric assessment, as traditionally carried out, has not been adequate for obtaining a valid profile of older people's functional status (Gallagher, Thompson, & Levy, 1980). The currently more acceptable approach to assessment of the elderly centers around the diagnostic interview that is standardized and structured relative to format and/or content.

Gurland (1973) notes that there is a movement for psychiatry to apply more of the methods of psychology, with the trend being in response to the unreliability of psychiatric diagnosis and the traditional clinical interview. Chacko (1982) used the *Diagnostic and Statistical Manual of Mental Disorders,* third edition of the American Psychiatric Association (DSM-III) (APA, 1980) on admissions to a geriatric psychiatry clinic and determined that (a) a higher number of paranoid disorders were classified as atypical disorders; (b) many elderly patients experiencing major depressive disorders did not meet the criteria for melancholia yet responded to somatic therapies; and (c) schizophrenic disorders were reclassified because of criterion restrictions. Portnoi (1982) complains that, even in the face of growing data regarding psychiatric problems among the elderly, no section of the DSM-III describes a uniform and explicit classification on mental disorders in the elderly (resorting to criteria established for problem areas over younger populations). Moreover, this may produce confusion in communication even among professionals. Examples of significant classification problems were detailed.

Other problems with traditional diagnostic labeling relative to the elderly have been reported (Gurland, 1973). They include the following: (a) a unidisciplinary, unidimensional labeling process does not attend to the complexity (multiple deficits and supports) of behavior somewhat unique to this age; (b) in many instances the primary value of a formal diagnosis is administrative; (c) clinicians are often reluctant to apply certain diagnoses to the elderly; (d) a diagnosis lightly regarded is probably poorly implemented; (e) the labeling process and its negative connotations often discourage interventions; (f) misdiagnosis is more likely in acute conditions; (g) there are difficulties in using labeling criteria in differentiating certain pathologies; (h) personal values and ageism do intrude; and (i) there is poor interrater reliability, particularly across discipline and across treatment sites.

Hesse, Campion, and Karamouz (1982) found that psychiatric conditions and attitudinal problems frequently interfered with the rehabilitation of aged clients in that too many conditions were ascribed erroneously to dementias, progression of disease, or "poor motivation." It would appear that strict, symptom-oriented diagnostic procedures relative to the elderly are not reliable and useful to the clinician or the client, that they permit cultural attitudes to intrude, and that they inadequately represent important classes of behavior vital to the older person's well-being and adaptation to his or her environment. Also, besides being subject to interviewer bias, the traditional diagnostic interview adheres essentially to one model: the medical model. Multiple deficits experienced by the elderly provide a strong argument for a multifunctional, and often multidisciplinary, diagnostic appraisal. Social, psychological, and physical domains all need attention (Birren & Renner, 1981; Gaitz, 1969; Gaitz & Baer, 1970; Gurland, 1973; Gurland et al., 1976, 1977—1978; Lawton, Whelihan, & Belsky, 1980; Pfeiffer, 1975; Sundberg, Snowden, & Reynolds, 1978).

The Importance of Recognizing Person–Situation Interaction

With the aged, expressed problems are more likely to be a result of losses and/or behavioral deficits (i.e., deficits not compensated for by the environment or individual). Environmental factors gain in importance in controlling behaviors as the individual's competence (everyday adaptive skills) decreases (Lankford & Herman, 1978). And because environments differ in the degree to which they support altered perceptual and cognitive behavior, the daily behavior of the perceptually and cognitively impaired elderly varies highly. Thus, ideally, adaptive behavior of an older person should be assessed relative to actual daily living tasks (Goodstein, 1980; Lawton et al., 1980). The delineation of specific behavioral/environmental deficits should demonstrate the type and degree of support needed for maintaining residence in the "community" in which the person is assessed. Further, it may be necessary to identify residence changes to find situational requirements congruent with the person's capabilities (Lawton, 1970).

The essential diagnostic product is an indication of the older person's capacity to do things required in his or her own environment. And because major life areas interact, deficits or supports in one area must be examined and interpreted in the context of the whole (Lawton, Moss, Fulcomer, & Kleban, 1982). For example, in a very supportive environment, memory deficit may not be related to an incapacity to cope with the demands of one's own milieu. Some environments require more self-management than others. Also, assessment is better conceptualized as being more oriented toward issues of problem solving: how might one acquire skills necessary to resolve a deficit or compensate for it via acquiring environmental supports. An ecological model of adaptation and aging (Gallagher et al., 1980) is more productive in the sense that context-relevant and necessary care can be determined. Sundberg et al. (1978), in a review of literature dealing with the assessment of personal competence and incompetence in life situations, determined that if assessment of ecological competence is to be useful, it must (a) promote attitudes toward clients that recognize their potentialities based on their current coping skills and ability to learn; (b) develop "age-free" assessment approaches recognizing competence in the elderly; and (c) assess the person along with assessment of present and potential environments.

Lawton (1972, 1978) has developed a useful model that conceptualizes behavior as falling within a number of domains. This model organizes assessment under the construct of *competence* such that most behaviors necessary to living successfully in the real world can be placed within it. It appears to be a blending of an ecological approach within behavior analysis. A pathology-oriented approach to the assessment of aging is more consistent with traditional psychiatric and psychological approaches. Yet, even within this latter model, the trend relative to the elderly is toward structured diagnostic interviews. Here there is emphasis on the need for a comprehensive (and multidimensional) approach that alerts the diagnostician to significant life domains, particularly the influence of situational variables (Fleiss, Gurland, & Des Roche, 1976; Gaitz, 1969; Gaitz & Baer, 1970; Gurland et al., 1970, 1976; Whelihan, 1979). Thus, even though the two models approach assessment from somewhat opposite perspectives, both emphasize similar needs relative to proper and thorough assessment of the significant and interdependent domains of the elderly.

In summary, there are at least four reasons for appraising individual person–situation interactions (with the attendant behavioral/environmental deficits and supports): (a) to match the functioning of the person with requirements of a particular environment; (b) to determine the need for particular types of services (support); (c) to prescribe interventions to be used to improve the level of functioning; and (d) to measure change in functioning over time (Patterson & Eberly, 1983).

The Value of Age-Free, Behavioral Interviewing

Within the behavior analysis perspective, human behavior is considered to be alterable (or reversible) until it is empirically demonstrated not to be. Such an approach is necessary with the elderly. It attends to concrete events (deficits/excesses, strengths/weaknesses, antecedents/consequences) as explanations for behavior rather than invoking constructs or labels. It does not place an overreliance on physical entities as the basis for behavior. The smallest units of analysis in relevant diagnostic interviewing of the elderly are the mutual and interdependent relations between the individual and his or her environment (Rebok & Hoyer, 1977). Mahoney (1975) asserts that it is more productive to examine the nature of the interdependence than to maintain that one's internal environment has greater priority in terms of behavior than the external environment. Even though physical changes may account for some part of any loss of environmental competence, using a strictly physical model of aging, and the diagnostic process based upon such an approach, is not appropriate. Indeed, it is biased against intervention with the elderly by assuming an irreversibility to behavior (purportedly based on aging-related, irreversible physical changes).

Ageism is pervasive and intrudes upon diagnostic procedures unless recognized or controlled. This can be countered by using structured diagnostic interviews that guide the clinician over specified life domains (Lawton, 1972), assisting the clinician to identify, understand, and "resolve" problem behavior on an age-free, problem-oriented basis. The fodder of intervention becomes empirically derived knowledge, rather than a collection of concepts and biases as to what should be causing nonadaptive behavior among the elderly. A comprehensive behavioral interview can generate information (deficits and supports) that more directly explains behavior, needing less specialized interpretations. Diagnostic data needing sophisticated interpretive comments often rely on "experts" and are much more open to professional biases as well as the intrusion of personal biases (ageism). Also, the diagnostic conclusion is based on secondary data, or norms, once again discounting the individuality of the aged. These also discount the uniqueness (effect) of the older person's behavior in his or her particular context.

Multimodal diagnostic interviews also diminish the need for diagnostic labels. Application of negative diagnostic labels has contributed to, or feeds into, the ageism problem. Labels often discourage intervention (e.g., chronic organic brain syndrome), have less utility in the total treatment of the elderly, and are rarely removed (just accumulated). Moreover, the narrow labeling process often prevents the clinician from seeing other major aspects of the older person.

In summary, any assessment approach relative to the elderly must ameliorate cultural and professional ageism, assess diverse, major areas of the older person's life, and highlight both internal and external antecedents for the expressed problem behaviors. Assessment must have an intended purpose—explanation and intervention. For the elderly, appropriate assessment is on a broader scale than for many younger populations, and positive change is definitely based upon a broad-based assessment of strengths and deficits. It is for these reasons that structured diagnostic interviewing is more reliable, valid, and *useful* with the elderly (Birren & Renner, 1981; Copeland *et al.*, 1976; Gaitz, 1969; Gaitz & Baer, 1970; Gallagher *et al.*, 1980; Gurland, 1973; Gurland *et al.*, 1976, 1977–1978; Lawton, 1970, 1972, 1978; Lawton *et al.*, 1980, 1982; Miller, 1979; Patterson & Eberly, 1983; Taylor & Bloom, 1974).

The Behavioral Incident Technique

The interviewer of the elderly person is often trying to assess the extent of the involvement of the client with a variety of people, medical, government, and charitable agencies, social organizations, and commercial establishments. Such involvements are often referred to as *social supports*. The authors find that the term *social supports* is a bit ambiguous. What is it that is being supported? What we are most often interested in measuring with regard to elderly clients is environmental interactions that "support" (i.e., prompt, reinforce, or otherwise help to maintain) maximally independent, organized, and generally adaptive behaviors. The reader should notice here that, consistent with our previous discussion, the focus is on person–environment *interactions*. This is quite different from more common approaches that treat the elderly person as a mere passive recipient of supports.

Focusing on the person–environment interaction means that both the activity of the elderly client and the source of support are crucial. For example, consider the candidate for home-delivered meals. How does this person normally feed himself or herself? Are the deficits causing the eating problem behavioral, financial, medical, or a combination of problems? What can the person currently do to obtain meals? What could he or she do better if given some assistance? What services are really needed?

Obtaining meals is actually a rather simple example compared with the problem of determining the nature and existence of supportive social relationships. Such social relationships are often considered to be of great importance to most people in maintaining a satisfactory personal life. Yet, the *nature* of these relationships is often barely touched on by those working with the elderly. It is sometimes determined whether or not the person in question does or does not have some type of contacts, and how often such contacts occur. However, this is minimal involvement, indeed. In the case where there is a relative or friend living nearby who visits and/or telephones regularly or who lives in the same house, this is almost always considered a "support." By the definition we are using, such frequent contact with accessible relatives or friends is not necessarily supportive. Frequency of contact tells little or nothing about the *quality* or effects of such contact.

Given the preceding considerations, how are social supports to be measured in the interview situation? Pascal and Jenkins (1961) contemplated similar issues with regard to other populations and developed the Behavioral Incident (BI) technique. This technique was closely modeled after techniques used by Kinsey, Pomeroy, and Martin (1948) and others. Kinsey and his co-workers were startlingly successful in getting ordinary American citizens to reveal many details regarding their sex lives, a difficult task indeed. The basis of the BI technique is to use behavioral shaping techniques to get the subject to describe *actual events* as opposed to opinions and generalities about events. This brief sentence says much that requires explication.

The focus of the interview is on an accurate description of events that reveal the presence or absence of a supportive interaction. Thus, a relevant question might be how a subject obtains weekly medical treatment. The interviewer in this situation would have the task of having the subject explain what he or she did to get the appointment, get transportation, what he or she discussed with the nurse, doctor, and pharmacist, and so on. The interviewer would then be in a position to judge whether or not there were problems or potential problems with a necessary support.

Perhaps a more difficult situation might involve the interaction of a depressed female client (who has many physical complaints) and her daughter who visits regularly. The relevant question would be, What is the daughter doing to maintain adaptive, nondepressed, noncomplaining behavior and what is she doing to maintain the opposite behavior? In this case, the BI would encompass the visit. The interviewer would seek to find out what the two did and what they talked about. Obviously, in this case, reports from both mother and daughter would be useful. From such information (and similar information from other visits), a properly trained interviewer would learn much about which aspects of these interactions were supportive and which were nonsupportive of desirable behavior.

Getting clients to describe actual events in this way sounds much simpler than it is. Most people are not trained to conduct interviews in this way. Indeed, many people are trained to ask for feeling statements and opinion statements rather than behavioral descriptions. Some training and practice in technique is needed.

Skillful use of verbal prompts and reinforcers is required to shape appropriate responses in the interview over predetermined content areas (Pascal & Jenkins, 1961; Witherspoon, deValera, Jenkins, & Sanford, 1973). For example, an interviewer may know that an elderly woman has a daughter living in the vicinity. When discussing relationships, the woman may persist in pointing out how wonderful her daughter is and how many interesting things she did as a child. The interviewer should recognize these statements (responding as minimally as necessary to maintain the contact) and as tactfully as possible ask specific questions, such as "When did your daughter last visit?" "How did she greet you?" "What did you talk about?" Responses to such questions regarding specific behaviors should be responded to with obvious interest by the interviewer in order to socially reinforce the interviewee's responding. In most cases, conscientious prompting and reinforcement will produce a sufficiently detailed portrayal of the interactions between the mother and daughter to enable the interviewer to determine what behaviors were being supported (prompted and reinforced) by the interaction. In many instances, interactions that might be considered "supportive" on the basis of relatively superficial information (such as frequency of contact) or on the basis of opinion statements may turn out to be destructive when BI information is obtained. The opposite is also true.

Although the BI is a very versatile technique and may be used to obtain many types of information, there are several areas of social support that should be of concern when trying to determine the assets and needs of elderly people. Some commonly useful items are discussed next.

Content Areas of the Behavioral Incident

Meals and Food Preparation. It should be determined how, and with what difficulties, the elderly person obtains meals on a regular basis. If the person prepares his or her own meals, then a detailed description of how he or she shops and prepares the food will be needed.

Economic Resources. The person should know where the money comes from, the amount, how the money is protected, and approximately how much the necessities (shelter, utilities, food, etc.) cost. In addition to the necessities, there is an economic deficit if there is no money for some small personal luxuries.

Social Relationships. Several types of social relationships are desirable: from the intimate to the superficial. By *intimate* we mean that clients know people with whom they can share their feelings and the important things in life: past, present, and future. Such relationships are supportive if there is an exchange that is mutually enjoyable and serves to reinforce adaptive behaviors. A relationship in which the client only complains or expresses the negative part of his or her life probably serves to promote poor life satisfaction and even depression. Also, the partner in such a relationship will probably find the interactions aversive, and this may serve to destroy the relationship.

At another level, it is important for clients to have people with whom they can share leisure activities or just enjoyable light conversation. Also required by the elderly are those individuals who can be called upon for occasional assistance when needed.

It is true that one or two people may provide all the previously mentioned interactions, but this is not a very desirable situation. Rather, it is desirable that the different kinds of interactions be maintained with several people.

Health Care. Elderly clients should have solutions to several situations involved in obtaining adequate health care. Obviously, they should have easy access to primary care physicians. Beyond this, they should know how to avail themselves of other public or private agencies providing care. They should know a pharmacist and be knowledgeable as to how to obtain and take needed medications.

Leisure Activities. It is useful for elderly people to enjoy leisure activities of more than one type several times a week. They should be aware of leisure activities that can be carried out *alone* as well as those with another person or a group. Witherspoon *et al.* (1973) designated hobbies in which one took pride as an important source of support.

The Residence. According to Witherspoon *et al.* (1973), it is important that a person exhibit interest, satisfaction, and even pride in his or her residence. This is evidenced behaviorally by efforts to maintain and decorate it, however simple these efforts may be (growing plants, displaying personal treasures, crocheting doilies, etc.).

Transportation. Support in this area requires that the client have ways of going to shopping sites, medical treatments, leisure activities, and to occasional unplanned places and events. Transportation is also needed for various ways of maintaining social contacts. More than one source of transportation is highly desirable.

An interview will now be presented that seeks to accomplish many of the desirable features of assessment as described before.

Case Illustration with Dialogue and Comments

The Interview

The person interviewed (Mrs. J.) is a 66-year-old divorced woman who was a regular client of the day treatment component of the behavioral treatment program described extensively by Patterson, Dupree, Eberly, Jackson, O'Sullivan, Penner, and Dee-Kelley (1982). This program assesses elderly people, particularly in regard to social skills and daily living skills. The results of these assessments are then used to indicate what types of skills training are needed in order to enhance the life of elderly clients.

This is an *initial* interview in that the interviewer (I) and the patient (P) had never met. Further, the interviewer was not involved clinically in the case. The reader should note that although the interviewer is seeking specific information in the specific categories described previously, the interview was treated as a relatively free-flowing process. To reiterate, the person talking is exhibiting operant behavior. The interviewer has the task of shaping this behavior by proper use of prompts and reinforcers; but the information must and should be free flowing according to the way the client presents it. It would be a great mistake to try to adhere rigidly to a particular order or style of obtaining the information, such as would be done with most standardized psychological tests and questionnaires. Such adherence to order or style would greatly limit the amount of information obtained. The present interviewer prefers to begin by talking about leisure-time activities, because this area is easy to discuss casually. Also, much information about social activities, family, and friends may be given very readily in connection with leisure activities. This occurred in the present interview.

I: What kind of things do you do for fun?

P: Lately, not much [opinion statement].

I: What are some things you have done recently?

P: Visited the historical district, played cards with the ladies in the laundry room, went window shopping in the mall. I enjoyed going to the airport and people watching. I like to do things when I have the transportation, but I can't do too much because of respiratory problems. I get out of breath very easily. [Comment: The facts seem to contradict the opinion statement that she hasn't done much recently. This became more apparent as the interview continued].

I: Tell me about the last time you did something just for fun.

P: Well, that was last Friday. My friend and I went to the historical district—spent several hours there in the shops, and we had dinner there.

I: That's a nice outing.

P: It is, there's something there for everyone. There were antiques, there are crafts, and so forth. There are imports—It's a very enjoyable place for a person my age. There are places to get coffee and just sit.

I: Mostly what you did was to visit the shops, have coffee, and go to dinner?

P: Yes, the food was very good and reasonable. That's the last thing I did, other than visit with my daughter and grandchildren.

I: You've done that recently?

P: Yes, last Sunday—and then I went to their house for dinner the next day.

I: When was the last time you saw your daughter before then?

P: They dropped in for an hour a couple days before.

I: How long before then?

P: A week or so. They have two small children, and its hard for them to come by very often, but I call her. She doesn't call me very often, but I call her. And I had calls from my daughters in Michigan and Pennsylvania.

I: What did you talk about?

P: They were all snowed in and had brutal weather, but the one in Pennsylvania I was concerned about. She had marital problems. I was kind of worried, depressed about her. She told me that they had worked things out and had renewed their marriage vows. Things are going well, and that made me feel much better. Before, she had been calling me complaining about my son-in-law [She went on to explain the situation of the daughter and the son-in-law. Apparently, the client knew a great deal about what was going on in their lives, although they live more than 1000 miles away.] I had told my daughter that telling friends and family didn't help the problem. She had to discuss it directly with her husband. She did, and they were able to work things out. I feel good about them, and I feel better about myself. I've made several adjustments in the last month here.

I: What have you done?

P: I moved from a trailer in the boondocks back to the apartments where I used to live. I have nice neighbors.

I: Do you see your neighbors regularly?

P: When I go to the laundry or pick up my mail. Sometimes I see them going in or out, and we speak.

I: Tell me about the last visit you had with a neighbor.

P: It's not one of those visiting kind of things where I would go over and have coffee. Sunday, we played cards while doing our laundry in the apartment laundromat.

I; What did you talk about?

P: About how they're repairing the street, and how bad it was that the freeze killed the oranges, things like that.

I: Do you have anyone you see several times a week?

P: No. I have made a reacquaintance with my friend who took me to the historical district. I've seen her twice last week and once this week, and I'll see her again on Friday. She has suggested us going to different places. [Comment: The opinion statement *no* seems to be contradicted by the events described.]

I; She has a car and you don't?

P: That's right. Transportation is a problem for me.

I: Tell me about your friend. What did you talk about the last time you went out together?

P: She has a very authoritative manner and is very domineering—usually puts me down. I went through a bankruptcy thing and wasn't allowed to work. I used to live in her garage apartment. I felt that she made me feel worse, so I didn't see her for several months. Now we've become friends again.

I: Tell me what you said to each other when you were out together recently.

P: I talked about how the Rev. Jesse Jackson had just got the flier released and how good that was. She said that it was all political and racial and that I really don't understand these things. Well, I used to have a very responsible job, and I think I have some understanding of the world. I don't feel like a moron. I feel that I can discuss the news and current events intelligently. Before, when we were friends, I got so many negative comments from her that I began to doubt myself, whether I was really just plain dumb and didn't understand things. I started staying mostly in my room when I lived at her place. I told myself that I had to get out of there because I was damaging myself and getting more and more depressed.

I: That was the only friend you had?

P: Yes, the only close friend. I had had others at work, but when you lose your job you lose contact with them, unless you have a car and can keep up with them. If I were driving I could meet them the way I used to. I gave up driving after I had a stroke—and then I had a heart attack. That led to losing most of my friends.

I: The friend that you had a good time with recently—I guess your conversation was different than it used to be?

P: I explained to her that I had to leave and move for my own benefit. I think maybe it had an impact on her. Maybe she didn't realize what she was doing. We were in one shop the other night where they had things from France— the dresses were very expensive. I was looking through the rack, and she said, "There's no sense in you looking, because you can't afford them." I said, "No, but I can appreciate the workmanship and how beautiful they are." That seemed to stop that.

I: Hm-mmm.

P: It used to be always a put-down.

I: But I suppose you had some pleasant conversation, say, over dinner.

P: In the French shop was the only time during the day that she did that, and I stopped it right away.

I: Tell me some pleasant conversation you had with her, like, what did you talk about at dinner?

P: We talked about our grandchildren. We talked about Christmas; and of course we are both cat lovers and bird lovers; and we talked about the birds outside of the courtyard. We made plans to get out more often, and I think that was good, because once I asserted myself and let her know that the put-down business was getting to me, and that I didn't feel that I was that kind of person, I think that we got along better. I would never move back in with her. I think that it's her way to do the put-downs. I have to accept her that way.

I: Let me ask you about your daughter that lives close by. You saw her recently. Tell me what you did and what you talked about. Do you remember a conversation you had with her then?

P: Well, we talked about their plans. They were going to a friend's house for a party, and they were going to stay over. They took the children. I told them that was good. We made plans for them to come over the next day so that we could go out for supper. We have a fairly good rapport.

I: You share personal things?

P: Yes. We've shared many personal things. Things that have left deep personal scars on me, but you have to go on.

I: She has told you things that are important in her life?

P: Yes. I try to be fair and listen, but I don't try to interfere between husband and wife. I don't know if this is pertaining to what your interested in . . .

I: Yes.

P: [At this point she proceeded to tell how she had assisted her daughter financially and otherwise during a period of deep marital conflict. She confided that she has guilt feelings over this matter, because of the way she was involved. However, she revealed that now she is close to the daughter and her family as indicated by the recent visits as previously described.]

I: Now, let's talk about something else. You mentioned that you have transportation difficulties. How did you last get to the food store?

P: I called my daughter, and she took me.

I: Is that the only way you can get groceries?

P: Yes. I call her, and she takes me. I don't have any other way. I called Share-a-Van, but they only take people to medical appointments.

I: Any place you can walk to get small items?

P: No. Besides, right now I don't think I'll have even food stamps for this month because of moving. I have to reapply. By the time I pay my rent $240 a month, $50 a month rental on an oxygen concentrator—then I have my electric, I don't know how much that will be. My son-in-law supplies me with a telephone. It's on his bill. My daughter in Pennsylvania will try to send me $15.00 a month for my oxygen which will leave me 10 to $15 each month to spend. It's not much, but it helps. My children have troubles of their own and their own families; I can't expect much help from them. I'm not allowed to work. I'm too ill.

I: Do you have a regular doctor?

P: Yes, Dr. T.

I: Do you have any difficulties seeing him?

P: Well, my daughter used to take me. But she has to take the children to school. I used to make my appointments according to her schedule. She can't do that any more. Now I don't know what I'll do. I guess I'll call Share-a-Van.

I: Your doctor's office is only a block from here. Can you walk that far?

P: No, I can't walk that far. I can't even walk from here [the day treatment program] to the cafeteria. They serve my meals on the unit. I know I'm a pest.

I: We expect that some people will eat on the unit. It's normal procedure. Do you have anything you do just for fun when you're by yourself?

P: I'm an avid reader.

I: You read a great deal?

P: I read a tremendous amount of books, and I knit. I read more than anything, more than I watch TV.

I: Regularly . . . you read every day?

P: Every day I read.

I: Are you reading a book right now?

P: Yes. . . . It's a mystery by Mary Stuart. I just finished [goes on to describe several books she's read recently, and mentions authors she prefers and authors she dislikes].

I: That's a good hobby. Do you have any problem getting books?

P: Oh, no. A friend of my daughter goes to one of these half-price exchange places. She knows what I like and just brought me a grocery bag full [goes on to talk enthusiastically about books and authors she likes; then engages in a criticism of television, especially the violence].

I: I need to ask about how you take your medicine. I know you take several kinds. Do you have them with you?

P: Oh yes. [Reaches in her purse and pulls out several small plastic bags attached to each other.] I put my pills in these little bags and label them according to when I'm supposed to take them. See here? [Shows interviewer a labeled bag] I'll take this before lunch.

I: How did you get the medicines from the pharmacy the last time?

P: I called ahead, and the pharmacist had them ready when my daughter took me to the doctor. The pharmacy is in the same building. Of course, I'm not sure how I'll get to the doctor now. Maybe Share-a-Van . . .

I: How do you pay for your medicine?

P: It's paid by the county. There's no problem. I do have a problem with food, though.

I: How's that.

P: I have only $60 per month for food; but I'm a diabetic and have high blood pressure—so I'm supposed to eat mostly fresh vegetables and meats. They're expensive.

I: What did you eat this morning?

P: I had some cereal. Of course, when I come here, I have a good lunch which is prepared according to my diet. That's my main meal of the day.

I: What do you plan to eat this evening?

P: I have some canned soup and rice. I have a bag of fruit which my neighbor brought me. I love fruit, and could eat it all the time.

I: How will you prepare your meal?

P: I have some small pans, but not enough utensils. I don't have any problems opening and heating canned food, or macaroni, or rice, or things like that.

The interview was terminated at this point because the interviewer thought he had obtained sufficient information to complete the assessment.

Summary of the Interview

The interview information will now be summarized and briefly discussed according to each major topic.

Meals and Food Preparation. Mrs. J. has several problems in this area. She does not have the money to buy the kinds of foods she needs, nor does she have money to buy utensils. This problem is currently exacerbated because of the temporary interruption in food stamps. Transportation might be somewhat of a problem because she is dependent upon her daughter for shopping. She is unable to buy casual incidentals on her own. Food preparation does not seem to be a problem.

Economic Resources. Mrs. J. has her money carefully budgeted, including a small amount for personal luxuries. There is some contradiction here with problems in buying food. It would be highly desirable for her to have money for taxis, but she does not.

Transportation. The daughter seems to be the sole source of regularly available transportation, and even this is limited. There is a deficit here.

Social Relationships. Mrs. J. apparently has maintained solid relationships with her daughters. She seems to have maintained her role as someone the daughters trust and can turn to in time of need. It is probable that these relationships are important to Mrs. J. in that they may maintain her opinion of herself as an important and useful person. However, these relationships also involve her in the daughters' difficulties. It might be that additional details about interaction with the daughters over an extended period might reveal aspects of the relationships that are not so supportive and might relate to the depression. More than an initial interview would be required for such a determination.

There seems to be a deficiency with regard to friends. Mrs. J. has only one close friend, and the relationship with this friend has been at least partially nonsupportive. It seems that this friend has helped to prompt and reinforce Mrs. J.'s negative self-image. Other than this friend and the daughters, only the most casual relationships were mentioned. These relationships, however, are apparently very supportive of normal, casual, social interactions and are of considerable importance to Mrs. J.

Health Care. Mrs. J. has very high-level skills at taking medicine. Also, other than the problem with transportation as previously mentioned, she has no problems with the doctor or the pharmacy. Maintaining a proper diet is not a problem.

Leisure Activities. Mrs. J. has kept amazingly busy considering her handicaps and economic limitations. She seems to be able to enjoy casual activities with others (the card games and conversation at the apartment and the activities she planned with her friend) as well as when she is alone. Reading is obviously an important pastime, and one in which she takes pride. The limitations here are those of transportation and health.

The Residence. Mrs. J. seems to be very pleased with her new apartment and considers it a great improvement over her previous two residences.

In the preceding case illustration, the interviewer's style is not apparent, except as noted by its product. The interviewee freely produced information that is pertinent, specific, and intimate. Thus, the interviewer's style and appropriate use of the chosen interview format appeared to result in cooperation from the client. A useful assessment was obtained that accurately portrays defined domains of the individual's life. These results were not accidental but planned. The interviewer knew both how to use his diagnostic instrument and how to interview an older person. A valid and useful assessment is a product of the chosen assessment approach, the interviewer's knowledge of the elderly, and his or her interview style in response to that knowledge.

Do's and Dont's of Interviewing the Elderly

Excellent articles have been written noting techniques for communicating with (and ultimately assessing) older people (Blazer, 1978; Goodstein, 1980; Gurland et al., 1977–1978; Pfeiffer, 1980). Gurland et al. (1977–1978) focus on limiting stress in the elderly that is elicited by an assessment interview. This leads to a fuller exploration of problems, enhances interviewee cooperation, and more likely leads to a completed interview. Also, limiting stress within the interview setting reduces the likelihood of prompting deficits in behavior suggestive of organic conditions (e.g., apparent memory impairment and disorientation). Potential sources of interview stress for the elderly include (a) fatigue as a result of lengthy and/or confusing questions; and (b) "the embarrassment of disclosing symptoms which suggest psychiatric disorder or cognitive incapacity (as well as the interviewee's fear that this information might initiate or prolong his hospitalization or stay in an institution)" (Gurland et al., 1977–1978, p. 22).

Goodstein (1980) notes that comprehensive evaluation is enhanced via certain interpersonal considerations: (a) address the older client by title and last name; (b) sit alongside the older client so that he or she can see your face and hear what you say; (c) be respectful, hopeful, and honest; (d) offer friendly nonverbal cues, such as looking in the older client's eyes when talking to him or her; (e) differentiate sympathy and empathy (sympathy makes older people feel like children, whereas understanding [empathy] is favored); (f) share something of yourself (sharing mutual interests may facilitate the process); (g) do not hesitate to discuss intimate data if presented; (h) permit physical contact (shake hands, pat on back for support); and (i) know your feelings about aging and how they affect your performance.

Blazer (1978) and Pfeiffer (1980) also have delineated effective techniques for communicating with the elderly during the diagnostic interview (some of which overlap those suggested by Goodstein). Patient/client factors as well as clinician factors that influence each other are presented. Patient factors include anxiety, sensory deprivation, cautiousness, unrealistic views and/or expectations of the clinician, and the tendency to concentrate upon presenting certain ideas or themes (such as somatic concerns, discussion of losses, a review of life, fear of losing control, and death). Pfeiffer (1980) and Blazer (1978) recommend that the clinician (a) approach the older interviewee with respect (greet the patient by title and surname); (b) position himself or herself near the interviewee so as to be able to touch the client if desired; (c) speak clearly and slowly with appropriate volume and use simple sentences; (d) inquire actively and systematically (such as with a behavioral interview) across major life areas (e.g. Lawton, 1972); (e) pace the interview, giving the older interviewee enough time to respond to questions (a slow and relaxed pace also reduces anxiety); and (f) pay attention to nonverbal communications that may give clues to changes in emotional state. Also, touch is indicated as a potentially effective way to relax the older interviewee. Finally, it is suggested that the interviewer focus on the "here and now" in a realistic but hopeful manner.

In summary, inadequate performance on the part of the interviewer can markedly impact on the information produced, which in turn can generate an inaccurate picture of the client's deficits and/or supports (and level of performance). Once an appropriate interview approach is formulated, much of the choice of accurate versus distorted indexes of performance are left to the style of the interviewer (whether or not the interviewer is aware of such). It would appear that a clearer picture of the older interviewee is obtained by using a broad-based, structured interview in the hands of an interviewer that communicates well with the elderly by recognizing and using the previously mentioned interview requisites.

References

American Psychiatric Association. (1980). *Diagnostic and statistical manual of mental disorders* (3rd ed.). Washington, DC: Author.

Baltes, M. M., & Barton, E. M. (1977). New approaches toward aging: A case for the operant model. *Educational Gerontology, 2*, 383–405.

Birren, J. E., & Renner, V. J. (1981). Concepts and criteria of mental health and aging. *American Journal of Orthopsychiatry, 51*, 242–254.

Blazer, D. (1978). Techniques for communicating with your elderly patient. *Geriatrics, 33*, 79–84.

Butler, R. N. (1969). Age-ism: Another form of bigotry. *The Gerontologist, 9*, 243–246.

Butler, R. N. (1975). Psychiatry and the elderly: An overview. *The American Journal of Psychiatry, 132*, 893–900.

Butler, R. N. (1980). Ageism: A foreword. *Journal of Social Issues, 36*, 8–11.

Butler, R. N., & Lewis, M. I. (1973). *Aging and mental health*. St. Louis: C. V. Mosby.

Butler, R. N., & Lewis, M. I. (1977). *Aging and mental health* (2d ed.). St. Louis: C. V. Mosby.

Chacko, R. C. (1982). Diagnostic dilemmas in geriatric psychiatry. *The Gerontologist, 22*(5), 240.

Copeland, M. J., Kelleher, M. J., Kellett, J. M., Gourlay, A. J., Gurland, B. J., Fleiss, J. L.,

& Sharpe, L. (1976). A semi-structured clinical interview for the assessment of diagnosis and mental state in the elderly: The Geriatric Mental State Schedule. I. Development and reliability. *Psychological Medicine, 6,* 439–449.

Dupree, L. W., O'Sullivan, M. J., & Patterson, R. L. (1982). Problems relating to aging: Rationale for a behavioral approach. In R. L. Patterson, L. W. Dupree, D. A. Eberly, G. M. Jackson, M. J. O'Sullivan, L. A. Penner, & C. D. Kelly (Eds.), *Overcoming deificits of aging* (pp. 7–21). New York: Plenum Press.

Fleiss, J., Gurland, B., & Des Roche, P. (1976). Distinctions between organic brain syndrome and functional disorders: Based on the Geriatric Mental State Interview. *International Journal of Aging and Human Development, 7,* 323–330.

Gaitz, C. M. (1969). Functional assessment of the suspected mentally ill aged. *Journal of the American Geriatrics Society, 17,* 541–548.

Gaitz, C. M., & Baer, P. E. (1970). Diagnostic assessment of the elderly: A multifunctional model. *The Gerontologist, 10,* 47–52.

Gallagher, D., Thompson, L. W., & Levy, S. M. (1980). Clinical psychological assessment of older adults. In L. W. Poon (Ed.), *Aging in the 1980's* (pp. 19–40). Washington, DC: American Psychological Association.

Goodstein, R. K. (1980). The diagnosis and treatment of elderly patients: Some practical guidelines. *Hospital and Community Psychiatry, 31,* 19–24.

Gurland, B. J. (1973). A broad clinical assessment of psychopathology in the aged. In C. Eisdorfer & M. P. Lawton (Eds.), *The psychology of adult development and aging* (pp. 343–377). Washington, DC: American Psychological Association.

Gurland, B. J., Fleiss, J. L., Cooper, J. E., Sharpe, L., Kendell, R. E., & Roberts, P. (1970). Cross-national study of diagnosis of mental disorders: Hospital diagnosis and hospital patients in New York and London. *Comprehensive Psychiatry, 11,* 18–25.

Gurland, B. J., Fleiss, J. L., Goldberg, K., Sharpe, L., Copeland, J. R. M., Kelleher ,M. J., & Kellett, J. M. (1976). A semi-structured clinical interview for the assessment of diagnosis and mental state in the elderly: The Geriatric Mental State Schedule. II. A factor analysis. *Psychological Medicine, 6,* 451–459.

Gurland, B., Kuriansky, J., Sharpe, L., Simon, R., Stiller, P., & Birkett, P. (1977–1978). The comprehensive assessment and referral evaluation (CARE)-rationale, development and reliability. *International Journal of Aging and Human Development, 8,* 9–42.

Health Care Financing Administration. (January, 1981). *Long-term care: Background and future directions.* Washington, DC: U.S. Government Printing Office.

Hesse, K., Campion, E. W., & Karamouz, N. (1982). Psychiatric stumbling blocks to geriatric rehabilitation. *The Gerontologist, 22,* 240.

Hoyer, W. J. (1973). Application of operant techniques to the modification of elderly behavior. *The Gerontologist, 13,* 18–22.

Ingersoll, B., & Silverman, A. (1978). Comparative group psychotherapy for the aged. *The Gerontologist, 18,* 201–206.

Kendrick, D. C. (1982). Why assess the aged? A clinical psychologist's view. *British Journal of Clinical Psychology, 21,* 47–54.

Kinsey, A. C., Pomeroy, W., & Martin, C. (1948). *Sexual behavior in the human male.* Philadelphia: Saunders.

Lankford, D. A., & Herman, S. H. (1978, May). *Behavioral geriatrics: A critical review.* Summary of paper presented at the Nova Behavioral Conference on Aging, Port St. Lucie, Florida.

Lawton, M. P. (1970). Assessment, integration, and environments for the older people. *The Gerontologist, 10,* 38–46.

Lawton, M. P. (1972). Assessing the competence of older people. In D. P. Kent, R. Kastenbaum, & S. Sherwood (Eds.), *Research planning and action for the elderly.* New York: Behavioral Publications.

Lawton, M. P. (1978, October). *What is the good life for aging?* Kesten Lecture, University of Southern California, Ethel Percy Andrus Gerontology Center.

Lawton, M. P., Whelihan, W. M., & Belsky, J. K. (1980). Personality tests and their uses with older adults. In J. Birren & R. B. Sloane (Eds.), *Handbook of mental health and aging* (pp. 537–553). Englewood Cliffs, NJ: Prentice-Hall.

Lawton, M. P., Moss, M. S., Fulcomer, M., & Kleban, M. H. (1982). A research and service oriented multi-level assessment instrument. *Journal of Gerontology, 37,* 91–99.

Mahoney, M. J. (1975). The sensitive scientists in empirical humanism. *American Psychologist, 30,* 864–867.

Marcer, D. (1979). Measuring memory change in Alzheimer's disease. In A. I. M. Glen & L. J. Whalley (Eds.), *Alzheimer's disease: Early recognition of potentially reversible deficits* (pp. 117–121). Edinburgh: Churchill-Livingstone.

Miller, E. (1980). Cognitive assessment of the older adult. In J. E. Birren & R. B. Sloane (Eds.), *Handbook of mental health and aging* (pp. 520–536). Englewood Cliffs, NJ: Prentice-Hall.

Miller, L. (1979). Toward a classification of aging behaviors. *The Gerontologist, 19*(3), 283–289.

Palmore, E. B. (1973). Social factors in mental illness of the aged. In E. W. Busse & E. Pfeiffer (Eds.), *Mental illness in later life* (pp. 41–52). Washington, DC: American Psychiatric Association.

Pascal, G. R. & Jenkins, W. O. (1961). *Systematic observation of gross human behavior.* New York: Grune & Stratton.

Patterson, R. L. (in press). Senile dementias. In R. Daitzman (Ed.), *Diagnosis and intervention in behavior therapy and behavioral medicine.* New York: Springer.

Patterson, R. L., & Eberly, D. A. (1983). Social and daily living skills. In P. M. Lewinsohn & L. Teri (Eds.), *Clinical geropsychology* (pp. 116–138). New York: Pergamon Press.

Patterson, R. L., & Jackson, G. M. (1980). Behavior modification with the elderly. In M. M. Hersen, R. M. Eisler, & P. M. Miller (Eds.), *Progress in behavior modification* (Vol. 9) (pp. 205–239). New York: Academic Press. (a)

Patterson, R. L., & Jackson, G. M. (1980). Behavioral approaches to gerontology. In M. L. Michelson, M. Hersen, & S. M. Turner (Eds.), *Future perspectives in behavior therapy* (pp. 295–315). New York: Plenum Press. (b)

Patterson, R. L., Dupree, L. W., Eberly, D. A., Jackson, G. M., O'Sullivan, M. J., Penner, L. A., & Dee-Kelly, C. (1982). *Overcoming deficits of aging: A behavioral approach.* New York: Plenum Press.

Pfeiffer, E. (1975). *Functional assessment: The OARS Multidimensional Functional Assessment Questionnaire.* Durham, NC: Duke University Center for the Study of Aging and Human Development.

Pfeiffer, E. (1980). The psychosocial evaluation of the elderly patient. In E. W. Busse & D. G. Blazer (Eds.), *Handbook of geriatric psychiatry* (pp. 275–284). New York: Van Nostrand Reinhold.

Portnoi, V. A. (1982). Underrepresentation of geriatric mental health disorders in DSM-III: Need for revision. *The Gerontologist, 22*(5), 239.

Rebok, G. W., & Hoyer, W. J. (1977). The functional context of elderly behavior. *The Gerontologist, 17,* 27–34.

Reisburg, B., & Ferris, S. H. (1982). Diagnosis and assessment of the older patient. *Hospital and Community Psychiatry, 33,* 104–110.

Rodin, J., & Langer, E. (1980). Aging labels: The decline of control and the fall of self-esteem. *Journal of Social Issues, 36,* 12–29.

Schaie, K. W. (1974). Translations in gerontology—from lab to life: Intellectual functioning. *American Psychologist, 29,* 802–807.

Schaie, K. W. (1976). *Competence and intelligence.* Paper presented at the annual meeting of the Western Psychological Association, Los Angeles.

Schaie, K. W. (1978). External validity in the assessment of intellectual development in adulthood. *Journal of Gerontology, 33,* 695–701.

Schaie, K. W., Chatham, L. R., & Weiss, J. M. A. (1961). The multiprofessional intake assessment of older psychiatric patients. *Journal of Psychiatric Research, 1,* 92–100.

Sundberg, N. D., Snowden, L. R., & Reynolds, W. M. (1978). Toward assessment of personal competence and incompetence in life situations. *Annual Review of Psychology, 29,* 179–221.

Taylor, H. G., & Bloom, L. M. (1974). Cross-validation and methodological extension of the Stockton Geriatric Rating Scale. *Journal of Gerontology, 29,* 190–193.

U.S. Department of Commerce, Bureau of the Census (1978). *Statistical abstract of the United States.* Washington, DC: U.S. Government Printing Office.

U.S. President's Commission on Mental Health (1978). *Task panel reports* (Vol. 3, Appendix). Washington, DC: U.S. Government Printing Office.

Whelihan, W. (1979, March). *Dynamics of the team interaction in geriatric assessment.* Paper presented at the Conference on Geriatric Assessment, VA Medical Center, St. Louis.

Witherspoon, A., deValera, E., Jenkins, W., & Sanford, W. *Behavioral interview guide.* (1973). Montgomery, AL: Rehabilitation Research Foundation.

Index

Affect, 30–31, 44–45
Affective disorders
  primary versus secondary affective
    disorder, 82, 88
  as a result of medical-neurological dis-
    ease, 83–84
  as a result of personality disorders,
    96–100, 104–105
  retarded versus agitated depression,
    103
  subtypes, 83–100
  See also Anxious depression; Bipolar
    depression; characterologic dys-
    phoria; Cyclothymic disorder;
    Dysthymic disorder; Major
    depression
Aggressive client, 20
Agoraphobia
  concurrent symptomatology, 60
  presence or absence of panic, 60
Alcohol breath–test procedures, 168
Alcoholism
  alcohol use versus abuse, 164–165
  classification of drinking patterns, 163
  minimizing self-report distortion, 168–
    169
Anorexia nervosa, 244–245
Antisocial personality, 137–140
  concurrent depressive symptoms, 96–
    97, 104
Anxiety disorders
  differential diagnosis based on
    panic symptoms, 60
  response to drug treatment, 60
  somatic complaints, 58–59
Anxious depression, 86–88, 103

Aphonia, 34
Apotemnophia, 215
Attention deficit disorder with hyperac-
    tivity, 322–326
Avoidant personality, 149–150

Bestiality, 216
Behavioral incident technique, 345–348
Binge–purge syndrome. *See* Bulimia
Bipolar disorder, 81, 90–93, 105–106
Borderline personality, 142–146
Bulimia, 245–247, 252
Bulimic anorectic, 255. *See also* Eating
    disorders

Characterologic dysphorias, 96–100,
    104–105
Children
  categories of childhood disorders, 313
  child interviews, 317–318
  issues in interviewing, 311–313
  parent interviews, 315–317
  special concerns in diagnosis, 332–333
  teacher interviews, 318
Circumstantiality of speech, 32
Clang associations, 32
Compulsive personality, 147–149
Confabulation, 33, 42
Confidentiality, 7–9
  age considerations, 8
Coprolalia, 221
Cyclothymic disorder, 81, 93–94

Delusions, 35–37
Dependent personality, 149–150
Depersonalization, 35

Derealization, 35
Diagnostic settings, 4–7
Drug abuse
  concurrent psychiatric symptoms,
    200–201
  stages of, 183–185
Drug dependence, 184–185
Drug preoccupation, 184
Drug tolerance, 184
Dysthymic disorder, 80, 94–96

Eating disorders. See also Anorexia ner-
    vosa; Bulimia; Obesity
  behavioral factors, 254–255
  cognitive and emotional factors, 255–
    256
  familial factors, 256–257
  medical and physical status, 253–254
  social factors, 256
Echolalia, 33
Echopraxia, 33
Ego-dystonic homosexuality, 233–236
Elderly
  assessment of ecological competence,
    342–343
  negative attitudes toward, 339
Emergency diagnosis, 4–6
Endogenous depression. See Major
    depression
Essential hypertension, 276–281
Ethnic factors
  in diagnosis, 12–13
  in interviewing, 9–12
Exhibitionism, 219

Family therapy
  family functions, 291–292
  overcoming resistance to treatment,
    296–298
Fetishism, 214–215
Flight of ideas, 32
Food records, 249–250
Formal thought disorder, 46–47
Frigidity. See Inhibited sexual excitement
Frottage, 221–222
Functional analysis of fear, 74–75
Functional dyspareunia, 208
Functional vaginismus, 208

Ganser syndrome, 43–44
Geriatric population. See Elderly

Hallucinations, 37–39
Hebephilia, 217
Histrionic personality, 134–137
  concurrent depressive symptoms, 98–
    100
Hypomania, 81, 90–91. See also Bipolar
    disorder

Illusion, 37
Impotence. See Inhibited sexual
    excitement
Incest, 218–219
Infantile autism, 326–329
Inhibited female orgasm, 207
Inhibited male orgasm, 207
Inhibited sexual desire, 206–207
Inhibited sexual excitement, 207
Intellectually deficient clients, 19–20
Interview schedules, 13. See also Struc-
    tured interviews
Interviewer behavior, 15–19

Loose associations, 32–33, 46, 119

Major depression, 80, 84–86, 89–90. See
    also Affective disorders
Mania, 81, 91–93. See also Bipolar
    disorder
Masked depression, 85
Melancholia. See Major depression
Mental status examination
  affect and mood, 30–31, 44–45
  appearance and behavior, 27–29
  attention, 40
  concentration, 40
  intelligence, 42–43
  memory, 40–41
  orientation, 39–40
  perceptual disturbances, 37–39
  psychomotor activity, 29–30
  reliability, judgment, and insight, 43–
    44
  speech and thought, 31–37
Migraine headache, 271–276
Mitral valve prolapse, 60
Mood, 31

Narcissistic personality, 140–142
Neologisms, 32–33

Obesity, 247–248, 250–252

Pain patients, 20–21
Panic attacks, 60, 87
Paranoid personality, 152–154
Partialism, 215
Passive–aggressive personality, 149, 150–152
Pedophilia, 216–217
Perseveration, 33
Personality disorders. *See* Antisocial personality; Avoidance personality; Borderline personality; Compulsive personality; Dependent personality; Histrionic personality; Narcissistic personality; Passive–aggressive personality
Physically disabled clients, 20
Premature ejaculation, 207–208
Psychomotor agitation, 29
Psychomotor retardation, 29–30
Psychophysiological disorders
  critical information for diagnosis, 281–284
  need for medical evaluation, 266–267
  symptom diary, 268, 274
  types of, 264

Racial factors
  in diagnosis, 12–13
  in interviewing, 9–12
Rape, 222
Retardation of thought processes, 33

Schizoid personality, 152, 154–155
Schizophrenia
  differentiation from
    affective disorders, 112, 114
    organic disorders, 112, 114
    personality disorders, 156
Schizotypal personality, 152, 155
Schneiderian symptoms, 36, 115
Sexual deviation
  deviant versus nondeviant arousal, 231–232
  interview precautions, 223–225
  multiple diagnoses, 231
  See also Apotemnophia; Bestiality;

Sexual deviation (*Cont.*)
  Coprolalia; Ego-dystonic homosexuality; Exhibitionism; Fetishism; Frottage; Hebephilia; Incest; Partialism; Pedophilia; Rape; Sexual masochism; Sexual sadism; Telephone scatalogia; Transvestism; Voyeurism; Zoophilia
Sexual dysfunction, 206–214. *See also* Functional dyspareunia; Functional vaginismus; Inhibited female orgasm; Inhibited male orgasm; Inhibited sexual desire; Inhibited sexual excitement; Premature ejaculation
Sexual masochism, 220
Sexual sadism, 220–221
Simple phobia, 61–62
Social phobia, 61
Sociopathic personality. *See* antisocial personality
Somatoform disorders, 283–284
Structured interviews
  schedules for affective disorders, 100–101
  schedules for alcoholism, 169–170
  schedules for children, 319–320
  schedules for drug abuse, 191
  schedules for schizophrenic disorders, 116
  schedules for the elderly, 344
Substance abuse. *See* Drug abuse; Alcoholism
Synesthesia, 37

Telephone scatologia, 221
Thought block, 33
Transvestism, 215–216
Tripartite model of anxiety, 57–58

Vorbeireden. *See* Ganser Syndrome
Voyeurism, 220

Zoophilia, 216